Psychiatric Nursing

made
Incredibly
Easy! WITHDRAWN

Second Edition

Clinical Editors

Carolyn Gersch, PhD (Candidate), MSN, RN, CNE
Nicole M. Heimgartner, MSN, RN, COI
Cherie R. Rebar, PhD, MBA, RN, FNP, COI
Laura M. Willis, MSN, APRN, FNP-C

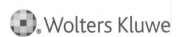 Wolters Kluwer

Philadelphia · Baltimore · New York · London
Buenos Aires · Hong Kong · Sydney · Tokyo

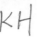

Executive Editor: Shannon W. Magee
Product Development Editor: Maria M. McAvey
Senior Production Product Manager: Cynthia Rudy
Editorial Assistant: Zachary Shapiro
Design Coordinators: Elaine Kasmer and Joan Wendt
Creative Services Director: Doug Smock
Senior Marketing Manager: Mark Wiragh
Manufacturing Coordinator: Kathleen Brown
Prepress Vendor: Absolute Service, Inc.

2nd Edition

Copyright © 2016 Wolters Kluwer

9 8 7 6 5 4 3 2 1

Printed in China

Library of Congress Cataloging-in-Publication Data

Psychiatric nursing made incredibly easy! (Lippincott Williams & Wilkins)
  Psychiatric nursing made incredibly easy! / clinical editors, Carolyn Gersch, Nicole M. Heimgartner, Cherie R. Rebar, Laura M. Willis. — 2nd edition.
     p. ; cm.
  Includes bibliographical references and index.
  ISBN 978-1-4511-9255-1
  I. Gersch, Carolyn J., editor. II. Heimgartner, Nicole M., editor. III. Rebar, Cherie R., editor. IV. Willis, Laura, 1969- , editor. V. Title.
  [DNLM: 1. Mental Disorders--nursing. 2. Psychiatric Nursing--methods. WY 160]
  RC440
  616.89'0231—dc23
                                                                                                        2014021539

WW.COM

9/23/16

RRS1503

Contents

Contributors

Dorit Breiter, DNP, ARAP, PMHNP-BC
Director
Psychiatric and Mental Health Nurse Practitioner Program
College of Nursing and Health Professions
Drexel University
Philadelphia, Pennsylvania

Barbara Broome, RN, PhD, CNS
Associate Dean
Kent State University College of Nursing
Kent, Ohio

Chien Yin Cepeda, RN
Nurse
Ancora Psychiatric Hospital
Hammonton, New Jersey

Virginia Conley, PhD, APRN, CS, FNP, PMHNP
Clinical Associate Professor
College of Nursing
University of Iowa
Iowa City, Iowa

Linda Carman Copel, RN, PhD, CS, DAPA
Associate Professor
Villanova University College of Nursing
Philadelphia, Pennsylvania

William J. Lorman, PhD, MSN, PMHNP-BC, CARN-AP
Vice President, Chief Clinical Officer
Livengrin Foundation, Inc.
Assistant Clinical Professor
College of Nursing and Health Professions
Drexel University
Philadelphia, Pennsylvania

Elizabeth Lynch, MS, PMHNP-BC
Psychiatric Nurse Practitioner
Blanton-Peale Institute and Counseling Center
New York, New York

Gilda Mark, APRN
Family Psychiatric Nurse Practitioner
Indian Health Service
Fort Collins, Colorado

Dana Murphy-Parker, MS, CRNP, PMHNP-BC
Track Director
Psychiatric/Mental Health Nurse Practitioner Program
Assistant Clinical Professor of Nursing
College of Nursing and Health Professions
Drexel University
Philadelphia, Pennsylvania

Donna Sabella, MD, BSN, PhD, MSN
Director of Education, National Research Consortium on
    Commercial Sexual Exploitation
Director, Global Studies
Director, Office of Human Trafficking
Assistant Clinical Professor
Drexel University
Philadelphia, Pennsylvania

Janet Somlyay, APRN, PMHNP
Child and Adolescent Psychiatry Practitioner
Laramie Behavioral Health Clinic
Laramie, Wyoming

Matthew Sorenson, RN, PhD
Associate Professor
Associate Director, Master's Entry to Nursing Practice
    Program
DePaul University
Chicago, Illinois

Kathleen R. Tusaie, RNCS, PhD
Associate Professor
University of Akron School of Nursing
Akron, Ohio

Previous edition contributors

C. Judith Birger, RN, CS, MS

Barbara Broome, RN, PhD, CNS

Colleen C. Burgess, RN, MSN, APRN, CS, NCSAC

Linda Carman Copel, RN, PhD, CS, DAPA

Joseph T. DeRanieri, RN, PhD, BCECR, CPN

Candace Furlong, RN, MSN, CNS

Sudha C. Patel, RN, MN, MA, DNS

Barbara C. Rynerson, RNC, MS, CS

Matthew Sorenson, RN, PhD

Phyllis Hart Tipton, RN, MSN

Kathleen R. Tusaie, RNCS, PhD

E. Monica Ward-Murray, SRN, RMN, BSN, MA, EdD

Preface

Welcome to the second edition of *Psychiatric Nursing Made Incredibly Easy!* It has been more than a decade since the first edition, a remarkable contribution to the field of psychiatric-mental health nursing, was published. This second edition continues in that tradition; it provides important fundamental knowledge of and care related to various psychiatric/mental health concerns. Although we have made remarkable progress in our understanding of mental health disorders over the past decade, the recognition and management of mental health and substance abuse disorders needs our utmost attention at this time. Not only does this book offer a quick overview, but it also helps nurses in all healthcare settings provide patients with the best possible care.

This revised and updated edition is available at a time in which two significant events impacting mental health are occurring. In the United States, the Affordable Care Act (ACA) gave millions of Americans different access to health care. Funds have been earmarked to help community health centers establish new services, and expand existing services, for people with mental health concerns. Nurses, as the largest group within the health care workforce, and their integrative and holistic approach toward patients, are essential to helping this population manage their mental health care needs. Currently, one in five Americans is known to suffer from depression and anxiety. And the majority of deaths related to suicide, homicide, and accidents can be traced to mental and substance abuse disorders. This underscores the importance of recognizing and understanding mental health disorders across the life span. The second significant event is the publication of the new edition of *Diagnostic and Statistical Manual of Mental Disorders*, 5th Edition (*DSM-5*), in 2013. Changes in the *DSM-5* concentrate on a developmental approach to psychiatric/mental health disorders and also allow a broader scope of flexibility in understanding that mental disorders occur with varying levels of severity. The *DSM-5* changes are covered at a fundamental level throughout this second edition.

Organized into 13 chapters, *Psychiatric Nursing Made Incredibly Easy*! covers patient and family advocacy, health promotion and teaching, psychopharmacology, interdisciplinary team approach, and ethical and legal perspectives of mental health care. Lighthearted humor with cartoons emphasize concepts, whereas quick scan tables, flow charts, and illustrations help to enhance the reader's understanding of material. Specific icons define:

Advice from the experts—offers tips and how-to's from experienced psychiatric nurses.

Myth busters—distinguishes facts from myths about people with mental health concerns and focuses on the proper care approaches.

Bridging the gap—offers overviews of unique beliefs and needs within specific groups.

Meds matters—focuses on the psychopharmacologic and/or alternatives remedies for psychiatric concerns.

Psychiatric Nursing Made Incredibly Easy! delivers concepts essential to a better understanding of mental health concerns across the life span and helps nurses in all health care settings provide the best possible care.

Carolyn Gersch, PhD (Candidate), MSN, RN, CNE
Associate Director, Division of Nursing
Chair, BSN Completion Program
Kettering College
Kettering, Ohio
President, Connect: RN2ED
Beavercreek, Ohio

Nicole M. Heimgartner, MSN, RN, COI
Associate Professor
Division of Nursing
Kettering College
Kettering, Ohio
President, Connect: RN2ED
Beavercreek, Ohio

Cherie R. Rebar, PhD, MBA, RN, FNP, COI
Director, Division of Nursing
Chair, Prelicensure Nursing Programs
Kettering College
Kettering, Ohio
President, Connect: RN2ED
Beavercreek, Ohio

Laura M. Willis, MSN, APRN, FNP-C
Associate Professor
Division of Nursing
Kettering College
Kettering, Ohio
President, Connect: RN2ED
Beavercreek, Ohio

Introduction to psychiatric nursing

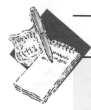

Just the facts

In this chapter, you'll learn:

♦ the nurse's role in caring for patients with psychiatric conditions

♦ ways to enhance therapeutic communication with patients

♦ therapies used to treat psychiatric conditions

♦ components of the nursing assessment of the patient with psychiatric conditions

♦ ethical and legal issues in caring for patients with psychiatric conditions

A look at psychiatric nursing

Like all people, patients with psychiatric conditions use all medical settings. These patients use medical clinics for wellness and follow-up care and are susceptible to medical illness or injury that requires hospitalizations. Any patient in a medical setting may be distressed because of their illness or confused as a result of a long hospitalization. Anxiety, depression, and confusion are commonly seen in the general population. With the increase in longevity, dementia is not uncommon.

To work effectively with any patient, it is essential to consider not only the physical concerns but also the psychological issues that may, or may not, be reported.

> You don't need to work on a psychiatric unit to encounter patients with psychiatric conditions.

Goal: More beautiful minds

It is estimated that 6.9% of national health care spending is directed toward mental health care (U.S. Department of Health & Human

Services, 2014). Understanding psychiatric illness has grown significantly over the past decade and the link between physical and mental health is better understood. Additionally, the care for patients with psychiatric conditions has evolved from inpatient hospitalization to outpatient community-based programs. Advocacy programs, assertive community treatment programs, and assisted outpatient treatment programs provide follow-up care and monitoring of patients with psychiatric conditions in the community. Programs are available to provide support and education regarding numerous situations or circumstances, including substance abuse programs, bereavement support, victims of violence groups, and shelters.

Real situations that make us think

Psychiatric concerns are more reported now than ever before. We have seen a number of tragedies reported in the media related to shootings in schools, universities, and community settings caused by untreated or poorly monitored individuals with psychiatric conditions. These senseless tragedies remind us of the seriousness of untreated illness. Additionally, many books on coping and mindfulness have become best sellers. Advertisements on television tout the latest antidepressant or other medication that is available to control symptoms of anxiety, pain, or sadness.

> Scientists are learning more and more about what makes our minds tick.

Upgrading our understanding

Through research, our understanding of neurobiology has improved exponentially. This growth in knowledge has expanded the awareness of the physiologic foundation of neurologic function and its relation to mental illness. Genetic testing can be used to improve our understanding of how medications impact our brains based on individual DNA. With this increase in knowledge, diagnosis and treatment of psychiatric illness has improved, particularly in the use of drug therapy (Stahl, 2013). It is essential for psychiatric and mental health nurses to remain current with the changing developments in diagnosis, treatment, and neurobiology.

Holism in the house

Our education as nurses, and particularly in psychiatry, teaches us to look holistically at our patients. We know through our research and nursing practice experience that emotional stability and resiliency improves outcomes in recovery from medical illness as well as psychiatric illness. Psychiatric consultations are now more readily ordered when health care professionals observe and recognize symptoms early in the process of delivering care.

Social factors

Today, researchers continue to explore the continuing increase of mental illness. They have identified increased stressors related to the changes in family dynamics. Our exposure to national trauma on September 11, 2001 and subsequent military conflicts have contributed to military personnel and veterans struggling with posttraumatic stress and depression related to the trauma, injury, and loss. Financial uncertainty, social isolation, and personal losses experienced by individuals continue to challenge the mental health care system to respond quickly and appropriately to the ever-expanding needs. (See *Links between stress and disease*, page 4.)

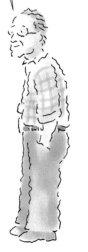

Elderly, fearful, and isolated— boy, am I depressed!

Angst through the ages

Psychiatric conditions affect all socioeconomic populations, all ages, and both genders. The teenage and elderly population are at the highest risk of depression and suicide. Substance use is reported even in young children. Alcohol and substance abuse and dependence are increasing, whereas services have challenges keeping up with access.

Classifying mental disorders

To successfully understand patients and respond to their needs, it is important to understand the language of psychiatry. The American Psychiatric Association (APA) developed a classification system to provide guidelines to diagnose psychiatric illness. This classification system has been updated over the years, most recently in 2013, with the recent edition of the *Diagnostic and Statistical Manual of Mental Disorders*, 5th Edition (*DSM-5*). *DSM-5* updates the prior edition of the *Diagnostic and Statistical Manual of Mental Disorders* (4th ed., text rev.; *DSM-IV-TR*) in an attempt to provide improved consistency to better diagnose and treat our patients. This latest edition is focused on viewing patients in a holistic and multidimensional manner so that their needs are more appropriately addressed. Social stressors are evaluated and noted as in the past (Kupfer, Kuhl, & Regier, 2013). (See *Understanding the DSM-5*, page 5.)

The *DSM-5* is a must-read for all psychiatric nurses.

Links between stress and disease

Hans Selye, a pioneer in stress research, found a link between the environment and biological response. He noted that emotional and physical stress cause a pattern of responses that unless treated, lead to infection, illness, disease, and eventually even death. Selye called this set of responses the *general adaptation syndrome* and identified three stages—alarm reaction, resistance, and exhaustion.

Alarm reaction

During this stage, any type of physical or mental trauma triggers immediate biological responses designed to counter the stress. These responses depress the immune system, which lowers resistance and makes the person more susceptible to infection and disease. Unless the stress is severe or prolonged, though, the person recovers rapidly.

Resistance

This stage begins when the body starts to adapt to prolonged stress. The immune system shifts into high gear to meet increased demands. At this point, the person becomes more resistant to illness.

However, the perception of a threat lingers, so the body never reaches complete physiologic equilibrium. Instead, it stays aroused, which places stress on body organs and systems.

Because adaptation appears to work initially, a person in the resistance stage may become complacent and assume he's immune to the effects of stress—and thus fail to take steps to relieve it.

Exhaustion

With chronic stress, adaptive mechanisms eventually wear down and the body can no longer meet the demands of stress. Immunity and resistance decline dramatically and illness is likely to set in. The point at which exhaustion occurs differs among individuals.

Interrupting the stress response

Selye's work laid the foundation for the use of relaxation techniques in interrupting the stress response, thereby reducing susceptibility to illness and disease (Townsend, 2014).

Role of psychiatric nurses

Psychiatric nursing is recognized by The American Nurses Association (ANA) as a specialized area of nursing practice. Psychiatric nursing incorporates the science of nursing based on clinical assessment skills and nursing diagnoses with the art of "therapeutic use of self" in establishing a professional, therapeutic relationship based on empathy. Psychiatric nurses continue to perform in the traditional role of nurses with the administration of prescribed treatments, monitoring the efficacy of those treatments, and educating their patients. Additionally, psychiatric nurses engage

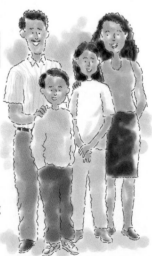

Understanding the *DSM-5*

The APA's *DSM-5* defines a mental disorder as a clinically significant behavioral or psychological syndrome or pattern associated with at least one of the following criteria:
• current distress (a painful symptom)
• disability (an impairment in one or more important areas of functioning)
• a significantly greater risk of suffering, death, pain, and disability
• an important loss of freedom.

The syndrome or pattern must not be merely an expected, culturally sanctioned response— such as grief over the death of a loved one. Whatever its original cause, it must currently be considered a sign of behavioral, psychological, or biological dysfunction.

The *DSM-5*

The *DSM-5* has eliminated the multiaxial system used by the *DSM-IV-TR* for the purpose of addressing the interrelationship of disorders formerly outlined in Axes 1, 2, and 3. Combining these Axes allows clinicians to integrate cognitive, developmental, and physical disorders to improve diagnosis based in neuroscience and psychiatry. It continues to address the psychosocial stressors formerly addressed in Axis 4 while incorporating improved cultural impact and functional disability—formerly Axis 5.

The structure of the *DSM-5* is now based on three sections. Section 1 describes the "Basics" of the new text in understanding the structure and use of the *DSM-5*. Section 2 describes the "Diagnostic Criteria and Codes" and uses a chapter structure to define criteria for illness combining like disorders based on symptoms. Section 3 describes "Emerging Measures and Models" to provide a road map for future development based on research leading to better understanding of the interrelationship of physical and cognitive function.

The hope of the *DSM-5* is that it will be more useful not only for psychiatrists but also for primary care physicians as a reference to assist their patients (Kupfer et al., 2013).

their patients and families in conversation based on therapeutic models to improve understanding of their illness and to improve function.

Psychiatric nursing is present in all health care settings such as inpatient, outpatient, community health care centers, mental health clinics, and visiting nurse services. Practice is as diverse as the settings. Therapeutic relationships are present in all nursing interactions as are the principles of psychiatric nursing. (See *The versatile nurse*, page 6.)

To work with patients with psychiatric conditions, a psychiatric nurse brings calm to the storm. Our patients bring challenges as complicated and distinct as the individual. The creativity and compassion of our interactions helps to establish the therapeutic relationship from which healing can occur (Townsend, 2014).

The versatile nurse

The psychiatric nurse will have one or many of the following roles depending on his or her skills, educational background, and experience:
- staff nurse/nurse leader
- primary provider of care
- administrator
- consultant
- in-service educator
- clinical practitioner
- researcher
- program evaluator
- liaison between the patient and other health care team members
- patient advocate.

Nurse: Know thyself

To effectively work as a psychiatric nurse, we must become aware of our own biases and beliefs. Taking an inventory of what drives us to make the decisions that we make allows us to more fully understand ourselves. Although it is impossible to completely separate from our core beliefs, it is essential to set aside our biases and accept the fact that our patients may feel differently than we do and ultimately make different decisions than we would. Giving patients the autonomy to which they are entitled reinforces our duty as nurses to provide accurate health information from which they can choose or decline.

Knowing yourself will help you care more effectively for patients with psychiatric conditions.

Scope of practice

The nurse practice act of each state is enacted by the state legislature and describes the scope of practice for all nurses working within their borders. It is important to familiarize yourself with your nurse practice act so that you work based on those laws. Other common standards of practice include:
- professional practice standards
- education and experience
- certification
- practice setting
- personal initiative.

Nurse practice acts

Each state regulates the scope of a nurse's practice through the nurse practice act. This act regulates and defines nurse practice for that state. It sets the minimum standards for entry into the practice of nursing, outlines the scope of practice for the nurse, and describes the requirements for advanced practice nurses. Additionally, it sets the requirements for licensure, license renewal, and any other conditions necessary for practice within the state. It is important to become familiar with your individual nurse practice act so that your practice follows the laws of your state.

Professional practice standards

Although nursing practice is regulated by each state, professional practice standards developed by the ANA provides guidelines for practice and performance in an effort to assist in establishing some uniformity in care. The ANA initially developed these standards in 1973 and updated them most recently in 2014. (See *ANA standards of care for psychiatric and mental health nursing*, pages 8 and 9.)

Education and experience

Integrating behavioral health care into primary care practice has become more common and is creating opportunities for expanding the practice of psychiatric nurses. To answer this need, the psychiatric mental health nurse practitioner (PMHNP), currently a master's prepared advanced practice nurse certified in psychiatry, has been added to many clinical, hospital, and community mental health clinics. Because of the changes to our health care system, growing demands for mental health care will continue to expand the need for the PMHNP to new practice areas and new levels of doctoral education.

Certification

Organizations and places of employment are requiring and/ or encouraging psychiatric nurses to become certified as experts in their field. ANA and American Nurses Credentialing Center (ANCC; 2014) provide certification testing. To qualify for certification, a psychiatric nurse must meet certain standards set by the credentialing agency as an indication of nursing competence. Some of the standards include length of time in practice, evidence of continued education in psychiatric nursing, recommendations from peers, and passing of an examination. Certification can be obtained as a nurse generalist, PMHNP, or clinical nurse specialist.

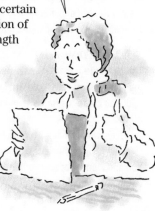

Acing the written test goes a long way toward gaining ANA certification.

Practice setting

Each practice setting shapes the type of care based on the philosophy and focus of the organization. In addition to the state's nurse practice acts, the administration's policies provide the guidelines for

ANA standards of care for psychiatric and mental health nursing

In 1973, the ANA issued standards designed to improve the quality of care provided by psychiatric and mental health nurses. Last revised in 2014, these standards apply to generalists and specialists working in any setting in which psychiatric and mental health nursing is practiced.

Listed below are the standards of care and standards of professional performance, along with rationales. *Note:* Standards Vh through Vh apply only to the advanced practice registered nurse in psychiatric and mental health (APRN-PMH) specialist.

Standards of care

Standards of care pertain to professional nursing activities demonstrated through the nursing process. The standards encompass assessment, diagnosis, outcome identification, planning, implementation, and evaluation.

The nursing process is the foundation of clinical decision making and encompasses all significant action taken by nurses in providing psychiatric and mental health care to all patients.

Standard I: Assessment
The psychiatric mental health registered nurse collects and synthesizes comprehensive health data that are pertinent to the health care consumer's health and/or situation.

Rationale: Collection of comprehensive patient information—which requires linguistically and culturally effective communication skills, interviewing, behavioral observation, database record review, and comprehensive assessment of the patient and relevant systems—enables the psychiatric and mental health nurse to make sound clinical judgments and plan appropriate interventions.

Standard II: Diagnosis
The psychiatric mental health registered nurse analyzes the assessment data to determine diagnoses, problems, and areas of focus for care and treatment, including level of risk.

Rationale: The basis for providing psychiatric and mental health nursing care is thorough assessment, recognition and identification of patterns of response to actual or potential psychiatric illnesses, mental health problems, and potential comorbid physical illnesses.

Standard III: Outcome identification
The psychiatric mental health registered nurse identifies expected outcomes and the health care consumer's goals for a plan individualized to the health care consumer or to the situation.

Rationale: Within the context of providing nursing care, the ultimate goal is to partner with the patient to improve health status and outcomes.

Standard IV: Planning
The psychiatric mental health registered nurse develops a plan that prescribes strategies and alternatives to assist the health care consumer in attainment of expected outcomes.

Rationale: A plan of care is used to guide therapeutic intervention, systematically document progress, and work with the patient toward planned outcomes.

Standard V: Implementation
The psychiatric mental health registered nurse implements the identified plan.

Rationale: Nurses use a wide range of interventions when implementing the plan of care. These interventions are designed to prevent mental and physical illness and to promote, maintain, and restore mental and physical health. They select interventions according to their practice level. At the basic level, nurses may select counseling, milieu therapy, self-care activities, psychobiological interventions, health teaching, case management, health promotion and maintenance, crisis intervention, community-based care, psychiatric home health care, telehealth, and various other approaches to meet the patient's mental health needs.

Standard Va: Coordination of care
The psychiatric mental health registered nurse coordinates care delivery.

Standard Vb: Health teaching and health promotion
The psychiatric mental health registered nurse employs strategies to promote health and a safe environment.

Standard Vc: Consultation
The psychiatric mental health advanced practice registered nurse provides consultation to influence the identified plan, enhance the abilities of other clinicians

ANA standards of care for psychiatric and mental health nursing *(continued)*

to provide services for health care consumers, and effect change.

Standard Vd: Prescriptive authority and treatment

The psychiatric mental health advanced practice registered nurse uses prescriptive authority, procedures, referrals, treatments, and therapies in accordance with state and federal laws and regulations.

Standard Ve: Pharmacologic, biological, and integrative therapies

The psychiatric mental health advanced practice registered nurse incorporates knowledge of pharmacologic, biological, and complementary interventions with applied clinical skills to restore the health care consumer's health and prevent further disability.

Standard Vf: Milieu therapy

The psychiatric mental health advanced practice registered nurse provides; structures; and maintains a safe, therapeutic, recovery-oriented environment in collaboration with health care consumers, families, and other health care clinicians.

Standard Vg: Therapeutic relationship and counseling

The psychiatric mental health advanced practice registered nurse uses the therapeutic relationship and counseling interventions to assist health care consumers in their individual recovery journeys by improving and regaining their previous coping abilities, fostering mental health, and preventing mental disorder and disability.

Standard Vh: Psychotherapy

The psychiatric mental health advanced practice registered nurse conducts individual, couples, group, and family psychotherapy using evidence-based psycho-therapeutic frameworks and the nurse–client therapeutic relationship.

Standard 6

The PMH registered nurse evaluates progress toward attainment of expected outcomes.

From American Nurses Association. (2014). *Psychiatric-mental health nursing: Scope and standards of practice* (2nd ed.). Silver Spring, MD: Author.

treatment and the parameters for the practice of the psychiatric nurse. This philosophy outlines the approach to care and the guidelines provide insight to the patient as well as the caregiver of what is expected within the practice.

Personal initiative

Each psychiatric nurse chooses how to perform within his or her scope of practice. He or she is prompted by educational experiences, awareness of biases and belief systems, ability to engage in therapeutic relationships, and clinical competence.

Theoretical basis of psychiatric nursing

Psychiatric nursing, as is true of all nursing specialties, is based on theoretical concepts and best practice supported by evidence. (See *Theoretical models of behavior*, pages 10 and 11.)

Theoretical models of behavior

Learning about the various models of human behavior gives you a better understanding of psychiatric disorders. These models are summarized below.

Remember, though, that human behavior isn't fully understood, so no model or theory is considered right or wrong or better or worse than any other. Commonly, psychiatric and mental health nurses use an eclectic approach, drawing on several theoretical models to inform their practice.

Psychoanalytic model (Freud)

According to the psychoanalytic model, the personality consists of the:
- id, encompassing the primitive instincts and energies underlying all psychic activity
- ego, the conscious part of the personality and the part that most immediately controls thought and behavior
- superego, the conscience.

During childhood, development occurs in five psychosexual stages—oral, anal, phallic, latency, and genital. Deviations in behavior result from unsuccessful task accomplishment during earlier developmental stages. Freud also proposed that behavior is motivated by anxiety, the cornerstone of psychopathology.

Understanding the psychosexual stages of childhood provides a framework for the nurse to understand adult behaviors. Also, the nurse can promote effective parenting by teaching parents about the child's needs during each psychosexual stage.

Interpersonal model (Sullivan, Peplau)

The interpersonal model holds that human development results from interpersonal relationships and that behavior is motivated by avoidance of anxiety and attainment of satisfaction.

Peplau drew on Sullivan's original theory to propose an interpersonal nursing theory, which advanced the practice of psychiatric nursing by defining it as an interpersonal process. She proposed that:
- nurses must promote the nurse–patient relationship to build trust and foster healthy behavior

- therapeutic use of self promotes healing
- the therapeutic relationship is directed toward meeting the patient's needs.

Social model (Caplan, Szasz)

The social model proposes that the entire sociocultural environment influences mental health. Deviant behavior is defined by the culture in which a person lives. Undesirable or abnormal behavior in one society may be considered normal in another. In addition, social conditions and interactions predispose people to mental illness.

Existential model (Frankl, Perls, May)

The existential model centers on a person's present experiences rather than past ones. It holds that alienation from the self causes deviant behavior and that people can make free choices about which behaviors to display.

Based on the existential model of behavior, nursing developed the concept that the nurse works to restore the patient to a state of "full life" from a state of "self-alienation."

Nursing model (Rogers, Orem, Sister Roy, Peplau)

The nursing model emphasizes the person as a biopsychosocial being. This holistic approach focuses on caring rather than curing and promotes collaboration between the nurse and patient. It establishes the nursing process as the basis for providing care.

According to the nursing model, the patient's needs direct the therapeutic relationship and the patient's reactions to nursing interventions guide future interventions.

Medical model

The medical model holds that disease is the cause of deviant behavior. It focuses on diagnosis and treatment of the disease. Application of the medical model to mental illness has led to identification of neurochemicals as possible causes of deviant behavior. The medical model also accepts socioenvironmental influences as potential causes of deviant behavior.

Theoretical models of behavior *(continued)*

Communication models (Berne, Bandler, Grindler)

Communication theory proposes that all human behavior is a form of communication and that the meaning of behavior depends on the clarity of communication between sender and receiver. Unclear communication produces anxiety, which results in behavior deviations.

The communication pattern used with individuals, families, and social and work groups identifies the causes of the behavioral deviation. When communication improves, so does behavior.

Nurses draw on the communication model when they teach patients effective communication techniques.

Behavioral model (Skinner, Wolpe, Eysenck)

According to the behavioral model, all behavior—including mental illness—is learned. Unlike other models, which focus on the patient's emotions, behavioral theory focuses on the patient's actions.

Behaviorists believe that behavior that's rewarded will persist. Desired behaviors can be learned through rewards and negative behaviors can be eliminated through punishment. Thus, people can learn to behave in socially desirable ways.

Humanistic model (Maslow)

In the humanistic model, understanding human behavior requires familiarity with a hierarchy that has six levels of need.

- Level 1: physiologic survival (food, oxygen, and rest)
- Level 2: safety, security, and self-preservation
- Level 3: love and belonging (developing fulfilling relationships)
- Level 4: esteem and recognition (feeling like a worthwhile, contributing member of society, appreciating one's own uniqueness)
- Level 5: self-actualization (self-fulfillment)
- Level 6: truth, harmony, beauty, and spirituality.

Nursing draws from the humanistic model by striving to meet patients' lower level needs before higher level ones. By performing a needs assessment, the nurse determines appropriate intervention strategies to help patients meet their needs (Townsend, 2014).

Nurse–patient relationship

In order to be successful in working with any patient, it is necessary to develop a therapeutic relationship with him or her. This relationship is based on trust, empathy, and caring. It is through your words and actions, as well as your silence, that you communicate to the patient that he or she is important and you are open to his or her needs.

A therapeutic relationship is one focused on the betterment of the patient. It is based on a purpose that leads toward a goal with a set time frame. It is a relationship in which both the patient and the nurse set the agenda—it is not done for the patient; it is a collaborative effort with him or her. It flows through four identifiable stages. (See *Phases of the nurse–patient relationship*, page 12.)

Memory jogger

To encourage your patient to trust you, think of the mnemonic TRUST.

T: Try expression

R: Reflection

U: Use silence

S: Set limits

T: Time with the client

Phases of the nurse–patient relationship

The phases of a therapeutic relationship include the preinteraction, orientation, working, and termination phases.

Preinteraction phase

During the preinteraction phase—which may last a few seconds or several weeks—the nurse assesses the patient for unresolved problems. The patient may not be actively involved at this point.

Orientation (introductory) phase

The orientation (getting-to-know-you) phase sets the tone for the relationship. Introductions are made and each person's roles are defined. Trust begins to develop.

Usually, the nurse initiates this phase, setting the limits of the professional relationship and establishing the focus for conversation based on assessment data.

Then the nurse and patient may make an agreement, write a contract, or discuss and establish goals. Be aware that some patients may be resistant during this phase, testing your true intent or denying that they have a problem.

Working (exploration) phase

During the working phase, the nurse and patient explore and evaluate problems and work toward achieving set goals. The nurse may take on the role of listener and facilitator, with the patient participating actively. The patient is free to examine problems while trying to gain insight or find solutions.

Termination (resolution) phase

During the termination phase, the nurse reviews and summarizes the patient's progress. Together, the nurse and patient determine if goals have been met—and, if not, why not.

Then the nurse formally ends the relationship, being sure to acknowledge the patient's feelings about termination. Be aware that the patient may feel hurt or angry at the nurse's "abandonment" (Townsend, 2014).

Effective communication

Effective, therapeutic communication is essential in psychiatric nursing. Verbal and nonverbal communication involves sending and receiving messages. "Body language" sends volumes of information both to and from your patient. It is important to be aware of the messages that you send.

Verbal communication

Communication exists in spoken, written, or unspoken language as in "body language." Nurses rely on multiple forms of communication to provide information to our patients. We often educate our patients on appropriate behaviors or treatment options and provide written documents to educate them on treatment upon discharge from the hospital.

Minimizing obstacles

It is important to remember that patients have biases and beliefs just as we do. In order to communicate effectively, it is important to understand cultural, ethnic, religious, and educational biases that are potential obstacles. Your sensitivity to your patient's beliefs can improve your ability to connect with your patient. (See *Factors that influence verbal communication.*)

Cutting through the fog

Developing a therapeutic relationship with a patient with psychiatric conditions can be challenging. Thought disorders, dementias, and mood dysregulation can impact your patient's ability to engage with you therapeutically. (See *Reducing communication barriers*, page 14.)

¿Habla usted inglés?

Not all patients speak the same language as the nurse. The Joint Commission (TJC) requires that hospitals provide interpreters to assist patients with communication. Many hospitals have interpreters on staff or use "language lines" when staff is not available. Sign language interpreters assist with hearing-impaired patients and various equipment, that is, paper and pencils and text telephone (TTY) machines, facilitate communication with these patients.

Patient patterns

It is important not only to listen to what the patient is saying but how the patient is saying it. Speech patterns, intensity of speech, and logic of the conversation provides a wealth of information about your patient and his or her health.

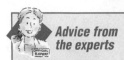

Advice from the experts

Factors that influence verbal communication

Various factors can hinder effective communication between the nurse and patient. Be sure to consider the patient's:
- native language
- culture or nationality
- sexual orientation or gender identity
- age and developmental considerations
- roles and responsibilities
- social background or status
- space and territoriality
- physical, mental, and emotional state
- values
- environment.

Nonverbal communication

We send messages to each other through our gestures, facial expression, posture, eye contact, clothing, touch, and appearance. In fact, most communication is nonverbal. Our body language communicates acceptance, joy, interest, as well as rejection, fear, and discontent.

Body talk

It is essential to be aware of how we approach our patients as much as we are aware of how our patient approaches us. We must monitor our body language to indicate that we are approachable, interested, and accepting of our patients.

Advice from the experts

Reducing communication barriers

Acknowledging and reducing communication barriers can promote a more effective relationship with psychiatric patients.

Language difficulties or differences
Use words appropriate to the patient's educational level. Avoid terms that he or she is unlikely to understand.

Be aware of words that may have more than one meaning. To some patients, for instance, the word "bad" may also be slang for "good."

If the patient speaks a foreign language or uses an ethnic dialect, obtain an interpreter to help you communicate. However, remember that a third person's presence may make the patient less willing to share his or her feelings.

Impaired hearing
If the patient can't hear you clearly, he or she may misinterpret your questions or responses. Check whether he or she is wearing a hearing aid. If so, is it turned on? If not, can the patient read lips? If possible, face the patient and speak clearly and slowly, using common words. Keep your questions short, simple, and direct.

If the patient has a severe hearing impairment, he or she may have to communicate in writing or you may need to collect information from his or her family or friends.

If the patient is elderly, speak in low-pitched tones. With aging, the ability to hear high-pitched tones deteriorates first.

Inappropriate responses
Avoid appearing to discount the patient's feelings, as by changing the subject abruptly. Otherwise, the patient may get the impression that you're disinterested, anxious, annoyed, or that you're judging him.

Thought disorders
If the patient's thought patterns are incoherent or irrelevant, he or she may be unable to interpret messages correctly, focus on the interview, or provide appropriate responses. When assessing, ask simple questions about concrete topics and clarify responses. Encourage the patient to express himself or herself clearly.

Paranoid thinking
Approach a paranoid patient in a nonthreatening way. Avoid touching, which may be misinterpreted as an attempt to enact harm. Also, keep in mind that a paranoid patient may not mean the things that he or she says.

Hallucinations
A hallucinating patient can't hear or respond appropriately. Show concern but don't reinforce hallucinatory perceptions.

Be as specific as possible when giving commands. For instance, if the patient says he or she is hearing voices, tell the patient to stop listening to the voices and listen to you instead.

Delusions
A deluded patient defends irrational beliefs or ideas despite factual evidence to the contrary. Some delusions may be so bizarre that you'll recognize them immediately. Others may be hard to identify.

Don't condemn or agree with delusional beliefs, and don't dismiss a statement because you think it's delusional. Instead, gently emphasize reality without arguing.

Delirium
A delirious patient experiences disorientation, hallucinations, and confusion. Misinterpretation and inappropriate responses commonly result. Talk directly, ask simple questions, and offer frequent reassurances. Delirium is reversible.

Dementia
The patient with dementia (irreversible deterioration of mental capacity) may experience changes in memory and thought patterns. Language may become distorted or slurred.

When interviewing, minimize distractions. Use simple, concise language. Avoid making statements that could be easily misinterpreted.

Using silence

Silence is an important tool for open communication. It allows a patient the time and space to communicate, think, evaluate, and process the challenges that brought them to you. Remember, even with silence, it is important to remain present in the conversation. Using body language sends the message that you are listening and engaged in the conversation.

Listening attentively

Engaging your patient using eye contact, touch (when appropriate), and gestures sends the message that you are actively listening to what he or she has to say. Responding appropriately confirms that you value and accept your patient.

Checking for congruence

One of the roles of a psychiatric nurse is to assess our patients for congruence of mood—how a patient describes how he is feeling—and affect—how a patient physically appears. If a patient is describing a distressing occurrence, the nurse would assess for the appropriate affect—the patient might appear sad and may be tearful during the conversation. Conversely, if the patient describes something happy or exciting, his or her affect should reflect this with a smile or a pleasant demeanor. If this is not what is observed, the patient is described as incongruent with mood.

> Rolling your eyes certainly qualifies as nonverbal communication!

Therapeutic communication

The use of self is the psychiatric nurses' tool. It is the development of the therapeutic relationship between himself or herself and the patient and, by using that relationship, is able to complete assessments and patient teaching, facilitate therapeutic conversations, and listen to the concerns that your patients bring to you. It encourages the development of insight and allows patients to evaluate and develop problem-solving strategies. Therapeutic relationships are established through therapeutic communication. Techniques that help to establish a therapeutic relationship include open-ended questions, validating feelings, reframing feelings and events, clarifying, refocusing, collaborating ideas, and providing information.

Blunderin' and bunglin'

Alternatively, communication that is nontherapeutic may impede and slow a patient's ability to engage in a trusting relationship with psychiatric nursing staff. (See *Nontherapeutic ways of communicating*, page 16.)

Advice from the experts

Nontherapeutic ways of communicating

Nontherapeutic techniques hinder an effective nurse–patient relationship. Avoid the following pitfalls when interacting with patients.

Attacking or defending
- Getting angry or arguing with the patient
- Challenging the patient's beliefs
- Being defensive

Casting judgment
- Judging or criticizing the patient
- Giving approval or disapproval

Interrogating (or demanding)
- Asking the patient "why" questions
- Asking excessive, inappropriate, or leading questions
- Probing sensitive areas or making the patient feel uncomfortable

Minimizing
- Stereotyping the patient
- Not listening
- Not taking the patient's beliefs seriously
- Failing to maintain eye contact
- Changing the subject inappropriately
- Working on a task while the patient is talking to you
- Letting your mind wander during a conversation
- Using clichés

Giving advice
- Giving advice
- Offering false reassurance

Pressuring
- Trying to talk the patient into accepting treatment

Running off at the mouth
- Talking on and on
- Not letting the patient respond
- Repeating a point you just made
- Interpreting or speculating on the dynamics of patient problems
- Making inappropriate comments

Rushing
- Responding to the patient before he or she finishes speaking
- Finishing sentences for the patient

Taking sides
- Joining attacks led by the patient
- Participating in criticism of staff members

Using open-ended questions or statements

Asking open-ended questions allows your patient to provide information. It requires engagement in the conversation rather than a "yes" or "no" answer. Examples include "Tell me more about that." and "How do you think you could have handled this differently?"

Conversational cul-de-sacs

Close-ended questions, questions that can be answered with a yes or no response, cut off conversation and provide little meaningful information.

Validating

The practice of validating reviews and restates what a patient has reported and allows the patient to correct any misunderstanding. It also assures the patient that he or she has been heard and understood. It also encourages your patient to continue his or her story and provides you with more insight into what is of concern to him or her.

Clarifying

At times, a patient may give confusing or contradictory information. Asking the patient to explain what he or she means allows your patient to clarify what is being described. Responses such as "I don't understand what you're telling me. Would you tell me about this again?" allow you to evaluate your patient's thought process, fosters the therapeutic relationship, and provides more detailed information in understanding what is of concern to your patient.

Sharing impressions

It is important to review what you have heard and reflect back your impression of what your patient is thinking and feeling. Encourage your patient to correct any misunderstanding that may have occurred. A response such as "Tell me if this is what you are saying" conveys that you are listening and wish to fully understand your patient's thoughts and feelings.

Share—don't challenge

Sharing, like restating, allows your patient to correct any confusions or misunderstandings and provides insight into his or her thoughts and feelings. It is important to monitor your response to share not challenge your patient.

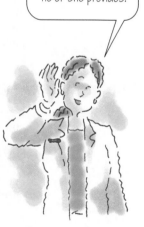

Ask the patient to clarify any confusing or vague information that he or she provides.

Restating

Restating, as with validating, reviews the information that your patient has shared but summarizes the information in your own words to confirm that you understand what he or she has said. This allows your patient to correct any misunderstanding, reinforces that you are interested in listening, encourages continued conversation, and may open an opportunity to provide education on a particular issue. An example of restating includes "If I understand you correctly, you are saying that you don't like taking medication several times a day."

Focusing

At times, patients can be disorganized and confused. Helping a patient to focus by asking a question such as "Can you tell me more about what is bothering you?" allows your patient to address a particular situation.

Providing information

Psychiatric nurses educate patients regarding medications, interventions, and treatment options. Providing information in a way that patients can understand based on their level of health literacy supports a therapeutic alliance and provides meaningful guidance to help them manage their condition. Be cautious not to provide advice while providing education (Townsend, 2014).

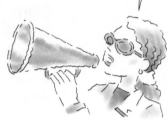

Allow the patient to make his or her own choices; practice listening rather than directing.

Assessment

Assessment is the basis of the nursing process. Psychiatric nursing, like other nursing specialties, is an evidence-based practice that involves evaluating our patients physically, emotionally, and psychosocially to identify assets and deficits. It is essential in initiating and evaluating treatment strategies and broadly informs nursing practice.

Testing—one, two, three

Accurate assessment techniques provide important updates on the physical, emotional, and behavioral changes of our patients. Appropriate assessment scales (Melancholia Scale [MES], Young Mania Rating Scale, World Health Organization Disability Assessment Schedule 2.0, etc.) are helpful in evaluating changes in a patient's presentation over periods of time.

Nursing interview in psychiatric mental health nursing

A systematic interview gathers broad information that helps you to:

- assess the patient's psychological functioning

- identify the underlying or precipitating cause of the patient's current concern

- understand the patient's coping methods and their effect on psychosocial growth

formulate the care plan

gauge progress and the effectiveness of treatments.

What's the point?

It is important to help our patients understand the importance of gathering important information in a systematic way to identify concerns. We must also communicate the benefits of addressing those concerns in an organized and appropriate manner.

General guidelines

In patient interviews, nurses ask a lot of personal and sensitive information. It is important to follow guidelines to ensure privacy.

Ensure privacy

Under the federal Health Insurance Portability and Accountability Act of 1996 (HIPAA) law, it is essential that we maintain a patient's confidentiality and protect his or her information from being shared unnecessarily. Interviews should be completed in a private, albeit safe, setting that will limit interruptions and provide a calm environment (U.S. Department of Health and Human Services, 2015).

Just the two of us

It is important that your patient understands that his or her privacy will be protected. Allow your patient to express who he or she feels should be involved during the interview process. There are many sensitive topics (e.g., sexual or substance activity) which he or she may be reluctant to share with family members present. It is appropriate to professionally ask them to leave the area while addressing those issues.

Show support and sensitivity

Patients with psychiatric conditions express themselves in many different ways. It is not uncommon to meet disorganized, psychotic, hypertalkative, withdrawn, or angry patients. Many are unwilling or unable to explain why they need treatment. It is important to make your patient feel safe and calm so that you are able to obtain an understanding of the concern through careful questioning, listening to responses, and objectively evaluating what you have learned. (See *Interview do's and don'ts*, page 20.)

Use reliable information sources

Some patients are "unreliable reporters" because of their psychotic or emotional presentation at the time of their first interview. It is important to identify collateral sources that know the

Advice from the experts

Interview do's and don'ts

When interviewing patients with psychiatric conditions, follow these guidelines.

Do set clear goals
An assessment interview is a systematic approach to obtain a history of the present illness (concern), prior episodes of psychiatric treatment, the presentation of symptoms—depressive or psychotic, history of self-harmful behaviors—suicidal thoughts or plans, prior suicide attempts, self-harmful behaviors of cutting or burning, etc. These are important to evaluate for every patient.

Do heed unspoken signals
Listening and observing each patient provides important clues in evaluating the health of your patient. Is the conversation organized and logical? Is speech rapid and pressured? Is he or she hyperverbal or with speech latency? Does the patient provide a lot of detail or seem dismissive? Does he or she appear anxious or depressed? Is he or she dismissive, anxious, grandiose, or depressed? How does the patient describe his or her mood, and does that mood description match your objective assessment (mood/affect congruity)?

Do check yourself
Patients often trigger an emotional response from their provider, such as aggression causing a fear response or anxiousness causing an anxiety response. These feelings of countertransference may occur when a patient sparks an underlying emotional feeling in the provider of care. It is important to be aware of your response to patients to avoid any interference in your ability to work therapeutically and professionally.

Don't rush
Take your time completing the interview. This is a time to gain information and, just as importantly, to establish a therapeutic relationship with your patient.

Don't make assumptions
It is important to ask questions about how situations affected your patient and what meaning he or she gives to each of those events. For one patient, the death of a beloved pet may trigger feelings of deep loss, sadness, and guilt, whereas for another, the response may be of anger and frustration. The importance of the event depends on how each patient internalizes his or her loss. It is dangerous to assume that because we feel a certain way, everyone else feels that way also.

Don't judge the patient
It is important to understand yourself and your biases so that you do not impose these beliefs on your patient. Remaining professional and "nonjudgmental" is essential to developing a therapeutic relationship. Your patient may have different beliefs than you have, but it is the appropriateness and logic of those beliefs that matter, not whether they share the same thinking as you.

patient well and are able to provide a better understanding of the history of the patient's concern. It is necessary, however, to obtain permission from our patients prior to interviewing the identified resources.

Consider the patient's culture

It is important to recognize that our patients come from diverse backgrounds and cultures. Being aware of our biases is essential to avoid misunderstandings and foster acceptance of all of our patients. (See *Abnormal—or just unfamiliar?*, page 22 and *Culture and Conduct*, page 23.)

Beginning the interview

Introduce yourself and explain the process and purpose of the interview. This often eliminates confusion and reduces the anxiety of your patient. Ask your patient how he or she would like to be addressed, and take the time to answer questions to begin the process of developing a therapeutic relationship.

Can you tell me about Mr. Smith? He gave me permission to talk with you, and I'd like to understand what has been happening.

Listening post

To put your patient at ease, speak in a private—but safe—area, keep a safe distance, sit so that you face the patient and make eye contact, talk in a calm and professional manner, and explain the process. For example, you may state "I'm going to be writing this information down because it is important that we understand what is happening as you describe it." Encourage your patient to provide pertinent details of onset, symptoms, prior treatment, etc.

Biographic data

Determine the patient's age, sex, ethnic origin, primary language, birthplace, religion, and marital status.

Socioeconomic data

Asking your patient for their highest degree/grade completed, employment status, source of income, housing, relationship status, and relationship with family and friends allows you to evaluate your patient's resources, support systems, and outside interests. Increased socioeconomic stressors may increase symptoms of illness.

Primary concern

Quote what the patient reports prompted him or her to seek treatment. What symptoms were they having, and what made them decide that today was the day to seek care? For example, a patient may report "I was feeling more depressed and anxious that usual." Be aware that some patients do not report having mental illness, others deny problems, and some are unclear of why they are seeking treatment.

History of present illness

The history explores the primary concern addressing:

    onset of symptoms—gradually or sudden onset

    types of symptoms—auditory/visual hallucinations, paranoia, delusions, etc.

    whether this is the first time the patient has experienced these symptoms or if he or she has experienced them in the past

    how severe the symptoms are—mild, moderate, or severe

    whether there is a trigger for the symptoms

    if the symptoms get better or worse with medication, treatment, and/or lifestyle changes

    whether the symptoms affect activity of daily living/employment

    if there are any unusual/bizarre presentations

You sure there's no problem?

During your assessment, it is important to evaluate any medical issues that a patient may have. Many medical problems mimic psychiatric concerns, such as hypothyroidism/depression, hyperglycemia/psychosis, etc. Many severe or chronic illnesses may cause an onset of depression or anxiety. Some medications, such as steroids, can cause an onset of psychosis (West & Kenedi, 2014).

Great expectations

It is important for each patient to be part of the treatment plan. The patient may have expectations about what he or she would like to accomplish through treatment; for instance, the patient may want

Bridging the gap

Abnormal— or just unfamiliar?

Cultural awareness is very important when working with psychiatric patients. Identifying cultural beliefs early in the assessment avoids confusion and mislabeling of symptoms. It is important to include consultants when evaluating unusual or unclear cultural beliefs. For example, patients from the Sea Islands (those of the Gullah culture) may report that "hoodoo" may have been used against them causing the current problem (Blue, 2012). It is important for the nurse to understand the underlying cultural beliefs that may support the patient's fears.

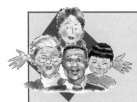

Bridging the gap

Culture and conduct

Culture and conduct
Be aware that several cultures respond differently to stressors. It is important to evaluate a patient's response with an awareness of cultural differences. For example, Chinese patients may be stoic, whereas Hispanic patients may express emotions outwardly.

Shame and stigma
Mental illness continues to carry a social stigma. Many patients feel shame because of their illness. Some cultures hide their mentally ill family members and rebuff questions about them.

Spiritual balance
Treatment options may be affected by a patient's cultural beliefs. Caribbean Island cultures may rely on spiritual or traditional remedies when making treatment decisions rather than Western treatment options.

to be free from auditory/visual hallucinations and delusions or achieve a stable mood. The more involved a patient in setting goals for treatment, the more likely he or she will work to achieve them.

Personal history

Was the patient born following a normal pregnancy that was full term? Did he or she hit all of the normal milestones? How did the family cope with change? Are there cultural traditions that are honored by the family? Are there any particular generational coping strategies? What was his or her family like? For example, who comprised the family? What were relationships in the family like? How many siblings does he or she have, and where does the patient fall in birth order? What is the highest grade level or degree that the patient has achieved? Does the patient work? What leisure activities or exercise does he or she enjoy? Does the patient have a legal history?

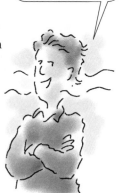

Go ahead. Ask me about my talents and accomplishments.

Psychiatric history

This is a review of all past psychiatric/psychological treatment, including any history of inpatient or outpatient treatment, symptoms of illness, number of hospitalizations, medication trials, and any periods of full remission of symptoms; history and treatment for of suicidal/homicidal ideation, suicide attempts, self-harmful behaviors—cutting/burning, and violence; and any history of alcohol, tobacco, or substance use or abuse, including amount, last use, and route.

Reluctant responders

Many patients are reluctant to answer, or they provide incomplete answers to the questions that we ask. Remind patients that it is important to provide complete information to avoid problems such as dangerous withdrawal symptoms. Many patients feel alone or weak related to the stigma attached to psychiatric disease. Providing empathetic support to patients helps them to see these problems as an illness with available treatment rather than a character flaw.

Psychosocial history

A psychosocial history includes the patient's spiritual and cultural beliefs and practices, coping skills, diet, lifestyle, committed relationships, social networks, and sleep patterns.

Upheaval index

Reviewing difficult life changes and how these changes affected the patient gives insight into coping strategies. Learning how the patient managed significant change, such as a recent marriage, birth of a child, divorce, acclimating to a new job or job loss, illness, or death of a loved one, gives insight into resiliency. Ask about coping methods, support systems, and resources used to gain a full understanding of how the patient reacts in stressful circumstances.

> Inquire about how the patient coped with a recent marriage, divorce, or other major life change.

It's all relative

Psychiatric illness may have a genetic component. Because of this, it is important to ask about relatives with diagnosed or suspected psychiatric illness. Additionally, if a family member has been treated successfully for a psychiatric illness, the medication/treatment used to stabilize that family member may be effective in stabilizing your patient. Becoming aware of substance or alcohol problems within the family may indicate a potential problem for abuse. Even if this is not a problem at this time, it may provide an opportunity to educate your patient on the increased risk of abuse because of a family history of abuse. Successful family suicides or suicide attempts is a significant red flag for potential suicide risk for your patient. Additionally, child abuse and violence often follow in families and need to be evaluated.

Medication history

Many medical disorders can mimic psychiatric illness. It is important to evaluate your patient for any physical disorders, particularly diabetes mellitus or thyroid disorders. These disorders require a full evaluation because a perceived "psychiatric disorder" may be one of organic origin. Stabilize the medical problem and the psychiatric symptoms disappear. Additionally, be aware that many medications, including over-the-counter nutritional and herbal supplements, can impact mental health and cause drug–drug interactions and need to be reported (Gurok, Mermi, Kilic, Canan, & Kuloglu, 2014).

Review the patient's medication history for therapeutic drug effects and adverse reactions.

Compliance check

It is important to have a complete list of all of your patient's prescribed medications (including over-the-counter nutritional and herbal supplements), a history of treatment adherence, and notation of any side effects that were experienced from medication. Additionally, under TJC guidelines, medication reconciliation of home medications is completed on admission to, and discharge from, the hospital. Throughout the hospitalization and on discharge, medication education and review is provided to the patient and written documentation is provided for reference.

Physical illnesses

Many chronic medical conditions may mimic psychiatric symptoms. It is important to have a full review of systems and physical examination complete upon admission to rule out psychotic changes related to a medical condition. Some symptoms commonly associated with medical conditions, as well as psychiatric conditions, include disorientation, thought distortions, and mood dysregulation. Kidney or liver failure, infection, thyroid disease, metabolic disorders, or increased intracranial pressure are often to blame.

Mental status evaluation

The mental status examination (MSE) is an objective review of a patient's cognitive functioning. MSE is a structured, objective approach to describe the physical and cognitive function through multiple areas on a given day.

The areas of review with normal findings are:

appearance: appears stated age, no acute distress, dressed appropriately for weather and season

attitude, calm, cooperative

speech: normal rate, volume, rhythm, tone

orientation: alert and oriented to date, time, location, and circumstance

motor: no psychomotor agitation/retardation

mood: "I'm good."

affect: full range and congruent with mood

thought process: linear, logical, goal directed

thought content: denies auditory/visual hallucinations, denies suicidal/homicidal ideation, denies paranoid thoughts and delusions, and no thought distortions evident

insight: appropriate

judgment: appropriate

eye contact: appropriate

Master of the MSE?

Nurses frequently complete MSEs to observe for changes from the patient's baseline. Careful observation of a patient helps us to determine when to change the plan of nursing care.

Level of consciousness

Evaluating a patient's level of consciousness (LOC)—a basic brain function—assesses the amount of stimulation necessary to arouse a patient. Some medical and psychiatric illnesses present with a reduced LOC, such as catatonia. Additionally, changes in LOC may indicate a change in condition, a change in liver function, acid-base imbalances, new or changing medical conditions, or a serious side effect from mediation which requires an immediate evaluation or a rapid response.

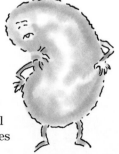

Oh dear. Kidney failure can cause an altered LOC.

General appearance

A patient's general appearance gives physical clues to help evaluate mental status. As in the MSE, a patient's appearance is measured against what is considered normal. When evaluating a patient's physical appearance, it is important to answer the following questions:

Is the patient dressed appropriately according to age, sex, and season?

Is the patient dressed in clean clothing?

Is the patient appropriately groomed, with clean hair, nails, and teeth?

Does the patient use cosmetics appropriately?

If your patient is disheveled, in appropriate clothing, poorly groomed, with excessive or bizarre makeup, it may indicate an increase in psychiatric symptoms or destabilization of mood.

Touchy subjects

It is important to measure a patient's height and weight on admission. Many medications can affect the metabolic rate, so baseline measurements are essential to monitor change. Assessing the color, condition of the skin, and any physical impairments or deformities provide clues to physical health. Unpleasant odors may indicate poor hygiene or infection.

Slouches, slumps, and substances

Assessing a patient's gait and posture on admission is important to evaluate for physical deformities, mood dysregulation, or fatigue. Changes in gait may indicate a patient is using substances or alcohol and may need to be monitored for withdrawal and other safety concerns. Poor posture or gait may place a patient at a higher risk for falling and safety precautions may need to be implemented. A shuffling, lurching, or unsteady gait may indicate neurologic problems.

Facial facts

Assess your patient's facial expression and response. Is he or she alert with an appropriate affect? Are eyes tracking appropriately? Do pupils respond appropriately and of equal size? Does he or she avoid eye contact? Unequal pupils can indicate head trauma with an undiagnosed subdural hematoma.

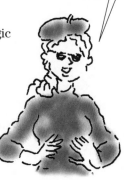

Are the sunglasses merely a fashion statement—or a way to avoid eye contact?

Reality check

Assess your patient's understanding of his or her psychiatric symptoms and what brought him or her to the hospital. It is important to compare the patient's understanding with your observations. Document incongruities.

Behavior

Assess your patient's attitude and presentation. What is the patient's mood? Does he or she report feeling happy, sad, or euphoric? Is he or she hyperactive, restless, or calm? Is he or she cooperative, irritable, or mute? Are there any reports of inappropriate hypersexual or violent behaviors? Does he or she interact appropriately with staff and peers? Document your findings.

Gestures

Evaluate any gestures noted. Are gestures appropriate or inappropriate? Is he or she gesturing as if interacting with someone? If so, your patient may be experiencing auditory or visual hallucinations.

Mannerisms

Does your patient have any rhythmic, repetitive mannerisms? Could these be tics or tremors? Are they restless movements, fidgety, pacing—tardive dyskinesia or akathisia?

Attitude

Evaluate the patient's attitude. Is he or she calm and cooperative or aggressive, hostile, or violent?

Activity level

An increased level of activity, decreased sleep, restlessness, and increased anxiety, coupled with rapid and pressured speech, may indicate a bipolar manic episode. A decrease in activity, increased sleeping, poor interaction with staff and peers, poor appetite, and poverty of speech may indicate an episode of depression.

Speech

Assessing speech patterns, content, rate, volume, rhythm, and tone give clues to a patient's level of function. This is also assessed in the MSE. It is important to note the characteristics of speech patterns to determine whether they reflect:
- illogical choice of topics
- irrelevant or illogical replies to questions
- speech defects, such as stuttering
- excessively fast or slow speech
- sudden interruptions
- excessive volume or barely audible speech

- altered vocal tone and modulation
- slurring
- excessive number of words (overproductive speech)
- minimal, monosyllabic responses (underproductive speech).

Sign language

Multiple modalities are available for hearing-impaired patients while in the hospital. American Sign Language interpreters, TTY machines, call relay services, etc. are available by appointment and by telephone. It is important to determine if a patient is hearing impaired or if his or her behavior is related to a psychotic event.

Time warp?

Does your patient struggle with poverty or latency of speech? This should be noted and evaluated.

Where's the logic?

Assess speech characteristics to evaluate changes in thought process. These alterations should be evaluated and noted.

- illogical or irrelevant replies to questions
- minimal or monosyllabic responses
- convoluted or excessively detailed speech
- repetitious speech patterns
- flight of ideas
- sudden silence for no apparent reason.

Mood and affect

To assess a patient's mood, ask a patient how he or she is feeling in concrete terms. Mood is a prevalent feeling but may change over the course of the day. Manic patients exhibit labile moods reporting alternating happiness and sadness throughout the day. An affect, on the other hand, is what is objectively observed: happiness = laughter, smiling, whereas sadness = depressed, tearfulness. The relationship between mood and affect is described as mood congruence—does the mood match the affect?

I think you got the better end of this mood swings deal.

Mood control

Mood changes may indicate a physiologic problem as well as a psychiatric problem. Acid/base levels, dehydration, alcohol, substance, stress, and medication side effects as well as mania may cause mood lability. Mood lability can be associated with poor sleep, hyperactive behaviors, periods of happiness, and irritability. Inconsistencies of mood or mood incongruity may be observable during these periods and should be documented as such. These inconsistencies need to be evaluated and monitored to rule out metabolic or endocrine problems.

Flighty or flat?

Assess and monitor for indicators of mood fluctuations:
• lability of affect—rapid, dramatic fluctuation in the range of emotions
• flat affect—an unresponsive range of emotion, which may signify schizophrenia or Parkinson disease
• inappropriate affect—inconsistency between affect and mood, as when the patient smiles when discussing an anger-provoking situation.

Intellectual performance

Intellectual ability, the ability to reason abstractly, make judgments, and problem solve, is affected in emotionally unstable patients. Multiple tests have been developed to evaluate the distressed patient. These simple tests also identify organic mental syndrome. Using the Mini-Mental Examination (MME) provides an easy assessment tool to evaluate intellectual performance through:

Orientation: person, place, time, and circumstance

Immediate/delayed recall: List three items and have your patient repeat them immediately and again in 5 to 10 minutes.

Remote memory: Assess the ability of the patient to recall distant events that were important in his or her life and can be collaborated.

Attention level: Evaluate the ability to concentrate and complete a task over a reasonable period of time. If a patient is found to have a short attention span, simple directions may assist in maintaining a patient's independence.

Comprehension: Evaluate the ability to read, grasp the content, recall, and explain a news or magazine article.

Concept formation: Ask your patient to explain the proverb "Birds of a feather flock together."

    a. Aspire for the abstract: If he or she is able to report that people who think or behave the same way often are found together, the patient is exhibiting abstract thinking.

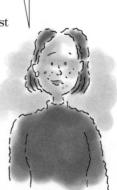

I'm only 12, but I'm old enough to think abstractly.

b. Confoundingly concrete: If the patient reports that birds fly in a group, then he or she is demonstrating concrete thinking—found in organic mental syndrome, mental retardation, severe anxiety, or schizophrenia.

General knowledge

To evaluate "common knowledge," it is appropriate to ask questions such as "Who is the president of . . ." or "What day of the week is it?"

Judgment

To evaluate a patient's understanding of illness and the ability to make appropriate decisions, it is important to assess judgment. While reviewing educational material on your patient's illness, you can ask "How do you know that some of the symptoms may be coming back and you need to call your doctor?" An appropriate response for a bipolar patient might be "I'm not sleeping as well. Instead of sleeping 7 hours per night, I'm only able to sleep 5 hours."

Insight

To evaluate the insight of your patient, it is appropriate to ask "What do you think is causing the problem with your sleeping pattern?" An expected response would be, "I had a stomach virus for 1 day and may not have taken all of my medication."

Degrees of insight

Assessing degrees of insight is important to understand risks to your patient and the need for further education. For example, a patient with bipolar disorder may blame his or her inability to take a morning dose of lithium to skipping breakfast and not wanting to take lithium on an empty stomach. Continuing to educate this patient may help to improve medication adherence. A patient who lacks insight may be psychotic.

Perception

Asking a patient to copy a simple drawing can assess perception. This exercise requires that your patient uses multiple senses to complete this task (Zimmerman, 2013).

All in the interpretation

There is an ongoing debate of the impact of "nature versus nurture" when considering psychiatric illness. Many experts believe that both impact mood and function. Psychoanalysts and psychopharmacologists often view mental illness as a combination of unresolved conflict as a result of a real or perceived loss than may cause change within the neurobiology of the brain. For instance, posttraumatic stress disorder is the result of a real or perceived life-threatening event which changes the neurobiology in the brain on how this memory is encoded and the physiologic response to an event that triggers the memory. Both psychoanalytic and psychopharmacologic approaches work together to understand the underlying trigger through therapy and decrease the physiologic response via medication to control the symptoms of this disorder.

Sensory perception disorders

Sensory perceptions are described as hallucinations or illusions. Hallucinations are perceptions that appear real but occur in a patient's mind, whereas illusions are a distortion of how the brain analyzes sensory information.

Hallucinations can be auditory, visual, tactile, olfactory, or gustatory. Auditory and visual hallucinations are often reported in psychiatric disorders, whereas tactile, olfactory, or gustatory hallucinations are more commonly observed in organic disorders.

Illusions can occur with a misinterpretation of any of the senses, but the most common are "optical illusions." "Heat mirages" are a common type of illusion experienced by people who drive on a hot, dry, black highway. Illusions are not necessarily a psychiatric disorder.

Patients with a variety of psychotic disorders report auditory and/or visual hallucinations that can lead to disorganized and illogical behaviors. Patients in severe alcohol withdrawal may experience auditory, visual, tactile, or olfactory hallucinations that resolve over time. At times, patients report command auditory hallucinations (CAH) that tell them to do certain things. CAH can be as benign as walking in a particular pattern or as serious as jumping from a bridge or stabbing someone with a knife.

Thought content/thought process

During your assessment, it is important to note any thought distortions that become apparent. Is conversation linear, logical, and goal directed? Does he or she perseverate about a particular thought or idea, report auditory or visual hallucinations, and/or report paranoid thoughts of being followed or monitored?

Delusions

Delusions are fixed, false beliefs that have no basis, or a tangential basis, in reality. Grandiose delusions such as "You work for me. I own this hospital and I'll fire you if you don't do what I want" or religious delusions such as "God sent me to tell people about the coming flood. He gave me special powers" are commonly seen in patients with schizophrenia.

Check the references

Ideas of reference are those in which a patient interprets an innocuous event to be of personal significance. For example, a patient may believe that a television newscaster is reporting news directly about the patient himself or herself. The terms *ideas of reference* and *delusions of reference* are often used interchangeably.

Obsessions and compulsions

Obsessive and compulsive behaviors can create havoc in a patient's life. Obsessions, the thought or preoccupation with a particular aspect of life, may lead to compulsions to act on the obsession. For example, an obsession about safety may lead to constantly checking that the doors are locked or the gas is turned off on the stove. The creation of these rituals can severely impact activities of daily life. It requires considerable effort, often coupled with therapy and medication, to control these obsessions and compulsions.

Morbid thoughts and preoccupations

Assess the patient for:

 suicidal, self-destructive, violent, or superstitious thoughts

 recurring dreams

 distorted perceptions of reality

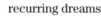 feelings of worthlessness.

Sex drive

It is important to evaluate changes in the sex drive of your patient. This can provide important insight into an emotional assessment. A nonjudgmental approach to sexual issues, or other sensitive topics, allows patients to engage in what can be perceived as an awkward discussion. Not all patients will share the same sexual orientation or beliefs that you have. Be aware of your own biases or discomfort when addressing sexuality with a patient.

Competence

Does your patient have insight into his or her illness and need for treatment? Does he or she have any appreciation of the problems that exist, or may develop, from a lack of treatment? Are his or her thoughts based in reality, and is he or she is aware of the effects of personal behaviors?

Be careful about competence

Assume that your patient is competent unless his or her thoughts or behavior strongly suggest otherwise. Ultimately, it is a judge's responsibility to evaluate and rule on competency and, if necessary, to assign a guardian.

> Only a judge can declare a person incompetent.

Defense mechanisms

Defense mechanisms are coping strategies used to reduce stress and to protect ourselves. We all use these strategies when we are in challenging situations. These strategies can be adaptive or maladaptive and are often unconscious responses.

Name that defense mechanism

Defense mechanisms include denial, regression, displacement, projection, reaction formation, and fantasy. It is important to evaluate patients' use of defense mechanisms.

(For common defense mechanisms you may encounter, see *Defining defense mechanisms*.)

Potential for self-destructive behavior

It is essential to evaluate patients for self-harmful behaviors. Asking the patient if he or she is suicidal will not cause the patient to become suicidal but provides important information about risk for self-injury. It is important to be aware that not all self-harmful behaviors necessarily mean that a patient is suicidal. Some patients engage in behaviors, such as cutting, burning, or mutilation, which they report help them to "feel" through the release of endorphins or reduce what they perceive as overwhelming distress.

Death wish

Some suicidal patients report that they would rather be dead than to continue with the ongoing pain of depression or other mental illnesses. If we are able to reduce the symptoms of their illness through medication and therapy, we may empower them to better manage their symptoms. Remember, patients with depression struggle to find positives in their life, whereas patients with schizophrenia may have command hallucinations telling them to harm themselves and patient with bipolar disorder may behave impulsively. Recognizing the risk of suicide can be challenging and it is better to err on the side of caution when creating an environment of safety. With any change in presentation, or an increase of symptoms of helplessness, hopelessness, or worthlessness, a suicide assessment should be completed immediately.

(See *Recognizing and responding to suicidal patients*, page 36.)

Defining defense mechanisms

People use defense, or coping, mechanisms to relieve anxiety. The definitions below will help you determine whether a patient is using one or more of these mechanisms.

Acting out

Acting out refers to repeating certain actions to ward off anxiety without weighing the possible consequences of those actions.

Compensation

Also called *substitution*, compensation involves trying to make up for feelings of inadequacy or frustration in one area by excelling or overindulging in another.

Denial

A person in denial protects himself or herself from reality—especially the unpleasant aspects of life—by refusing to perceive, acknowledge, or face it.

Displacement

In displacement, the person redirects impulses (commonly anger) from the real target (because that target is too dangerous) to a safer but innocent person. For example, a patient may yell at a nurse after becoming angry with his or her mother for not calling. The nurse is the "safer, innocent" person, whereas the mother is the "real target."

Fantasy

Fantasy refers to creation of unrealistic or improbable situations as a way of escaping from daily pressures and responsibilities or to relieve boredom. For instance, a person may daydream excessively, watch TV for hours on end, or imagine being highly successful when actually feeling unsuccessful. Fantasy helps the patient feel better momentarily.

Identification

In identification, the person unconsciously adopts the personality characteristics, attitudes, values, and behavior of someone else (such as a hero that is emulated and admired) as a way to allay anxiety.

Intellectualization

Also called *isolation*, intellectualization refers to hiding one's emotional responses or problems under a façade of big words and pretending there's no problem.

Introjection

A person interjects when he or she adopts someone else's values and standards without exploring whether they are personally fitting.

Projection

In projection, the person attributes his or her own unacceptable thoughts, feelings, and impulses to others.

Rationalization

Rationalization occurs when a person substitutes acceptable reasons for the real or actual reasons that are motivating his or her behavior. The rationalizing patient makes excuses for shortcomings and avoids self-condemnation, disappointments, and criticism.

Reaction formation

In reaction formation, the person behaves the opposite of the way he or she actually feels. For instance, a loved one may be treated with hatred, whereas a hated enemy is treated with kindness.

Regression

Under stress, a person may regress by returning to the behaviors used in an earlier, more comfortable time in life.

Repression

Repression refers to unconsciously blocking out painful or unacceptable thoughts and feelings, leaving them to operate in the subconscious.

Sublimation

In sublimation, a person consciously transforms personally or socially unacceptable drives into constructive ambitions and actions. For instance, a person who lost a friend to alcohol abuse may channel his or her anger into organizing a local chapter of Alcoholics Anonymous.

Undoing

In undoing, the person tries to undo the harm he or she feels he or she has inflicted on another. A patient who says something bad about a friend may try to undo the harm by saying nice things about the friend or by being kind and apologizing.

Withdrawal

Withdrawal refers to growing emotionally uninvolved by pulling back and being passive.

Recognizing and responding to suicidal patients

Assess your patient for the following indications of suicidal ideation (thoughts of suicide):
• withdrawal from others (social isolation)
• signs and symptoms of depression—crying, sadness, fatigue, helplessness, poor concentration, reduced interest in sex and other pleasurable activities, constipation, and weight loss
• overwhelming anxiety (the most common trigger for a suicide attempt)
• saying farewell to friends and family
• putting affairs in order
• giving away possessions
• conveying covert suicide messages and death wishes
• making overt suicidal statements, such as "I'd be better off dead."

Responding to a suicide threat

If you believe the patient intends to attempt suicide, assess the seriousness of intent and the immediacy of the risk. A patient with a chosen method and who plans to commit suicide in the next 48 to 72 hours should be considered a high risk.

Tell the patient you're concerned, and urge him or her to avoid self-destructive behavior until the staff has an opportunity to help. Then consult with the treatment team about arranging for psychiatric hospitalization or a safe equivalent such as having someone be present with the patient at home.

Safety precautions

If you believe the patient is at high risk for suicide, initiate the following safety precautions:

• Provide a safe environment. Check for and correct any conditions that pose a danger. Look for exposed pipes, windows without safety glass, and access to the roof or open balconies.
• Remove dangerous objects—belts, razors, suspenders, light cords, glass, knives, scissors, nail files, and clippers.
• Supervise the patient when shaving, taking medication, or using the bathroom.
• Make the patient's specific restrictions clear to staff members.
• Plan for observation of the patient.
• Clarify day staff and night staff responsibilities.

Stay close

Helping the patient build appropriate emotional ties to others is the ultimate means of preventing suicide. Besides observing the patient, maintain personal contact with him or her. Encourage continuity of care and consistency of primary nurses.

When to keep secrets

A patient may ask you to keep his or her suicidal thoughts confidential. Remember that such requests are ambivalent—a suicidal patient typically wants to escape the pain of life but also wants to live.

Tell the patient you can't keep secrets that endanger life or conflict with treatment. You have a duty to keep the patient safe and ensure the best care (Townsend, 2014).

Crisis control

If you have identified a patient at risk for suicide, it is essential to provide a safe environment to protect him or her from self-harm. With treatment, it is anticipated that this patient will be able to identify people important in his or her life and positive reasons for continuing to live. Unfortunately, we are not always able to save everyone.

Personality and projective tests

There are many assessment tools used to evaluate potential problems with patients. Several that are commonly used include the MSE, the MME, Beck Depression Inventory, Hamilton Depression Scale (Ham D), Bipolar Depression Rating Scale (BDRS), Assessment of Involuntary Movement Score (AIMS), CAGE questionnaire, and the ESPRIT questionnaire. Psychological testing provides additional information that give insight into intellectual functioning, focusing problems, or personality-related issues. Some of these screening tools are performed routinely during nursing assessments; however, many are scored and evaluated by the provider.

Physical examination

As discussed earlier, many physical illnesses present with similar symptoms as psychiatric illness. It is important that each patient is fully evaluated with a complete physical examination—including diagnostic studies—prior to any diagnosis.

Diagnosis

As nurses, we do not provide psychiatric or medical diagnoses, but we do choose applicable nursing diagnoses based on our evaluation and assessment. These nursing diagnoses assist us in planning effective care.

Planning

As an integral part of the treatment team, nurses are involved in creating and implementing a plan of care (see *Who's who on the interdisciplinary care team*, page 38). This plan is based on nursing diagnoses, the patient's diagnosis that is determined by the provider, and orders given by the provider. It is important to prioritize goals based on the severity of the problem—safety is always a priority—and how significant the impact is on the patient's life.

Effective planning must:

• focus on specific patient needs
• consider the patient's strengths and weaknesses
• encourage the patient to help set achievable goals and participate in his own care
• include feasible interventions
• be within the scope of applicable nursing practice acts.

Who's who on the interdisciplinary care team

Professionals from varying disciplines and backgrounds may be involved in the care of patients with psychiatric condition. The chart below identifies the education and responsibilities of each member of the interdisciplinary team.

Team member	Education	Responsibilities
Physician	Medical doctor or doctor of osteopathy, with a residency in psychiatry	Diagnosis and treatment of mental disorders
Psychologist	Master of science (MS) or doctor of philosophy (PhD)	Diagnosis of mental disorders, psychological testing, psychological treatments such as psychotherapy
Social worker	MS	Diagnosis of mental disorders; psychosocial therapies such as family, couple; also linked with community resources
Counselor	MS or PhD	Counseling
Occupational therapist	MS or occupational therapy doctorate (OTD)	Functional independence in tasks of living
Recreational therapist	Bachelor of science (BS)	Leisure-related activities
Nutritionist	MS	Nutritional therapy, education, maintaining balanced diet
Speech therapist	MS	Communication disorders
Expressive therapist (visual, musical, dance)	Master of arts (MA)	Expressive therapy through art, music, or dance
Pastoral counselor	Master of theology (or equivalent); ecclesiastical endorsement by faith group	Determination of spiritual and faith assets of each patient in the healing process
Vocational counselor	BS	Evaluation of student abilities, interests, talents, and personality characteristics so that they can develop realistic academic and career goals
Nurse generalist	Bachelor of science in nursing (BSN)	Provision of nursing care to patients in inpatient settings, offering direct and indirect care through the nurse–patient relationship
Clinical specialist	Master of science in nursing (MSN)	Provision of individual, family, and group psychotherapy in inpatient, outpatient, and community health settings and in private practice
Advanced practice nurse	MSN or doctor of nursing practice (DNP); certification in specialty (e.g., psychiatric nurse practitioner)	Provision of psychiatric mental health consultation to other nurses, patients, and families in the hospital setting

Care plan

A care plan provides the structure for consistency of patient care. It is a document created by the interdisciplinary team that is reviewed and acknowledged by the patient that identifies problems, goals, and treatment strategies. It is the baseline for documentation and provides a benchmark for improvement of the patient. Each care plan is reviewed and revised based on a patient's progress.

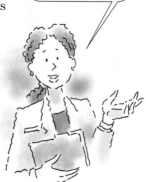

The care plan isn't a mere formality. It helps ensure continuity of care.

Groovy goals

Each goal must:
- relate directly the identified problem
- be measurable and realistic
- be stated as a desired outcome as a result of multidisciplinary care
- reflect the agreement of the patient and family
- be stated in a way that the patient and family can understand (Townsend, 2014).

Implementation

The treatment plan is implemented on admission and continues throughout treatment. The patient and family are involved in the development and application of the plan. They are including in the ongoing review and revisions of the plan in order to best meet the needs of the patient. Each plan is individualized based on continued assessments and evaluations to provide effective care. It is the goal of every treatment plan to provide a decrease or elimination of symptoms so that each patient will be safely discharged and achieve an optimal level of function.

Treatments

There is a vast array of treatment available for patients. The cornerstone of treatment remains medication and therapy based on individual needs. Nurses work with a diverse community and many treatments are available to address particular issues including psychiatric illnesses, drug/alcohol withdrawal and detoxification, traumatic brain injury, and cognitive loss.

Drug therapy

Medications target particular symptoms by affecting neurotransmitters in the brain. These medications are carefully titrated to therapeutic levels to avoid uncomfortable or serious side effects and must be carefully monitored for efficacy, adverse effects, and adherence. Education about medication therapy is an ongoing role of the psychiatric nurse.

Counseling and other therapies

Nurses are an important part of the interdisciplinary health care team. Psychologists; psychiatrists; and occupational, recreational, and art therapists may all be involved in patient care.

Psychotherapy

Psychologists, psychiatrists, and licensed social workers provide treatment through a broad range of therapeutic approaches designed to engage patients in identifying and modifying maladaptive attitudes, feelings, or behaviors. Psychologists are also involved in psychological testing that reflects underlying problems that impact treatment and treatment plan modifications. (See *Types of psychotherapy*.)

Behavior therapy

Behavioral therapy identifies problematic behaviors presumed to be learned and used in response to "triggers." Several therapeutic models look at the maladaptive responses, attempt to identify the trigger, and then challenge the response with the goal of changing the maladaptive behavior. Cognitive behavioral therapy (CBT) and dialectical behavioral therapy (DBT) are widely used therapeutic models to address problematic behaviors. (See *Drawing a bead on behavior therapy*, page 42.)

Milieu therapy

Controlling the therapeutic environment is the core of milieu therapy. The therapeutic milieu is more than the physical area of the unit. It is the community that is established by the staff and patients to promote a calm, healing environment. This occurs on locked or unlocked inpatient units as well as in outpatient treatment sites. It is one of many tools used to foster recovery through appropriate behavior. It requires the shared responsibility of staff and patients in their roles in conforming to the rules and policies of the community to maintain a therapeutic environment.

Out of uniform

Frequently, staff that care for patients with psychiatric concerns wears street clothing rather than uniforms while working in mental health settings. This provides an environment that feels "normal" instead of "clinical."

Types of psychotherapy

The therapist may act as a neutral observer or active participant. The success of therapy depends largely on patient–therapist compatibility, treatment goals, and the patient's commitment to therapy.

Individual therapy

Individual therapy involves a series of counseling sessions, which may be short- or long-term. After working with the patient to establish appropriate goals, the therapist mediates the patient's disturbed behavior patterns to promote personality growth and development.

Group therapy

Guided by a psychotherapist, a group of people (ideally 4 to 10) experiencing similar emotional problems meets to discuss their concerns. The duration of group therapy may vary from a few weeks for acute conditions requiring hospitalization to several years for chronic conditions. Group therapy can be especially useful in treating addictions.

Cognitive therapy

According to cognitive theory, depression stems from low self-esteem and a belief that the future is bleak and hopeless. The goal of cognitive therapy is to identify and change the patient's negative generalizations and expectations—and thereby reduce depression, distress, and other emotional problems.

The therapist assigns homework, such as making lists of pleasurable activities to reduce or replace automatic negative thoughts and conclusions.

Family therapy

Family therapy aims to alter relationships within the family and change the problematic behavior of one or more members. Useful in treating childhood or adolescent adjustment disorders, marital discord, and abusive situations, family therapy may be short- or long-term.

Crisis intervention

Crisis intervention seeks to help patients develop adequate coping skills to resolve an immediate problem. The crisis may be developmental (such as a marriage or the death of a family member) or situational (such as a natural disaster or an illness).

Therapy focuses on helping the patient resume the precrisis functional level. It usually involves just the patient and therapist but sometimes includes family members. It may consist of one session or of multiple sessions over several months.

Detoxification

Many patients have primary or co-occurring problems with drugs or alcohol. Programs that are designed to safely withdraw patients from drugs or alcohol use frequent monitoring and medication to avoid uncomfortable and/or life-threatening complications of detoxification. These inpatient or outpatient programs provide a safe alternative to a "cold turkey" self-withdrawal following long-term misuse of substance. During and following medical monitoring of withdrawal, therapy is offered to help patients understand the risks associated with continued substance use and referrals for ongoing treatment are provided.

Drawing a bead on behavior therapy

Behavioral therapy is appropriate for children and adults and may be used for individual or group therapy. It is used to change patterns of behavior and multiple therapeutic modalities fall under its umbrella, including assertiveness training, aversion therapy, desensitization, flooding, positive conditioning, response prevention, thought stopping, thought switching, and token economy.

Assertiveness training

Assertiveness training increases self-esteem by encouraging patients to appropriately stand up for themselves while respecting the rights of others (Townsend, 2014). It teaches the patient ways to express feelings, ideas, and wishes without feeling guilty or demeaning others.

You can help the patient by providing examples of appropriate behavior and role modeling responses that are assertive rather than nonassertive, aggressive, or passive-aggressive.

Aversion therapy

In aversion therapy, a technique based on classical and operant conditioning, an unwanted stimulus is used to change unwanted habits (Varcarolis, 2013). For example, a patient who abuses alcohol may be prescribed disulfiram (Antabuse), which makes the individual extremely ill if they ingest alcohol (Varcarolis, 2013).

Systematic desensitization

The treatment of choice for phobias, desensitization involves teaching the patient techniques that promote relaxation and then slowly introducing exposure to the thing that is feared (Varcarolis, 2013). For example, a patient who has a fear of flying in airplanes may be taught deep breathing and other relaxation techniques and then gradually introduced to a series of stimuli related to flying (e.g., visualization of an airplane; thinking about walking onto the plane to be seated; and eventually, taking an actual flight).

During desensitization therapy, provide the patient with reassurance and review relaxation techniques.

Monitor responses to each anxiety-producing situation, and emphasize that the patient need not proceed to the next one until he or she feels ready.

Implosion therapy

Also called *flooding*, implosion therapy involves direct exposure to an anxiety-producing situation. However, instead of using relaxation techniques (as in systematic desensitization), this approach is based on the assumption that fast, direct confrontation helps the patient overcome fear (Townsend, 2014).

Implosion therapy is contraindicated in patients who has fragile psyches and for those who may have medical conditions (e.g., heart dysrhythmias) that could be exacerbated during treatment (Townsend, 2014).

Operant conditioning

Operant conditioning involves behavioral modification based on a system of positive or negative reinforcement (Varcarolis, 2013). Positive reinforcement encourages behavior to occur more frequently, whereas negative reinforcement discourages behavior from occurring.

Thought stopping

Thought stopping helps the patient control inappropriate expressions of feelings (Boyd, 2012) by saying a phrase such as "stop" and then redirecting attention on another activity or thought. It can be helpful to teach the patient to visualize an actual stop sign when saying "stop" (Boyd, 2012).

Token economy

Using token economy, selected acceptable patient behavior is rewarded by giving out tokens, which the patient uses to "buy" a privilege or object, such as television viewing time, or special snacks (Boyd, 2012).

During this type of treatment, monitor the patient's behavior and provide or withhold rewards consistently and promptly (Boyd, 2012).

Drugs and dual diagnosis

Substance abuse and/or dependence continue to be an ever-increasing problem, and psychiatric illness does not preclude a patient from using alcohol or street drugs. These items are easy to obtain and readily available; are highly addictive; and may cause significant, permanent damage to the brain tissue. *Dual diagnosis* is a term that is used to describe individuals with psychiatric conditions who have coexisting problems with alcohol or drug use (National Association on Mental Illness [NAMI], 2014).

Patients with dual diagnosis are less likely to follow treatment plans than those with only a psychiatric diagnosis. They are at higher risk for impulsive, violent, and suicidal acts (NAMI, 2014).

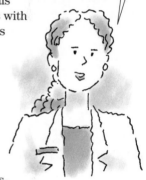

Many patients suffer from both mental illness and substance abuse.

Electroconvulsive therapy

Electroconvulsive therapy (ECT) has been used successfully to provide relief for patients with severe major depression or bipolar disorder that has not responded to other treatment methods (American Psychiatric Association [APA], 2010). ECT remains controversial as a result of preconceived beliefs and misinformation. It is important that nurses understand the risks and benefits of ECT to properly educate and support patients who choose this treatment option.

APA practice guidelines provide recommendations for the use of ECT, including education on the procedure with written and signed consent.

Procedure

ECT is performed in the operating room using general anesthesia. Small electrodes are placed on the head, either bilaterally or unilaterally, and a brief electrical stimulation of the brain is conducted (APA, 2010). ECT is typically administered two to three times per week for approximately 6 to 12 treatments, depending on the patient's symptom severity and responsiveness to treatment (APA, 2010).

The most common side effects of ECT that occur the day of treatment include nausea, headache, fatigue, confusion, and slight memory loss (APA, 2010). Patients may report some short-term memory loss and difficulty learning or remembering short-term events following ECT (APA, 2010). Short-term memory loss typically resolves within a few months.

Can't explain it

Although ECT is not completely understood, it is thought that the electrical impulse causes a neurochemical change in the brain that is effective, over time, in assisting to control symptoms.

Evaluation

Through continued assessment, the nurse can evaluate the effectiveness of treatment. Assessment and evaluation are processes that are ongoing and provide continued information on the patient's progress. Additionally, they provide needed data when reviewing and revising the plan of care to best meet the needs and expectations of the patient.

Documentation

Documenting interactions and observations completely, accurately, and in a timely manner is the legal and ethical responsibility of the nurse. It is essential for continuity of care as well as confirming that nurses have completed the necessary treatments ordered for patients. Documentation should objectively address assessments, the plan of care, interventions, and the patient's progress toward meeting identified goals.

> Documentation provides legal proof of the nature and quality of patient care.

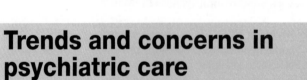

Legal duty

It is the legal duty of health care providers to document the details of the care provided to the patient. Unclear, insufficient, or subjective documentation may result in a denial of reimbursement for services provided or provide grounds for liability of the nurse, other provider of care, and/or facility for inadequate or improper care.

Trends and concerns in psychiatric care

In the American health care setting, there has been a steady decrease over the decades since the 1970s in the number of patients that have been admitted and maintained at the various state hospitals as care has moved back into the community setting. With the advent of the Affordable Care Act, it remains to be seen whether Americans will experience parity in the care of patients with psychiatric conditions. Reimbursement and funding dollars are often controlled by insurance companies that use case management algorithms designed to move patients to a lower level of care as soon as possible. Because of this, improved collaboration between inpatient, outpatient, community, residential, and ancillary services must improve.

Deinstitutionalization

Following the exposure of abuses to patients hospitalized in psychiatric facilities in the 1960s and 1970s, and with the advent of medications that better controlled the symptoms of psychiatric illnesses, state institutions discharged patients with psychiatric conditions more quickly. These discharged patients were to receive care within their communities in residential housing and outpatient treatment centers. Unfortunately, the quantity of services was not adequate for the number of patients that needed them. This failure has led to homelessness for some and the criminalization of mental illness for others.

Shame and stigma

Stigma and shame remain the most significant barriers to treatment for patients with psychiatric conditions. Advocacy groups continue to work to create public awareness and understanding for this vulnerable population while providing support and resources for the patient and family.

Legal and ethical issues

Professional standards established by the ANA describe the legal and ethical issues that structure the role of the psychiatric nurse. Professional psychiatric nurses must meet the same standards of "reasonable and prudent behavior" as deemed acceptable of other professional psychiatric nurses with the same experience and education preforming in the same capacity. Additionally, the nurse practice act of each state outlines the legal obligations of all nurses working with patients.

Rights of the mentally ill and developmentally disabled

The U.S. Constitution protects the rights of all citizens. Patients with psychiatric conditions or developmentally disabled citizens cannot be denied rights because of disability or dependency. A violation of rights, even unknowingly, could result in serious legal penalties.

Life and liberty

Patients with psychiatric conditions and developmentally disabled patients have a right to life, liberty, and control of their lives as much as they are able. Unless a patient represents a danger to self or others, impeding a patient's liberty and controlling his or her behavior is illegal. The protection of the freedoms for vulnerable populations are the result of historic abuses imposed on individuals within these populations and the commitment to prevent this from happening again.

Right to treatment

The Constitution has been interpreted by the courts and establishes the right to appropriate, humane treatment for patients via all available treatment options.

Discrimination elimination

The Americans with Disabilities Act of 1990 (revised in 2010) guarantees parity for the disabled citizen by affording a "national mandate for the elimination of discrimination against individuals with disabilities."

Mental health patient's bill of rights

A universal bill of rights for mentally ill patients was established in the Mental Health Systems Act of 1980. Congress outlined that treatment will be provided by:
• by adequate staff
• in the least restrictive setting
• in privacy
• in a facility that provides a comfortable bed, an adequate diet, and recreational facilities
• with the patient's informed consent before unusual treatment

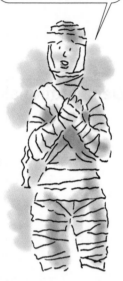

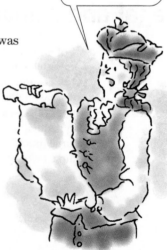

- with payment for work done in the facility, outside of program activities
- according to an individual treatment plan.

Keeping the patient informed

Nurses taking care of a patient with a psychiatric condition must assess and evaluate what the patient knows about his or her illness and the need for treatment. Discharge planning begins at the admission. Enlisting the patient in development of a treatment plan encourages him or her to consider important elements in maintaining health and may improve "buy in" while discharge preparations take place. If the patient is unwilling or unable to participate in formulating a comprehensive plan, it is important to document specific barriers.

Right to refuse treatment

Most patients are able to make informed decisions to refuse or postpone treatment if that is their choice. These patients are considered competent to make health care decisions for themselves. If a patient chooses to refuse or postpone treatment within the hospital setting, he or she is stated to be making decisions "against medical advice."

Order from the court

In some cases, the doctor or treatment team may determine that a patient presents a danger to self or others and requires medication, treatment, and a continued inpatient hospitalization. The laws governing retention of a patient against the patient's wishes vary from state to state. It is important to familiarize yourself with the laws in your specific state regarding this process. In most states, to retain a patient against his or her will, the hospital must petition the court to "hear" the argument from the hospital to retain the patient and listen to the patient explain the reason that he or she should be released from the hospital. If the court agrees with the hospital, then the patient will remain "committed" to the hospital for a specified period of time for treatment. If, however, the court agrees with the patient, the court will issue an order for the patient to be released from the hospital.

Rights of minors

It is essential for a hospital or facility to establish legal guardianship immediately upon the admission of a mentally ill or developmentally disabled minor. Generally, the minor is accompanied by a parent or an appointed legal guardian on admission.

Parental waiver

If the parents have surrendered responsibility for their minor child to an institution and the institution has provided the appropriate documentation to support this, the hospital may be responsible for decisions related to the care of the minor child.

Right to informed consent

It is not the nurses' responsibility to obtain informed consent from a patient; that responsibility falls to the primary provider of care. It is, however, the nurses' responsibility to provide important, pertinent information; clarify questions about the consent; and document any concerns the patient may identify. If a patient has additional questions regarding the actual treatment or procedure to be performed, the nurse must have the primary provider of care return to talk further with the patient. If the nurse answers "no" to any of the following questions, the mental health care team must be notified prior to initiating any treatment, so that clarification regarding the consent process can be further discussed.

Let's discuss your understanding of the procedure you're about to undergo.

- Can this patient consent in the same way as another patient to treatment?
- Does this patient have a complete understanding of the risks, benefits, or alternatives of this treatment?
- Is this patient able to give informed consent?

Satisfying answers

It is the responsibility for the treatment team to provide complete information to the patient or the legal guardian so that they can make an informed decision. Because of the relationship that a nurse has with his or her patient, he or she is often involved in answering questions, providing resources, and evaluating how well the patient or legal guardian understands the treatment option. The nurse may then enlist specific members of the health care team to address any confusion that may remain.

Get sued now, get sued later

It is important to remember that the role as a nurse is to advocate for patients. If informed consent is not obtained and the nurse chooses to participate in the procedure, the nurse—along with the primary provider of care and/or the facility—could be held liable. In many states, that statute may be until the minor becomes an adult (e.g., age 18). Obtaining consent or partitioning the courts for treatment over objection protects your patient as well as you, your team, and the facility.

Consent to medical research

Drastic, extreme, or questionable forms of treatment prompt many complicated questions and ethical considerations. Hospitals and organizations rely on their institutional review board (IRB) to review the risks, benefits, and needs of any patient that may be considered for these treatments that are part of research studies. Individuals should participate only when the potential benefits outweigh the risks and should be considered for a clinical trial. Patients or their guardians must fully understand the risks and benefits of any treatment and sign consent to participate in the study.

Ask the Feds

There are strict state and federal regulations that direct how clinical trials are implemented and require great care with the inclusion of mentally ill patients in a trial.

Right to privacy

Each of us has a right against unwarranted and unwanted intrusion into our personal lives. However, patients may have this right violated when health care providers carelessly discuss their private information in public areas. Be mindful of your environment, and protect your patient's privacy.

You must protect your patient's privacy and teach him or her about privacy rights.

Codes and bills

The federal HIPAA regulations, the American Hospital Association's Patient's Bill of Rights, and the ANA code of ethics provide information on how you share information, to whom you share information, and your responsibility in preserving your patient's right to keep personal health information private. In our role as health care providers, we are often informed of private, sensitive information and it is incumbent upon us to protect this information from unwanted disclosure. All records concerning care must be kept confidential unless the patient agrees to their disclosure. Remember that HIPAA is the law!

Teaching patients about privacy rights

As an advocate for patients, it is our responsibility as a nurse to behave in a professional, ethical manner as described by the nurse practice act of our state as well as other guidelines mentioned earlier. In this role, we rigorously protect our patient's privacy and educate him or her on his or her rights to privacy, not only while receiving treatment but also to personal medical records once treatment has been concluded. Within these rights, a patient is able to refuse the release of information, even to his or her family. Picture taking of a patient is prohibited in mental health facilities to avoid inadvertently including other patients in the picture and accidently breaching other patients' rights of confidentiality.

When you must disclose

The HIPAA regulations requires that hospitals maintain confidentiality for their patient except in four instances:

 suspected child abuse

 criminal cases

 government requests

when the public has a right to know

Reproductive and sexual rights

Reproductive and sexual rights of the mentally ill patients have been upheld by the U.S. Supreme Court. These rights include the right to:

 marry

 have children

 use contraception, abortion, or sterilization, if desired

 follow a lifestyle of their own choosing.

> Mentally ill patients have the right to marry and have children.

Legal guardianship

If the developmentally disabled or mentally ill patient is an adult, it is important for the facility to determine if this patient has or requires a legal guardian. The legal guardian should be identified in the patient's chart. The legal guardian may be a spouse, parent, or someone appointed by the courts and it is important for the facility to be aware of the contact information.

When parents have been found unfit or unable to care for their children by the courts, a legal guardian will be appointed to accept responsibility for the care of the minor. If, however, the courts have appointed no guardian, the state will act in this role.

Can't seem to agree

Disagreements about a patient's care may occur between the patient and a legal guardian. If that occurs, it is essential to alert the appropriate channels within the facility.

Competence

Just because a patient has a psychiatric condition, it does not mean that they are incompetent or lack capacity to consent to treatment. Sometimes, however, members of the interdisciplinary team question the competence of a patient even if the patient has not been judged to be legally incompetent. Sometimes, illness may cause temporary mental incompetence. In this situation, it is important to consult state laws to determine who is able to make health care decisions for the patient. Frequently, it is a family member or relative that would make these decisions, but if there is no relative legally designated, willing, or able to make these decisions, a court must authorize treatment or appoint someone to make these decisions.

Restraints and seclusion

Seclusion and restraints are used only to prevent a patient from injuring self or others and only when other less restrictive methods have failed.

Restrain yourself from punishing

Restraints are a short intervention, often coupled with medication, and/or used in an emergency to maintain safety. Seclusion and restraints are not used for punishment or convenience but are meant to allow a patient to be in a safe place and regain control.

Restraint policies

The use of seclusion and restraints is governed by facility policies and accrediting body guidelines, such as those from TJC. The orders are time limited with the patient on continuous observation with frequent documentation. Patients are assessed on a schedule for food, fluids, toileting, and safety. Seclusion or restraints are discontinued as quickly as the patient is able to regain control and agree to remain in control.

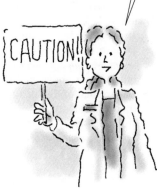

If you must restrain a patient, use the minimal amount of restraint necessary.

Orders from the primary provider of care

Many states require an order from a licensed independent practitioner (LIP) prior to the application of the restraints. However,
several states continue to allow an emergency application of
restraints to be followed by an order as soon as possible following
the application of the restraints. The use of restraints is time limited, and monitoring per TJC guidelines is required.

References

American Nurses Association. (2014). *Psychiatric-mental health nursing: Scope and standards of practice* (2nd ed.). Silver Spring, MD: Author.

American Nurses Credentialing Center. (2014). Retrieved from http://www.nursecredentialing
.org/

American Psychiatric Association. (2010). *Electroconvulsive therapy (ECT)*. Retrieved from
http://www.psychiatry.org/File%20Library/Mental%20Illness/Lets%20Talk%20Facts/
APA-ECT.pdf

American Psychiatric Association (2013). *Diagnostic and statistical manual of mental
disorders* (5th ed.). Arlington, VA: Author.

Blue, A. (2012). *Cultural competency*. Retrieved from http://academicdepartments.musc.edu/
fm_ruralclerkship/curriculum/culture.htm

Boyd, M. A. (2012). *Psychiatric nursing: Contemporary practice* (5th ed.). Philadelphia, PA:
Lippincott Williams & Wilkins.

Gurok, M. G., Mermi, O., Kilic, F., Canan, F., & Kuloglu, M. (2014). Psychotic episode induced
by St. John's wort (*Hypericum perforatum*). *Journal of Mood Disorders, 4*(1), 38–40.

Kupfer, D. J., Kuhl, E. A., & Regier, D. A. (2013). DSM-5—the future arrived. *Journal of the
American Medical Association, 309*, 1691–1692.

National Association on Mental Illness. (2014). *Dual diagnosis: Substance abuse and mental
illness*. Retrieved from http://www.nami.org/Content/NavigationMenu/Inform_Yourself/
About_Mental_Illness/By_Illness/Dual_Diagnosis_Substance_Abuse_and_Mental_
Illness.htm

Stahl, S. M. (2013). *Stahl's essential psychopharmacology: Neuroscientific basis and practical applications* (4th ed.). New York, NY: Cambridge University Press.

Townsend, M. C. (2014). *Essentials of psychiatric mental health nursing: Concepts of care
in evidence-based practice*. Philadelphia, PA: F.A. Davis.

U.S. Department of Health & Human Services. (2014). *Projections of health expenditures
for mental health services and substance abuse treatment: 2004-2014*. Retrieved from
http://store.samhsa.gov/shin/content//SMA08-4326/SMA08-4326.pdf

U.S. Department of Health and Human Services. (2015). *Health information privacy*. Retrieved from http://www.hhs.gov/ocr/privacy/index.html

Varcarolis, E. (2013). *Essentials of psychiatric mental health nursing: A communication
approach to evidence-based care* (2nd ed.). Philadelphia, PA: Saunders.

West, S., & Kenedi, C. (2014). Strategies to prevent the neuropsychiatric side-effects of corticosteroids: A case report and review of the literature. *Current Opinion in Organ Transplantation, 19*(2), 201–208.

Zimmerman, M. (2013). *Interview guide for evaluating DSM-5 psychiatric disorders and the mental health examination.* East Greenwich, RI: Psych Products Press.

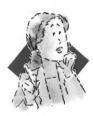

Quick quiz

1. The currently used system for classifying and diagnosing mental disorders was established by the:

    A.   American Nurses Association.

    B.   American Psychiatric Association.

    C.   state boards of nursing.

    D.   American Medical Association.

Answer: B. The American Psychiatric Association established the currently used system of classifying and diagnosing mental disorders. The latest version, published in *DSM-5*, emphasizes observable data and deemphasizes subjective and theoretical impressions.

2. The MSE assesses all of the following except the patient's:

    A.   LOC.

    B.   mood, affect, and perceptions.

    C.   medication side effects.

    D.   activities of daily living.

Answer: C. The MSE examines the patient's LOC, general appearance, behavior, speech, mood and affect, perceptions, intellectual performance, judgment, insight, and thought content.

3. Which nursing statement reflects the nontherapeutic communication technique of minimizing?

    A.   "If I were you, I would take this medication."

    B.   "Don't feel badly. Everything will work out fine."

    C.   "Why do you feel so depressed all of the time?"

    D.   "I think your sister is right about how bad of a temper that you have."

Answer: B. A reflects "giving advice," C reflects "interrogating," and D reflects "taking sides." B minimizes the patient's feelings by telling them that everything will be fine.

4.   Which test assesses a patient's orientation and recall?
   A.   Beck Depression Inventory
   B.   Thematic apperception test
   C.   Mini-Mental Status Examination
   D.   Millon Clinical Multiaxial Inventory III

Answer: C. The Mini-Mental Status Examination assesses the patient's orientation, registration, recall, calculation, language, and graphomotor function.

5.   A preoccupation that's acted out is called:
   A.   an obsession.
   B.   a compulsion.
   C.   a delusion.
   D.   a hallucination.

Answer: B. A compulsion is a repetitive behavior that the patient feels compelled to perform in response to an obsession.

Scoring

☆☆☆ If you answered all five items correctly, superb! Your psychiatric sagacity is spectacular!

☆☆ If you answered three or four items correctly, well done! You're obviously all psyched up about psychiatric disorders.

☆ If you answered fewer than three items correctly, don't despair! You have plenty of time to digest the material in this *Incredibly Easy* resource!

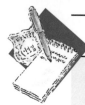

2

Disorders of children and adolescents

Just the facts

In this chapter, you'll learn:

♦ theories of growth and development

♦ characteristics of mentally healthy young people

♦ signs and symptoms of psychiatric disorders in children and adolescents

♦ treatment options for children and adolescents with psychiatric disorders.

A look at disorders of children and adolescents

Because children and adolescents are in a state of rapid change and growth, a wide range of behavior is considered normal. Nonetheless, many children and adolescents experience emotional and mental distress that is more severe than the normal highs and lows of growing up. Although some get better over time, others have serious and persistent problems that affect their daily activities and require professional help.

Between 10% and 20% of children and adolescents worldwide experience mental health problems (Kieling et al., 2011). These problems can start in early childhood and can affect how children achieve their expected developmental, cognitive, and emotional milestones. Unfortunately, undiagnosed and/or untreated mental health problems can impair the child's or adolescent's ability to function at home, in school, or within community settings and hinder the formation of healthy peer relationships. It is often hard to tell

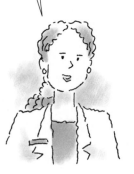

Some psychiatric problems may start in early childhood.

whether a child or adolescent has a psychiatric disorder. Often, a young person may first present with medical problems or demonstrate a range of normal to abnormal emotional behaviors. Most clinicians concur that a mental health problem exists if the persistent behavior is not age-appropriate, does not conform to the cultural norms, and produces impaired functioning in daily activities.

Illness inventory

This chapter discusses some of the most common psychiatric disorders affecting youths:
- attention deficit hyperactivity disorder (ADHD)
- oppositional defiant disorder (ODD)
- conduct disorder
- depression
- autism spectrum disorder
- intellectual disability (intellectual developmental disorder).

Surprising stats

According to the National Institute of Mental Health, about one in five children and adolescents in the United States suffer from mental illness severe enough to cause impairment across the lifespan. Furthermore, 50% of lifelong cases of mental illness begin by the age of 14. However, fewer than one in five receives treatment, even though many of these disorders can be treated effectively with psychotherapy and drug therapy (Kieling, et al., 2011; Merikangas, et al., 2010).

Risk factors

Psychiatric disorders occur in children and adolescents of all social classes and backgrounds. Certain factors place a child at greater risk, such as:
- low birth weight
- physical health problems
- family history of mental or addictive disorders
- multigenerational poverty
- separation or lack of social support from caregivers
- abuse, neglect, or exposure to violence
- immigrant parents.

Psychosocial consequences

A child or adolescent with a psychiatric disorder has many challenges to overcome. Despite greater public awareness and understanding of mental disorders, these illnesses still carry a stigma that can affect the individuals and their families. Children who behave inappropriately may frighten or offend other children and people in the community, making themselves social outcasts (O'Driscoll, Heary, Hennessy, & McKeague, 2012; Turner, Finkelhor, & Ormrod, 2010).

Family discord

Family members may lack adequate knowledge of psychiatric disorders and may feel guilty or embarrassed at having a child who is perceived to be mentally unhealthy. If the family members do not understand or cannot cope with the child's behavior, they may become frustrated and withdraw or be overactive in their attempts to control the child's behavior. Ultimately, the parents' or guardians' exasperation may escalate to verbal or physical abuse of the child.

Placement issues

A child whose behavior severely disrupts the family or who can't be integrated into the family unit may require temporary or permanent placement in a structured facility. The placement decision may be influenced by social, financial, religious, and cultural considerations, as well as demographic availability of a facility.

Educational issues

Although most children and adolescents with psychiatric conditions can attend regular schools, those with severe disorders may derive more benefits when enrolled in special classes or special educational facilities. However, these classes may be out of reach financially or geographically for some families.

Childhood development

To understand childhood disruptions and the mental health problems that can result, nurses must be familiar with the patterns of normal child development. A child moves from infancy through childhood to adolescence in an orderly manner. As the child grows, the personality develops.

Nature plus nurture

Personality formation is influenced by genetic and environmental factors. Sigmund Freud, Erik Erikson, and Jean Piaget proposed developmental theories to describe the progressive stages of childhood and adolescence. (See *Theories of growth and development*, page 58.)

When nurses are familiar with theories of growth and development, they can apply them to clinical situations,

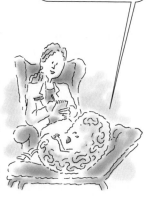

I could write a book about child development! Just call me Sigmunda Freud!

Theories of growth and development

As children grow, they develop intellectually, emotionally, sexually, socially, and spiritually. They learn to think abstractly and logically, to use language, and to explore the world around them. Several theorists, including Sigmund Freud, Erik Erikson, and Jean Piaget, explain how this growth occurs.

Freud: Psychosexual development

Freud theorized that the human mind consists of three major entities—id, ego, and superego. The id seeks instant gratification. The ego orients the person to reality, intercepting impulses from the id. The superego (conscience) develops during childhood—the product of rewards and punishments bestowed on the individual.

According to Freud, children must master each developmental stage before they can move on to the next one.

• **Oral phase (birth to 18 months):** The infant is totally dependent and narcissistic and starts to become aware of the self as an individual. Ego development begins.
• **Anal phase (18 months to 3 years):** The child learns to postpone immediate gratification and to manipulate surroundings. Episodes of negativity, rebellion, and conflict may occur. The superego begins to develop.
• **Phallic phase (ages 3 to 6):** The child develops an awareness of anatomic and sexual differences between males and females. The child identifies and adopts the characteristics of the same-sex parent. The skills of cooperation and early socialization occur.
• **Latency period (ages 6 to 12):** As the child identifies with peers, parents become less important. The child's focus is on developing new skills and knowledge and interacting with children of the same gender. Intellectual curiosity increases.
• **Genital (puberty to adult) (age 12 to 20):** The child moves emotionally away from the family and establishes close relationships with peers and the opposite gender. Energy is directed toward work, personal accomplishments, and interpersonal relationships. There is adolescent sexual experimentation. Successful resolution of this stage is seen by establishing loving and healthy relationships.

Erikson: Psychosocial development

Erikson's theory of human development indicates that major personality changes occur throughout the life cycle.

Passage from one stage to another depends on successfully gaining the skills of the preceding stage. Unlike many other theorists, Erikson suggests that new experiences may provide opportunities to cope with deficits in earlier stages.

• **Trust vs. mistrust (birth to 18 months):** The infant derives a sense of security from gratification of needs and develops basic trust in the consistent caregiver and later in others.
• **Autonomy vs. shame and doubt (18 months to 3 years):** The child begins to view the self as a person apart from the parents. Children are beginning to develop a sense of personal control and independence.
• **Initiative vs. guilt (ages 3 to 6):** The child starts to behave assertively as he or she's guided to explore and investigate the world. The child develops a beginning sense of purpose.
• **Industry vs. inferiority (ages 6 to 12):** Accomplishment occurs and a sense of responsibility develops as the child masters tasks and social skills. The child develops a sense of competence.
• **Identity vs. role diffusion (ages 12 to 20):** The adolescent develops a sense of self and personal identity.
• **Intimacy vs. isolation (ages 20 to 30):** The ability to establish a commitment to another person occurs. The young adult develops loving, intimate relationships.

Piaget: Cognitive development

Piaget's cognitive theory of development describes successive stages of mental activity that occur during childhood. By successfully encountering new experiences, the child adapts and progresses to the next stage.

• **Sensorimotor stage (birth to age 2):** The infant's world focuses on the self. An understanding of the world is experienced through the senses and by motor movements.
• **Preoperational stage (ages 2 to 7):** The child develops language, memory, and imagination. Now there is a distinction between the past and the future made by the child.
• **Concrete operations stage (ages 7 to 12):** The child develops logical thinking and can now use symbols, and abstract concepts such as time, space, categories, numbers, and justice are envisioned.
• **Formal operations stage (ages 12 to adult):** The adolescent begins to think abstractly and systematically and starts to foresee options and possibilities.

Advice from the experts

Characteristics of mentally healthy young people

When assessing a child for possible psychiatric conditions, the nurse needs a basis for comparison. A mentally healthy child or adolescent:
• trusts parents and appropriate caregivers
• views the world as a safe place where needs will be met
• has an age-appropriate sense of reality
• perceives the personal environment realistically

• demonstrates a positive sense of self
• handles age-appropriate stress and frustration effectively
• shows age-appropriate coping skills
• demonstrates mastery of developmental tasks
• communicates or expresses self adequately and appropriately
• has useful and satisfying relationships.

determining a child's developmental level and assessing the accomplishment of the tasks defined for each stage.

Recognizing the typical characteristics of mentally healthy young people also helps the nurse compare a child's or adolescent's behavior against the expected norm. (See *Characteristics of mentally healthy young people.*)

Communicating with children and adolescents

When caring for a child or an adolescent with a psychiatric condition, the nurse's first task is to establish rapport. To do this, the nurse must show empathy and understanding.

Keep in mind that children may be frightened at first during a first encounter with a health care provider. To break the ice, initiate conversation with the child by asking about toys, hobbies, pets, school, and other subjects that focus on the child's interests.

Communicating with children

To further enhance communication, follow these guidelines:
• Keep verbal communication brief and use simple language.
• Communicate with kindness.
• Ask direct questions when seeking specific information.
• Use body language to reinforce the conversation and help children express their ideas and feelings.
• Give feedback as appropriate based on the child's developmental stage.

- Talk about reality by focusing on the "here and now."
- Speak quietly but firmly when reinforcing behavioral limits.
- Avoid arguments.
- Make your expectations clear.
- Role-model effective ways of communicating.

Assessment

To fully assess a child or adolescent for a psychiatric condition, the nurse must evaluate the family as well. Begin by collecting biographic data, including the ages of all family members, from the primary caregivers (often the parents or grandparents). Gather information about the family's health, school, housing, economic situation, and religious, ethnic, and cultural background. (See *Emotional display in Asian Americans.*)

Document an objective description of the primary caregivers, including any communication difficulties, lack of knowledge on growth and development, and family issues and problems.

How do the primary caregivers feel?

Ask the primary caregivers what their concerns are. Ask them how they view the child's behavior, what they think contributes to it, and how they believe it can be resolved. Evaluate each caregiver's attitude toward the child and the child's present condition. Then obtain the child's developmental history. Find out which, if any, services and agencies are involved in the family's or child's care.

Then begin your interview of the child, including a mental status assessment. (See *Assessing the mental status of a child or adolescent.*)

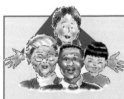

Bridging the gap

Emotional display in Asian Americans

When caring for an Asian American child, don't expect the child to display emotions openly and freely. In some Asian cultures, it's more acceptable for a person to withhold overt displays of emotion. A child who's reluctant to talk about feelings isn't necessarily uninterested, resistant, or noncompliant with treatment. The child may have been taught by the family to suppress emotional expression.

Shameful behavior?
Be aware, too, that in many Asian cultures, the actions of a disobedient child are seen as bringing dishonor to the family. Consequently, a child who has disobeyed may feel much shame and guilt.

Advice from the experts

Assessing the mental status of a child or adolescent

When evaluating the mental status of a child or adolescent, be sure to assess:
- physical appearance (including whether the patient looks age-appropriate)
- hygiene and grooming
- attention level and behavior during the interview
- understanding of his or her role in the interview
- speech or language development
- intellectual functioning
- judgment
- demonstrated strengths (e.g., eye contact, appropriate social skills)
- insight into self and the situation
- mannerisms, tics, and other involuntary movements
- mood and affect
- anxiety level
- obvious obsessive or compulsive behaviors
- frustration tolerance
- inability to listen, follow directions, concentrate, or focus
- ease of distraction
- impulsivity
- assigns blame to others for problems
- acting out or oppositional behavior
- verbal or physical aggression
- thought disorders, hallucinations, or delusions.

Especially for adolescents
- strengths
- depression

- anxiety
- communication problems
- difficulty expressing feelings and lack of understanding for other people's feelings
- low self-esteem
- unmet needs for attention and affection
- emotional closeness to peers and family members
- relationship difficulties
- overachievement or underachievement
- noncompliance with family or school rules, society's norms, and laws
- ineffective support system
- limited coping or problem-solving skills and blaming of others for difficulties experienced
- limited social skills
- impulsive behavior
- manipulative behavior
- procrastination
- lack of leisure skills or lack of time for leisure activities
- academic or employment problems
- discomfort with sexual feelings or inappropriate sexual behaviors
- money problems
- drug and/or alcohol use and/or disordered eating
- abuse or misuse of technology (e.g., cell phone, Internet, etc.)
- legal issues or problems

Diagnosis

A child with signs or symptoms of a psychiatric condition should be first evaluated by a physician or a nurse practitioner who specializes in pediatrics and mental health. Based on findings, the practitioner may recommend further evaluation by a specialist in child behavioral problems, such as a psychiatrist, psychologist, psychiatric mental health advanced practice nurse, or social worker.

Specialist, speak

When evaluating the child, the specialist considers the child's developmental level, social and physical environment, and reports from parents and teachers. The intent of the evaluation is to rule out other possible causes for the child's behavior.

If appropriate, the specialist makes a diagnosis according to the American Psychiatric Association's *Diagnostic and Statistical Manual of Mental Disorders*, 5th Edition (American Psychiatric Association, 2013).

Attention deficit hyperactivity disorder

A neurobiological disorder, ADHD is characterized by a pattern of inattention, impulsiveness, and hyperactivity, which is more severe than normally observed in children at the same developmental level. Unless identified and treated properly, ADHD may progress to conduct disorder, academic and job failure, depression, relationship problems, and substance abuse.

Most children with ADHD experience signs and symptoms by age 4. A few aren't diagnosed until they enter school.

Paying attention?

ADHD affects roughly 11% of children (ages 4 to 17) in the United States. This amounts to approximately 6.4 million children (Centers for Disease Control and Prevention, 2013).

Gender preference: Males

ADHD affects at least twice as many boys as girls. The child's behavior may cause problems at school, in the home, and in the community and may influence emotional development and social skills.

Historically, experts thought children outgrew ADHD by adolescence. We now know that ADHD continues into adulthood for many people. In fact, the disorder affects approximately 4% of adults (WebMD, 2014).

Causes

No known biological basis for ADHD exists. Research shows that the disorder tends to run in families, suggesting a genetic influence. For example, when one identical twin has the disorder, the other is likely to have it, too. Ongoing research on chromosome 16 may reveal additional genetic information about ADHD.

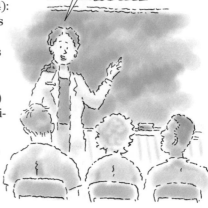

On average, three children in every classroom have attention deficit hyperactivity disorder.

Risk factors

Some scientists believe the following conditions may predispose a child to ADHD (Mayo Clinic, 2014):
• maternal use of drugs, alcohol, or substances while pregnant
• maternal exposure to environmental poisons while pregnant
• premature birth
• exposure to environmental toxins (e.g., lead)
• blood relatives with ADHD or another psychiatric condition.

Signs and symptoms

Signs and symptoms of ADHD fall into three categories:

  attention deficit/hyperactivity disorder, combined presentation

attention deficit/hyperactivity disorder, predominantly inattention presentation

attention deficit/hyperactivity disorder, predominantly hyperactive/impulsive presentation

Boredom

Commonly, these behaviors intensify when the child is bored, in an unstructured situation, or required to concentrate or focus on a task for an extended period.

Inattention

Children with ADHD have a short attention span, don't seem to listen, and have a hard time keeping their minds on any one thing. They get bored easily, tiring of tasks they do not enjoy after just a few minutes.

Difficulty concentrating

Although children with ADHD may give effortless attention to the things they enjoy, they have difficulty concentrating and focusing deliberate, conscious attention on organizing and completing a task or learning something new. Inattention causes them to disengage, lose things, be forgetful, and make careless mistakes.

Difficulty following through

Children with ADHD have difficulty following through on instructions, may not pay attention to necessary details, fail to finish tasks, and have trouble with organization. Easily distracted, they're reluctant to engage in tasks that call for sustained mental effort. (See *ADHD and psychosis: A possible link?*)

Impulsiveness

Children with ADHD have trouble controlling both their positive and negative immediate reactions. They act before they think. They interrupt others; for instance, they may blurt out remarks or answer a question before the person has finished asking it.

Difficulty waiting

Waiting for their turn and waiting for things they want are also challenging for children with ADHD. When upset, they may grab another child's toy or strike out physically to obtain what is it that they desire at that moment.

Hyperactivity

Children with ADHD are always in motion and can't seem to sit still. In school, they fidget or squirm in their seats, roam around the room, or talk excessively. They have trouble engaging in quiet activities and may find it very challenging to sit through a class. The activities they perform may be purposeful or meaningless. They often try to do several things at once and are frequently drawn to handle things that they should not touch.

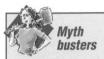

Myth busters

ADHD and psychosis: A possible link?

Myths and misinformation can cause needless worry in parents of children with ADHD. One myth involves the reputed link between ADHD and psychosis.

Myth: Children with ADHD can easily become psychotic.

Reality: Children with ADHD may seem disorganized because of their impulsiveness and distractibility. However, few have psychotic symptoms, such as delusions, hallucinations, or thought disorders.

Diagnosis

The child should undergo a complete medical evaluation, including a neurologic examination, along with hearing and vision screening. A psychiatric evaluation should be performed to assess intellectual ability, academic achievement, and potential learning disorder problems. Sometimes, speech and language evaluations are also necessary.

Pathway to the diagnosis

It is difficult to diagnose a child with ADHD before the age of 4. However, parents frequently report that the child was very active as a toddler. Typically, the child is identified with symptoms of ADHD in the early elementary school years. The first apparent symptom is usually hyperactivity if the child is in a preschool program, with inattention occurring upon entering elementary school. During adolescence, the outward signs of hyperactivity diminish and turn inward to feelings of restlessness, annoyance, and impatience. It is important to note that children with serious inattention-type symptoms tend to have academic difficulty and problems with peers and daily school activities. Children who demonstrate serious hyperactivity and impulsive behaviors are more likely to experience negativity from peers and accidental injuries (Barkley, 2013).

Treatment

Treatment focuses on coordinating the child's psychological and physiologic needs. Psychotherapy can reduce ADHD symptoms and teach the child and family ways to modify the inappropriate behaviors. Drugs like methylphenidate (Concerta) or lisdexamfetamine dimesylate (Vyvanse) help to ease inattention, impulsiveness, and hyperactivity. (See *Pharmacologic options for treating ADHD*, pages 66–69.)

The child also may benefit from an individualized educational plan, with special services that support and build strengths and minimize problems stemming from identified vulnerabilities.

> **Memory jogger**
>
> The word PEPS can help you recall the major treatment components for ADHD.
>
> **P**sychotherapy
> **E**ducation
> **P**harmacology
> **S**trengths

Nursing interventions

These interventions are appropriate for a child with ADHD:
- Maintain a safe, calm environment that minimizes stimulation and distractions and helps the child remain in control
- Develop a trusting and accepting relationship with the child.
- Encourage the child to talk about problems, difficulties, and feelings.
- Assess potential for risk of injury related to hyperactivity and gross motor behaviors.

Learn acceptable behaviors

- Help the child differentiate between acceptable and unacceptable behaviors. Discuss disruptive behaviors, patterns of losing control, and the consequences of these behaviors.
- Teach the child to make choices and select appropriate ways of behaving.
- Monitor the child's activities and assist the child to learn to set limits, stay calm, and take opportunities to control undesirable behaviors.

> Maintain a safe, calm environment for a child with ADHD.

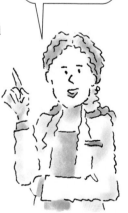

(Text continues on page 68.)

Meds matters

Pharmacologic options for treating ADHD

Central nervous system stimulants and nonstimulants have been used effectively to control symptoms of ADHD in both children and adults—lisdexamfetamine dimesylate (Vyvanse), methylphenidate (Concerta), atomoxetine (Strattera), and guanfacine (Intuniv). For many patients, these drugs dramatically reduce hyperactivity and improve their ability to focus, learn, and work.

Drug	Adverse reactions		Contraindications
Lisdexamfetamine dimesylate (Vyvanse)	• Anorexia • Anxiety • Decreased appetite • Weight loss or decrease in expected weight gain • Dry mouth • Insomnia • Gastrointestinal (GI) symptoms (upper abdominal pain, nausea, vomiting) • Psychotic or manic symptoms in patients with no prior history of such		• Use of monoamine oxidase (MAO) inhibitor therapy within previous 14 days (may cause a hypertensive crisis) • Hypertension • Individuals with cardiac abnormalities (cardiomyopathy, structural abnormalities, heart arrhythmias, coronary artery disease) • Pregnancy
Methylphenidate (Concerta, Ritalin)	• Anorexia • Nausea or vomiting • Weight loss or decrease in expected weight gain • Temporary growth delay or slow growth • Stomachache or abdominal pain • Dry mouth • Tremors	• Headache • Insomnia • Transient motor tics • Mild blood pressure elevation • Social withdrawal • Rebound hyperactivity or irritability • Metallic taste • Blurred vision	• Tourette disorder • Motor tics • Diabetes mellitus • Kidney disease • Cardiovascular disease • Use of MAO inhibitor drug within the past 14 days
Guanfacine (Intuniv)	• Insomnia • Irritability, confusion, or agitation • Nightmares • Depression • Nausea/vomiting • Abdominal pain • Stomachache • Chest pain • Syncope • Rebound effect	• Weight gain • Blood pressure alterations • Headache • Vision disturbance • Skin rash • Increased urination • Enuresis • Rhinitis • Dry mouth	• Children younger than 6 years old • Impaired renal function • Impaired liver function • Pregnancy

Nursing interventions

- Administer early in the day to avoid insomnia.
- Swallow without chewing or crushing.
- Discuss concurrent use of prescription and over-the-counter (OTC) drugs with child's primary health care provider.
- Monitor height and weight regularly.
- Monitor sleep patterns.
- Be aware that stimulant drugs have the potential for abuse.
- Use of caffeine will increase stimulant effect.

- Give oral dose with meals to minimize anorexia.
- Apply Ritalin patch directly upon opening pouch to a dry, clean hip area and alternate hips daily.
- Administer at least 6 hours before bedtime or 8 hours if extended release.
- Monitor growth and development regularly. Weigh the child two to three times weekly.
- Monitor growth parameters.
- Monitor vital signs.
- Monitor for tics.
- Monitor for depression.
- If using patch, monitor localized skin irritation.
- Advise parents about having the child take a drug "holiday" over vacations and holidays.
- Be aware that stimulant drugs have the potential for abuse.

- Give with food in the evening to minimize daytime sleepiness.
- Take extended-release tablets with liquids like water or milk but not with a high-fat meal.
- Tell parents that therapeutic effects take 3 to 4 weeks to appear.
- Monitor for signs of dehydration or overheating.
- Discuss concurrent use of OTC drugs with the child's primary health care provider.
- Advise parents about having the child take a drug "holiday" over vacations and holidays.
- Instruct parents not to abruptly stop the drug, but to wean off of it under prescriber's directions.

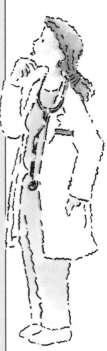

(continued)

Pharmacologic options for treating ADHD *(continued)*

Drug	Adverse reactions		Contraindications
Atomoxetine (Strattera)	• Anorexia • Nausea/vomiting • Weight loss or decrease in expected weight gain • Temporary growth delay • Stomachache or abdominal • Mood swings with crying • Dry mouth	• Urinary retention • Orthostatic hypertension • Headache • Muscle pain • Dermatitis • Irritability • Hypersensitivity reactions • Insomnia • Elevated liver enzymes • Jaundice	• Children younger than 6 years of age • Impaired cardiac function • Impaired liver function • Use of MAO inhibitors drug in the last 14 days (as it may cause a hypertensive crisis) • Pregnancy

Subdue the frenzy

• Schedule frequent breaks to help the child control his or her impulsiveness and minimize hyperactive behavior.
• Teach caregivers that hunger, thirst, fatigue, the need to urinate, and other physical problems may trigger hyperactivity.
• Instruct caregivers on the use of problem solving, time-outs, and natural consequences.
• Work with caregivers to communicate with the children's school to have an educational evaluation and develop a plan for needed services and specific student accommodations (e.g., untimed tests, review sessions, repeating or reviewing assignment instructions, tutoring, etc.).
• Teach caregivers to implement a healthy meal and snack plan, as poor nutrition may exacerbate ADHD symptoms.

Ease impulsivity

• Help the child learn how to take turns, wait in lines, and follow rules.
• Work with the child to divide tasks into doable steps in order to experience success in meeting identified goals.
• Give the child opportunities to participate in activities with peers.
• Provide the child with positive feedback for improvement and with encouragement to take steps to manage problematic behaviors.

Nursing interventions

- **Warning:** This drug may increase risk of suicide ideation in children and adolescents.
- Monitor client very closely for depression or suicidal thoughts.
- Give single dose in morning or give half the dose in the morning and the other half in early evening.
- Give with food to minimize anorexia and GI upset.
- Monitor growth and development regularly.
- Tell parents that therapeutic effects take 3 to 4 weeks to appear.
- Monitor vital signs.
- Discuss concurrent use of OTC drugs with the child's primary health care provider.
- Know that higher doses decrease seizure threshold.
- Advise parents about having the child take a drug "holiday" over vacations and holidays.
- Be aware that stimulant drugs have the potential for abuse.

Oppositional defiant disorder

All children sometimes talk back, argue, disobey, and defy their parents or teachers, especially when they're hungry, tired, or stressed. In fact, for toddlers and young adolescents, oppositional behavior may be a normal part of their development. It is essential to determine the frequency and tenacity of oppositional behavior in order to ascertain if it is within the normal range of behaviors or if it is symptomatic behavior.

Heightened hostility

Hostile, uncooperative behavior in a child may signal ODD if it's more consistent and severe than that of other children of the same age and developmental level and if such behavior affects the child's social, family, and academic life.

A child with ODD is consistently negative, disobedient, argumentative, and hostile. The child behaves in a provocative manner deliberately meant to annoy and upset authority figures. The child manifests an angry mood, defiant behavior, and vindictiveness.

No end to the argument

During an argument, children with ODD do not back down, even if they stand to lose privileges. To the child, the important thing is the struggle, which

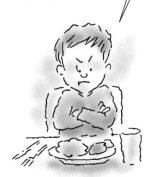

Defiant, disobedient, and hostile— could I have ODD?

overshadows the reality of the situation. If anyone objects to the behavior, the child views it as stimulation to continue the argument. ODD may be a precursor to conduct disorder (discussed in the following section).

A lot of ODD

Roughly 1% to 11% of school-age children have ODD. Onset generally occurs between ages 8 and 19 (Oppositional defiant disorder, n.d.).

Prior to adolescence, ODD is more common in males by a 1:4 ratio of males to females. After adolescence, it affects both genders equally.

Causes

The biological basis of ODD remains unknown. However, research on the metabolism of the neurotransmitters serotonin, norepinephrine, and dopamine and abnormalities found through brain imaging suggest chances in the prefrontal context and the amygdala occur in people with ODD.

Risk factors

Various biological, psychosocial, and environmental risk factors may play a role. These factors include (Mayo Clinic, 2012):
- child's natural disposition
- inconsistent, unsupervised child rearing
- excessive parental control with punitive discipline or limit setting
- abuse or neglect
- family conflict or power struggles
- imbalance in brain chemicals (e.g., serotonin)
- limitations or developmental delays in the child's processing of thoughts and feelings.

Signs and symptoms

Signs and symptoms of ODD usually occur in more than one setting, although they may be more noticeable at home or at school. They include:
- persistent or consistent pattern of defiant, disobedient, hostile behavior
- disobeying directly by not following rules
- disobeying indirectly by procrastinating and being sneaky
- refusing to cooperate
- being touchy and easily annoyed
- frequent bouts of anger and resentment
- persistent fighting

I'm not going to do that and you can't make me.

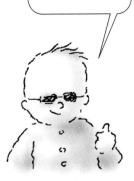

- excessive arguing
- stubbornness
- testing of behavioral limits
- temper tantrums
- deliberate attempts to upset or annoy people or animals
- vindictiveness
- blaming others for their misbehavior
- violating the rights of others.

Diagnosis

A child with suspected ODD should undergo a complete psychiatric evaluation. The family should be assessed, too, with particular attention given to family interactions, communication patterns, and disciplinary style.

Treatment

Treatment of ODD focuses on meeting the child's and family's psychological and psychosocial needs and preventing ODD from progressing to conduct disorder. The child may benefit from individual psychotherapy, with an emphasis on anger management.

Teach the caregivers

Caregivers may benefit from educational programs that teach them how to manage the child's behavior. Together, the caregivers and child may undergo family psychotherapy to improve communication, promote adaptive coping skills, and practice positive behaviors.

Usually, drug therapy is reserved for children who also demonstrate symptoms of anxiety or depression.

Nursing interventions

These nursing interventions are appropriate for a child with ODD:
- Convey a nonjudgmental attitude to help establish a trusting relationship with the child.
- Discuss what consequences will occur when limits are exceeded.

Negate the negativity

- Help the child address negative feelings, especially feelings of anger and resentment. Determine appropriate strategies for handling these feelings.
- Assist the child in addressing situations and issues that trigger negative thoughts and feelings.
- Discuss appropriate strategies to use for handling negative emotions (such as shame, blame, and anxiety) and the feelings of "wanting to get even."

Stop the plotting

- Help the child learn to accept responsibility for personal behavior rather than becoming defensive and plotting revenge.
- Teach the child how to express anger appropriately and methods of controlling temper.
- Identify and discuss the child's use of passive-aggressive behavior, evaluate its effect on others, and devise strategies to eliminate it.

Role-play and reinforce

- Teach the child problem-solving and communication skills. Provide role-playing opportunities in order to become comfortable and more self-confident when using these new skills.
- During interactions, convey acceptance of the child and separate the child's unacceptable behaviors from his or her worth and dignity as a person. Reinforce the child's acceptable behavior and positive behavior changes.
- Work with the child and family to address conflict, establish clear expectations, and improve communication skills.

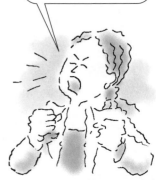

AARGH! This is one type of behavior you certainly shouldn't role-model!

Conduct disorder

Displaying aggressive physical behavior and violating the rights of others are the hallmarks of a conduct disorder. Children with this disorder initiate and react aggressively to people. They engage in fighting, bullying, intimidating people, deliberating destroying property, and assaulting others. Typically, the child has poor relationships with peers and adults and tends to perceive the intentions of other people as hostile and threatening even when this is not the case. Some of the identified personality characteristics of these children include poor self-control and frustration tolerance, outbursts of temper, suspiciousness, lack of sensitivity to consequences, and reckless behaviors. The child lacks feelings of remorse or guilt.

Future legal problems

Children with conduct disorder tend to become involved in behaviors, which violate the norms of society. Behaviors that may bring the child to the attention of the criminal justice system include assaults, theft, vandalism, truancy, substance use, running away, and prostitution. Violent behaviors may cause suspension or expulsion from school and the need for placement in foster care, a group home, or a juvenile detention center.

Gender preference

Conduct disorder affects both genders, but it is much more common in males, especially among males with childhood onset. Although conduct disorder may occur as early as the preschool years, it usually is diagnosed from middle childhood (about age 9) through early adolescence. Among teenagers in the United States, the prevalence of conduct disorder is approximately 2% to 9% (Bernstein, 2014). (See *Just a rambunctious child?*)

Consequences

A child with conduct disorder is at high risk for:
- school suspension or expulsion
- job problems
- risk-taking behaviors
- sexually transmitted diseases
- rape
- pregnancy
- physical injuries and accidents
- substance abuse
- legal problems
- anxiety
- depression with suicidal thoughts, suicide attempts, and suicide itself.

Causes

The cause of conduct disorder isn't fully known, but research indicates that it may be due to genetic and environmental factors. Research on chromosomes 2 and 19, the neurotransmitters serotonin and norepinephrine, and on the hormone, testosterone, may lead to information on the biological basis of the disorder. Studies of twins and adopted children suggest the disorder has both biological (including genetic) and psychosocial components. If the child has an adoptive parent or sibling with conduct disorder, there is an increased environmental risk.

Other considerations

Some children diagnosed with conduct disorder also have ADHD. These children also have minimal academic success and educators note that academic achievement is low for tested IQ and developmental age. These coexisting conditions may increase the use of drugs and alcohol and involvement in sexual activities at an early age.

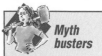

Myth busters

Just a rambunctious child?

All children misbehave now and then. In fact, misbehavior is so common in children that some people think it's normal. However, misbehavior that's persistent and pronounced is *not* normal.

Myth: A child with conduct disorder is just a rambunctious kid involved in normal mischief.

Reality: Conduct disorder is a serious mental health problem. A child with this disorder engages in dangerous behavior, which may lead to involvement with the juvenile justice system or even incarceration.

Social risk factors

Various social factors may predispose a child to conduct disorder. All of these factors can lead to lack of attachment to the parents or family unit and eventually to lack of regard for societal rules. They include:
- early caregiver rejection
- separation from parents, with no adequate alternative caregiver available
- aggressive behavior leading to unhealthy peer relationships and eventually peer rejection
- early institutionalization
- family neglect, abuse, or violence
- frequent verbal abuse from parents, teachers, or other authority figures
- parental psychiatric illness, substance abuse, or marital discord
- large family size, crowding, and poverty.

Other risk factors

Certain physical factors and other conditions also increase the risk of conduct disorder. These include:
- neurologic damage caused by low birth weight or birth complications
- under-arousal of the autonomic nervous system
- lower than average intelligence and learning disabilities
- insensitivity to physical pain and punishment.

Signs and symptoms

Signs and symptoms of conduct disorder include:
- fighting with family members and peers
- speaking to others in a nasty manner
- being cruel to people or animals
- vandalizing or destroying property
- cheating in school
- cutting classes
- running away
- smoking cigarettes
- using drugs or alcohol
- stealing or shoplifting
- engaging in precocious sexual activity
- abusing others sexually.

Diagnosis

Understanding the patterns of behavior that a child with conduct disorder uses to violate the rights of others requires a complete

---

Memory jogger

To remember the behaviors associated with conduct disorder, simply think of the term itself.

C: cheats

O: obnoxious

N: nasty in speech and behavior

D: drug and alcohol use

U: unpredictable behavior

C: cruel to people or animals

T: truant

D: destroys property

I: intimidates others

S: steals

O: onset of anti-social personality disorder

R: rages

D: disrespectful

E: esteem low

R: reckless or risky behavior

interdisciplinary team approach, including medical and psychiatric evaluations, feedback from caregivers, a school consultant's input, a case manager's plan, and a probation officer's report. A team approach is important because antisocial behaviors often go underreported.

What else may be going on?

Educational assessments must be reviewed to determine if the child also has cognitive deficits, learning disabilities, or problems in intellectual functioning. A neurologic examination may be needed if the child has a history of head trauma or seizures (Harvard Medical School, 2011).

Treatment

Treatment focuses on coordinating the child's psychological, physiologic, and educational needs. Psychotherapy can help the child learn problem-solving skills, social skills, how to decrease disruptive symptoms, and modify antisocial behavior. Drugs may be prescribed to treat neurologic difficulties or severe symptoms of anxiety and depression (Loy, Merry, Hetricks, & Stasiak, 2012). Educational strategies focus on encouraging and helping the child to succeed and continue to stay in school.

ID them early

Early identification of at-risk children is important because many signs and symptoms of conduct disorder emerge in the first years of life when the child's temperament or personality characteristics emerge and correlate with behavioral problems.

Parental vigilance is needed

Caregivers of an at-risk child should be taught how to set limits and stop the child's aggressive, defensive, and manipulative behavior. They need to learn to create healthy interactions and facilitate the child's self-worth.

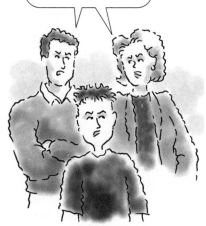

Caregivers must act and not overlook, deny, or make excuses for a child's inappropriate or aggressive behavior.

If persistent acting out . . .

Unfortunately, some children with conduct disorder seriously act out and eventually enter the juvenile justice system. Juvenile justice interventions provide structured rules and a means for monitoring and controlling the child's behavior.

Nursing interventions

These nursing interventions are appropriate for a child (or adolescent) with conduct disorder:
• Work to establish a trusting relationship with the child. Be sure to convey that you accept the child while you are setting limits and following through with actions to help him or her address inappropriate behavior.
• Provide clear behavioral guidelines, including consequences for disruptive and manipulative behavior.
• Talk to the child about making acceptable choices, handling anger, and coping with disappointments and frustrations.
• Teach and role-model effective problem-solving skills and have the child demonstrate them in return.
• Help the child identify personal needs and the best strategies for meeting them.
• Work with the child to develop and sustain healthy relationships.

Avert abuse

• Identify abusive communication, such as threats, sarcasm, and disparaging comments.
• Teach options and alternatives and have the child take responsibility to stop being verbally abusive.
• Teach him or her how to express difficult and negative feelings appropriately through constructive methods to release stress and frustrations.
• Monitor the child for anger as well as signs of internalizing anger, as shown by depression or suicidal ideation.

Rein in revenge

• Work on helping the child accept responsibility for behavior rather than blaming others, becoming defensive, and wanting revenge.
• Teach the child effective coping skills and social skills.
• Use role-playing to have the child practice ways of handling defensiveness and gaining skill and confidence in managing problematic situations.

Major depression

Everyone feels sad now and then. Mood changes are normal not only in adults but also in children and adolescents. Depression is a health problem, which can interfere with the person's ability to function. The continuation of a sad mood can cause difficulties in eating, sleeping, concentrating, and/or functioning.

Myth busters

Bipolar predisposition?

Many people think children who experience depression are likely to develop bipolar disorder later in life. This isn't true.

Myth: Children who experience childhood depression are highly likely to develop bipolar disorder as adults.

Reality: Only a small percentage of children with depression develop bipolar disorder as adults. However, a family history of both bipolar disorder and childhood depression, not just depression alone, makes bipolar disorder more likely.

Ripple effect

Depression can have widespread effects on a child's adjustment and functioning. Depressed children may feel unloved, pessimistic, or even hopeless about the future. They may think life isn't worth living. A depressed child is at increased risk for physical illness and psychosocial difficulties that persist long after the depressive episode resolves.

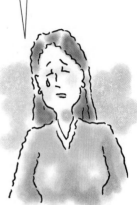

Depression puts children at risk for illnesses and lingering psychosocial problems.

The blahs and the blues

Major depression (also called *clinical* or *unipolar depression*) manifests itself as a depressed mood or a loss of interest in almost all usual activities. There is impaired functioning, a sad or irritable mood, disturbances in sleep and appetite, lethargy, and inability to experience pleasure. (See *Bipolar predisposition?*)

Two excruciatingly long weeks

Major depressive disorder is characterized by one or more major depressive episodes, defined as episodes of depressed mood lasting at least 2 weeks. About one-half of depressed patients experience a single episode and recover completely. The rest have at least one recurrence.

Agonizing episode

In children and adolescents, a major depressive episode lasts an average of 6 to 9 months. Depressed children and adolescents are sad and lose interest in activities that were enjoyable. They are often more irritable than sad, and their irritability may lead to aggressive behavior. They have difficulty making decisions and concentrating. They lack energy or motivation and may neglect their appearance and hygiene if not carefully monitored by a caregiver.

Many miserable kids

Approximately 11% of children and adolescents have a depressive disorder by the age of 18 (National Alliance on Mental Illness, 2014). Depression now has an earlier onset than it did in past decades.

For all too many children, early-onset depression persists, recurs, and continues into adulthood. Depression in youth may predict more severe depressive illness in adult life.

Substances and suicide

Depressed adolescents are at increased risk for substance abuse and suicidal behavior. Suicide attempts peak during the mid-adolescent years. The incidence of death from suicide increases steadily throughout the adolescent years. Among adolescents aged 15 to 19, suicide is the third leading cause of death (Centers for Disease Control and Prevention, 2014).

Causes

The multiple causes of depression are not completely understood. Research suggests possible genetic, familial, biochemical, physical, psychological, and social causes. In some patients, the history identifies a specific personal loss or severe stress that likely interacts with a person's predisposition for major depression. Factors such as childhood experiences, stressors, traumatic events, medical illnesses, and exposure to toxic substances can precipitate depression.

Biological tip-offs

Among depressed patients, researchers have found deficiencies in the major neurotransmitters, serotonin, norepinephrine, dopamine, acetylcholine, and gamma-aminobutyric acid (GABA). It is also known that computed tomography (CT) and positron emission tomography (PET) scans show abnormally slow activity in the prefrontal cortex and temporal lobes of depressed patients (Clark, Jansen, & Cloy, 2012).

Melancholy genes

Scientists believe depression can be an inherited disease. However, what is inherited is a vulnerability to depression. In twin studies, it has been found that if one twin develops depression, the other twin has only a 76% chance of developing the disorder. Research on genetic abnormalities involving chromosomes 4, 11, 18, and 21 has been linked to depression. A family history of depression also increases the risk of the disorder.

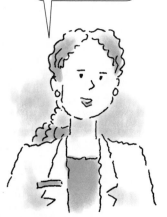

Depression may be linked to certain chromosomal abnormalities.

Medical miseries

Depression is also linked to certain medical conditions, such as:
• neurologic problems, such as brain tumor, brain trauma, multiple sclerosis, Parkinson disease, and Huntington disease
• cardiovascular disease
• acquired immunodeficiency syndrome
• electrolyte imbalances (especially calcium, magnesium, sodium, and potassium)
• endocrine disorders, such as Addison disease, Cushing syndrome, thyroid disorders, diabetes mellitus, and parathyroid disorders
• nutritional imbalances, such as deficiencies in B and C vitamins, iron, zinc, and protein.

Risk factors

Common risk factors associated with major depression include:
- family history of depression
- excessive stress
- abuse or neglect
- physical or emotional trauma
- loss of a parent
- loss of a relationship
- other psychiatric disorders
- chronic medical illness
- developmental, learning, or conduct disorders.

Signs and symptoms

Early diagnosis and treatment of depression is crucial for healthy emotional, social, and behavioral development. Assess the child for such signs and symptoms as:
- persistent sadness
- irritable, cranky mood
- physical complaints, such as headache or stomachache
- crying for no apparent reason
- inability to concentrate or make decisions
- withdrawal from peers and social situations
- restlessness, fidgeting, or frequent moving
- boredom with daily activities
- difficulty sleeping or sleeping more than usual
- disorganization with periods of agitation
- fatigue or lack of energy
- rejection of self or others
- not caring about self, others, or activities
- sense of worthlessness
- verbal or physical fights with others
- thoughts of death, suicidal ideation, suicide attempts, and other high-risk behaviors
- struggling with normal developmental adjustments
- absence of expected weight increase for growth and developmental stage.

Under the radar

All too often, depression goes unrecognized by the child's family, doctor, and teachers. Signs and symptoms may be mistaken for the normal mood swings typical of a particular developmental stage. Also, symptoms of depression may be expressed in varying ways depending on the child's developmental stage.

Memory jogger

To help remember the major signs and symptoms of depression in children and adolescents, think of SWAP.

S: school problems

W: withdrawal

A: alterations in sleep, appetite, and energy levels

P: physical health problems

Children and young adolescents may have trouble identifying and describing their emotional states. Instead of expressing their feelings, they may act out their feelings, which may be interpreted as misbehavior. Often, young people express irritability as the major symptom of their depression rather than a depressed mood (Eapen & Crncec, 2012).

Depression with a difference

Despite some similarities, childhood depression differs from adult depression in two key ways.

Psychotic features are less common in children and adolescents.

Anxiety symptoms (such as reluctance to meet people) and physical symptoms (such as aches and pains, stomachache, and headache) are more common in depressed children and adolescents.

Diagnosis

The diagnosis of depression can be made from patient self-reports, interviews, and observations. An interdisciplinary team approach is crucial. The team should include a medical and psychiatric evaluation, a school consultant's input, and feedback from caregivers.

Tool time

Certain tools may be useful in screening children and adolescents for major depression. Three such tools are:

Children's Depression Inventory 2 (CDI2) for ages 7 to 17

Beck Depression Inventory–Youth (2nd edition) (BDI-Y II)

Center for Epidemiologic Studies Depression Scale for Adolescents

Reynolds Adolescent Depression Scale 2.

A child who screens positive on one of these instruments should undergo a comprehensive diagnostic evaluation by a mental health professional. The evaluation should include interviews with the child, caregivers, and, when possible, other informants (such as teachers and social services personnel) (Carnevale, 2011).

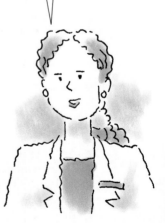

The child may be screened with the Children's Depression Inventory 2 or the Beck Depression Inventory–Youth II.

Treatment

Treatment of major depression may entail psychotherapy (particularly cognitive-behavioral therapy), medication, or a combination. Targeted interventions may involve the home or school environment.

Focus on Relationships

Interpersonal therapy may be another psychotherapy option. This type of therapy focuses on working through disturbed relationships that may contribute to depression.

Don't stop too soon

Continuing psychotherapy for several months after symptom remission may help patients and families strengthen the skills they learned during the acute phase of depression. It may also help them cope with depression's aftereffects, address environmental stressors, and understand how the child's thoughts and behaviors could contribute to a relapse.

Pharmacotherapy

Although antidepressant drugs can be effective treatments for adults with depressive disorders, their use in children and adolescents has been controversial. The National Institute of Mental Health recommends the use of antidepressants only when the benefits outweigh the risks. The U.S. Food and Drug Administration (FDA) issued a warning about the increased risk of suicide and suicidal thoughts in children and adolescents treated with selective serotonin reuptake inhibitor (SSRI) antidepressant medications (Moreland & Bonin, 2014). (See *Pharmacologic options for treating depression*, page 82.)

Medication is considered a first-line treatment for children and adolescents who have severe symptoms that make effective psychotherapy difficult, can't participate in psychotherapy, and have psychosis or chronic or recurrent depressive episodes.

Preventing a relapse

After symptom remission, the doctor may recommend that the child continue drug therapy because of the high risk that depression will recur. As appropriate, antidepressant medication may be discontinued gradually over at least 6 weeks or longer under the supervision of a health care provider.

Nursing interventions

These nursing interventions are appropriate for a child (or adolescent) with major depression:
- Structure and maintain a safe, secure environment.
- Sustain the child's typical routine.

Meds matters

Pharmacologic options for treating depression

A child or adolescent with major depressive disorder may receive an SSRI or serotonin and norepinephrine reuptake inhibitor (SNRI). The chart below details the general adverse reactions, contraindications, and nursing interventions for SSRIs and one SNRI.

Drug	Adverse reactions		Contraindications	Nursing interventions
SSRIs • Fluoxetine (Prozac) • Paroxetine (Paxil) • Sertraline (Zoloft) • Escitalopram (Lexapro)	• Anorexia • Nausea • Appetite changes • Dry mouth • Headache • Nervousness • Fatigue • Suicidal behavior or ideation	• Tremor • Dizziness • Seizures • Chest pain • Skin rash • Blurred vision • Flulike reaction	• Kidney problems • Liver problems • Diabetes mellitus • Suicidal ideation • Concurrent use of a MAO inhibitor	• Assess and supervise patients at risk for suicide. • Monitor weekly for weight changes. • Monitor for safety because drug may cause dizziness.
SNRI • Duloxetine (Cymbalta)	• Nausea • Dry mouth • Somnolence • Constipation • Decreased appetite • Suicidal ideation		• Kidney problems • Liver problems • Suicidal ideation • Concurrent use of a MAO inhibitor	• Assess and supervise patients at risk for suicide. • Monitor weekly for weight changes.

• Monitor the child for dangerous or self-destructive behavior.
• Work with the child to address his or her needs.
• Help the child to learn ways of becoming more social with peers.
• Provide appropriate times to eat, rest, sleep, and play or relax.
• Help the child develop a support system.

Put it in writing

• Develop an agreement or contract with the child to seek out staff if he or she feels desperate or suicidal.
• Teach the child to talk things out rather than act things out.

Addressing problems

• Discuss concerns and issues that are upsetting or bothersome.

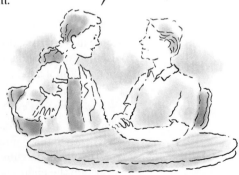

Do you have any concerns you'd like to discuss?

- Help the child talk about problems and stressors.
- Teach methods to express strong emotions appropriately.
- Identify techniques to combat self-defeating behaviors, negative verbalizations, and self-statements.
- Work on age-appropriate strategies for solving problems.
- Encourage the child to express feelings openly.
- If the child has suffered a major loss, talk about the loss, what it means, and ways of grieving.

Get physical

- Provide physical outlets for energy and aggression (such as sports, music, or art) to help the child express feelings and develop healthy coping skills.
- Teach techniques that help the child to be assertive, speak up, and ask for what is needed.
- Have the child identify supportive people that he or she can go to when conflict or stressors are experienced and how to talk to these people about feelings and needs.

Autism spectrum disorder

Autism spectrum disorder (ASD) is a term for a disorder, which includes autistic disorder, pervasive developmental disorder not otherwise specified, childhood disintegration disorder, and Asperger disorder. It begins during childhood and lasts throughout life. Each particular diagnosis is described by identifying its level of severity, child's age and developmental level, genetic problems, and level of intellectual disability. Severity is based on the degree of social impairment and restricted repetitive behaviors. The clinician will note the child's responses to the environment and impairments in language, communication, and social interaction.

There are three levels of severity for ASD:
Level 1: requires support
Level 2: requires substantial support
Level 3: requires very substantial support

At a loss for words

Typically, the autistic child has disordered thinking. He or she may have severe learning difficulties, intellectual differences, and difficulty understanding and using language. The child may withdraw or retreat into a fantasy world. People with autism often have trouble understanding the feelings of others and the world around them. Behaviors that are repetitive (e.g., rocking, body swaying) and self-injurious (e.g., head banging, biting self) may be demonstrated. Symptoms must be present in the early developmental stages and must significantly affect social, occupational, or other types of function (Autism Speaks, 2014).

Not interested in people

A child with ASD may appear aloof from others, is adverse to affection or physical touch, and lacks interest in social interactions. He or she seems to prefer inanimate objects to human companionship or friendships with other children and may grow inappropriately attached to such objects.

Five boys for every girl

ASD occurs four times more frequently in boys than in girls. According to the National Institute of Neurological Disorders and Stroke (NINDS; 2014), 1 in every 88 children has been diagnosed with an ASD. If girls do not have noticeable intellectual impairment or language delays, they may go unrecognized for a longer period of time. Couples with one child with ASD have roughly a 5% chance of having another child with ASD.

Causes

No known single cause for the disorders that encompass ASDs exists. Some studies suggest it may stem from abnormalities in brain structure or function. Brain scans show differences in brain shape and structure in children with ASD.

Other possible causes of ASD include medical problems, a genetic predisposition, environmental factors, and abnormal levels of serotonin or other neurotransmitters.

Signs and symptoms

ASD may cause symptoms during infancy. It is commonly discovered when caregivers notice their child doesn't continue to develop as expected, becomes withdrawn or aggressive, or loses language skills already acquired.

Sometimes, the child appears to develop normally until about age 2 and then regresses rapidly.

Mysterious crying

Young children with ASD usually have impaired language development and difficulty expressing their needs. They may laugh or cry for no apparent reason. Even those who gain rudimentary language skills cannot communicate effectively.

Manifested symptoms

Other signs and symptoms of ASD include:
- indifference toward others
- delayed and impaired verbal and nonverbal communication
- abnormal speech patterns, such as echolalia (repeating words or phrases spoken by others)

- lack of intonation and expression in speech
- repetitive rocking motions
- hand flapping or body swaying
- dislike of changes in daily activities and routines
- self-injurious behaviors, such as head banging, hitting, or biting
- unusual fascination with inanimate objects, such as fans and air conditioners
- dislike of touching and cuddling
- frequent outbursts and tantrums
- little or no eye contact with others
- increased or decreased sensitivity to pain
- no fear of danger.

Diagnosis

Usually, most children with ASD are diagnosed by age 3. However, no definitive diagnostic tool exists. Several other conditions, such as Rhett syndrome and selective mutism, may resemble the disorder, possibly complicating diagnosis.

ASD is usually diagnosed by age 3.

Narrowing the field

After ruling out other disorders (such as neurologic disorders, hearing loss, speech problems, and intellectual development disorder), a comprehensive evaluation is performed by an interdisciplinary team composed of a psychologist, neurologist, psychiatrist, speech therapist, and audiologist (NINDS, 2014).

Specialist's strategy

The interdisciplinary team uses various methods to identify the disorder, including a standardized rating scale to help evaluate the child's social behavior and language. The specialist also may test for certain genetic and neurologic problems. Typically, the caregivers are interviewed to elicit information about the child's behavior and early development and may be asked to videotape the child's behavior at home.

Screening for developmental problems

Developmental screening may reveal behaviors that suggest ASD, such as (NINDS, 2014):

- failure to babble or point by age 12 months
- failure to say single words by age 16 months
- failure to say two-word phrases on his own by age 24 months
- poor eye contact, no smiling, and lack of social responsiveness
- loss of language or social skills at any age. (See *Screening tools for ASD*, page 86.)

Screening tools for ASD

Although no single behavioral or communication test can detect ASD, several screening instruments can be used as aids in diagnosing ASD (National Institute of Mental Health, 2011).

Checklist for ASD in toddlers (CHAT)
This scale screens for ASD in children age 18 months. A short questionnaire, it has two sections, one prepared by the parents and the other by the child's doctor.

Autism screening questionnaire
This 40-item screening scale is used with children age 4 and older. It evaluates communication skills and social functioning.

Screening tool for ASD in two-year-olds (STAT)
This scale uses direct observation to study behavioral features in children younger than age 2. It identifies three skills areas important in diagnosing ASD: play, motor imitation, and joint attention.

Check the tape

Reviewing family videos, photos, and baby albums may help parents document when the child reached certain developmental milestones and when signs of ASD began to appear.

Diagnostic criteria

After evaluation and testing, the interdisciplinary team may arrive at a diagnosis based on clear evidence of:
• poor or limited social relationships
• underdeveloped communication skills
• repetitive behaviors, activities, and interests.

Treatment

A combination of early intervention, special education, family support, and, in some cases, medication may help some ASD children lead more functional lives. Early intervention and special education programs may increase the child's capacity to learn, communicate, and relate to others. This approach also may reduce the impaired social relationships, communication problems, and restricted activities and behaviors.

Biochemical boosts

Although no drug has been shown to treat ASD successfully, the FDA has approved risperidone (Risperdal) for children ages 5 to 16 and aripiprazole (Abilify) for children ages 6 to 17 when there is self-injury, severe mood changes, and disorganized or aggressive behavior. Stimulants such as methylphenidate may reduce inattentiveness, impulsivity, and overactivity in some ASD children. However, stimulant drugs also may increase the child's internal preoccupation, stereotypical behavior, and social withdrawal.

SSRIs may be useful in managing some symptoms, such as compulsive behavior, irritability, and withdrawal. Lithium, gabapentin (Neurontin), and carbamazepine (Tegretol) have been shown to reduce impulsiveness and sensory sensitivity associated with ASD. Other drugs including buspirone (BuSpar), propranolol (Inderal), and atenolol (Tenormin) may be used to treat severe aggression in children with ASD.

Comfort through coping

Family counseling can help the family better understand the disorder and assist them with coping strategies and behavior modification therapies.

In some situations, home care is available to assist with the child's physical or behavioral management in the home. If the child's disruptive behavior persists, alternative residential placement may be necessary.

Intellect, talent, and education

Intellectual differences are noted in people with ASD. Many children with ASD are good at drawing and using computers. Some children with ASD benefit from attending special schools that use behavior modification. However, many experts believe educational mainstreaming is preferable.

Nursing interventions

These nursing interventions are appropriate for a child with ASD:
• Supervise the child and establish safe environments at home, school, and in the community.
• Monitor the use of language carefully by effectively choosing appropriate words to use when speaking to the child. The child is likely to interpret words concretely and may interpret a harmless request as a threat. Be in tune to the child's nonverbal communication because the child may express needs this way.
• Offer emotional support and information to the caregivers. Suggest they meet with caregivers of other ASD children for support and advice on coping with daily life concerns and typical problems such as temper tantrums and toilet training.
• Promote effective communication by advising caregivers to have close, face-to-face contact with the child and learn about the child's communication style and verbal and nonverbal habits.

ASD symptoms start during the toddler period and caregivers need to be watchful of developmental delays and regression in social skills or language.

Routines and regularity

- Teach the child self-care slowly over time, using simple, concrete, and visual instructions based on what is reasonable for the child to accomplish.
- Teach the caregivers to maintain a regular, predictable daily routine, with consistent times for waking up, dressing, eating, attending school, and going to bed.
- Suggest that caregivers use a picture board, especially if the child is a visual learner, showing the activities that will occur during the day to help make transitions more easily.
- If the child's routine must be changed, instruct caregivers to prepare the child for the changes.

Decrease temper tantrums

- Teach caregivers to learn triggers to aggression and avoid situations known to stimulate outbursts.
- Teach caregivers how to recognize the behaviors that precede temper tantrums, such as increased hand flapping. Instruct them to intervene before a tantrum occurs.
- Help caregivers devise a plan to improve behavior by giving tangible rewards for desired behavior.

Strive for safety

- Instruct caregivers on ways to make the home safer (e.g., by installing locks and gates so the child can't wander unsupervised).
- If the child's behavior is self-injurious, teach caregivers ways to prevent injury by providing helmets and protective padding. Also, help caregivers connect increasing anxiety with tendency to self-injure.
- Instruct caregivers to intervene to stop anxiety from escalating and offer diversionary activities.
- Inform caregivers that punishment may worsen self-injurious behavior.

Intellectual disability (intellectual developmental disorder)

Intellectual disability (ID), referred to as *mental retardation* in the past, is a developmental disorder that is defined by limitations in general mental abilities and in performing usual activities of daily living. There are associated deficits in communication, social skills, self-care, and adaptive behavior.

ID affects roughly 1% to 3% of the population. Its onset occurs before age 18. Early intervention for babies and toddlers is recommended.

Learning process

A child with an ID has low intelligence, defined as an IQ below 70. Children with ID may take longer to speak, walk, and develop the skills to dress and fed themselves. They also have difficulty in school learning things. They can learn; however, it takes them longer periods of time to master a skill. Usually, problems arise from the child's inability to handle the expected activities of daily living appropriate for age and culture.

Degrees of impairment

The degree of impairment for children with ID varies with the classification. Severity levels for ID are classified as mild, moderate, severe, or profound. (See *Severity levels for persons with ID*, page 90.)

Causes

Scientists believe ID results from biological factors, psychosocial factors, or a combination. Such factors include:
• single dominant gene problems, such as neurofibromatosis or tuberous sclerosis
• chromosomal disorders, such as trisomy 21, fragile X syndrome, or Klinefelter syndrome
• inborn errors of metabolism, such as phenylketonuria (PKU), hyperglycemia, or Tay-Sachs disease
• problems during embryonic development, such as maternal illness (such as diabetes or toxemia) or maternal infection (such as rubella, herpes simplex, or human immunodeficiency syndrome)
• pregnancy and perinatal factors, such as prematurity, maternal-neonate blood group incompatibility, brain trauma, or oxygen deprivation
• infancy or early childhood problems, such as severe malnutrition, head trauma, meningitis, encephalitis, or poisoning from lead, medication, or toxic chemical exposure (prenatal or postnatal)
• environmental problems, such as poor parenting, abuse and neglect, inadequate nutrition, sensory deprivation, poor nurturance, or poor social or language development

Maternal infection is one possible cause of ID.

Streptococci, INC

Unanswered question

In roughly 40% to 50% of persons with ID, predisposing factors can't be determined.

Severity levels for persons with ID

The functioning level of a person with an ID varies with the degree of severity.

	Self-care ability	Educational level	Social skills
Mild (IQ 50–70)	The person may be able to live somewhat independently with monitoring or assistance with life changes, challenges, or stressors (such as personal illness or the death of a loved one).	The person can achieve sixth-grade reading skills and may master vocational training.	The person can learn and use social skills in structured settings.
Moderate (IQ 35–49)	Typically, the person requires supervision and needs to be monitored when performing certain independent activities.	The person can achieve up to second-grade skills and may be trained in skills to participate in a sheltered workshop setting.	The person has some speech limitations and difficulty following expected social norms which may impede peer relationships.
Severe (IQ 20–34)	The person requires complete supervision but may be able to perform simple hygiene skills, such as brushing teeth and washing hands.	The person rarely participates in academic training but may learn some simple skills.	The person has limited verbal skills and tends to communicate needs nonverbally or by acting them out.
Profound (IQ below 20)	The person requires constant assistance and supervision.	The person can't benefit from academic or vocational training but may master simple self-care skills.	The person has little speech development and little to no social skills.

Signs and symptoms

Family members may suspect ID if the child's motor, language, and self-help skills fail to develop or are developing much more slowly than those of the child's peers.

Typical indications of ID include:
- failure to achieve developmental milestones
- deficiencies in cognitive functioning such as inability to follow commands or directions
- failure to achieve intellectual developmental markers
- reduced ability to learn or to meet academic demands
- expressive or receptive language problems
- psychomotor skill deficits

Psychomotor skills	Living situation	Economic situation
The person can develop average to good skills but may have minor coordination problems.	The person must live with the family or in community housing as assistance with health care and legal decisions is needed.	The person may hold a job if closely supervised and can budget or manage money with guidance. Support would be needed to have a marriage and family.
The person has only fair gross motor skills and may have limited vocational opportunities.	The person typically lives in a structured situation for supervision and reinforcement of teaching activities of daily living.	The child may learn to handle a small amount of pocket money as well as how to make change but needs support with managing money.
The person has poor psychomotor skills, with limited ability to perform simple tasks even under direct supervision.	The person must live in a highly structured and closely supervised setting.	The supervised person may be taught how to use change and help with shopping.
The person lacks both fine and gross motor skills and needs constant care and supervision.	The person must live in a highly structured, closely supervised setting.	The person must depend on others for money management.

- difficulty performing self-care activities
- neurologic impairments
- medical problems such as seizures
- negativity and low self-esteem
- irritability when frustrated or upset
- depression or labile moods
- acting-out behavior
- persistence of infantile behavior
- lack of curiosity.

Just a quiet child?

Disruptions or limitations in adaptive behaviors reflect the severity of ID. For example, with a mild level of ID, the child may show lack of curiosity and quiet behavior.

Memory jogger

To remember the major signs of ID, think of the five Ds.

Decreased cognitive and intellectual functioning

Deficits in psychomotor skills

Difficulties in performing self-care activities

Degrees of neurologic impairment

Depressed or labile mood

With a severe level of ID, limited independent functioning may persist throughout life.

Diagnosis

Diagnosis centers on a comprehensive personal and family medical history, a complete physical examination, and thorough developmental assessment and intelligence testing.

> Screening tests measure the child's intellectual functioning and adaptive behaviors.

Adaptation and intellect

Developmental screening tests are used to assess age-appropriate adaptive behaviors. To measure intellectual functioning and learning ability, a standardized IQ test, Denver Developmental Screening Test, or Bayley Scale of Infant Development is given.

The child also undergoes standardized tests for measuring social maturity and adaptive skills, such as the Vineland Behavior Scales (VABS) or the Adaptive Behavior Scale (ABS) or the Scales for Independent Behavior–Revised (SIB-R).

In addition, the child should be examined for underlying organic problems, including neurologic, chromosomal, and metabolic disorders. When discovered early, conditions such as hyperthyroidism and PKU can be treated and the progression of disability can be stopped or, in some cases, partially reversed. If brain injury or another neurologic cause is suspected, the child may be referred to a neurologist or neuropsychologist for testing (Barry et al., 2013).

Treatment

Treatment focuses on coordinating the child's psychological and physiologic needs. Drugs rarely are indicated unless the child has an overlapping mental disorder.

Key components of treatment for persons with ID include:
- behavior management
- environmental supervision
- monitoring of the child's developmental needs and problems
- programs that maximize speech, language, cognitive, psychomotor, social, self-care, and occupational skills
- ongoing evaluation for overlapping psychiatric disorders, such as depression, bipolar disorder, and ADHD

• family therapy to help caregivers develop coping skills and deal with guilt or anger.

Basic skills training

Many states have early intervention programs for children younger than age 3 with ID. Day schools may be available to train the child in basic skills, such as bathing and feeding. Extracurricular activities and social programs help the child gain self-esteem and learn social behaviors.

Independent living

Training in independent living and job skills typically starts in early adulthood (depending on the degree of disability). Many persons with mild disability can gain the skills they need to live independently and hold a job. Persons with moderate to profound disability usually need supervised community living. (See *Settings for those with ID.*)

Nursing interventions

These nursing interventions are appropriate for a person with ID:
• Determine the child's strengths and abilities and develop a plan of care to maintain and enhance capabilities.
• Monitor the child's developmental levels and initiate supportive interventions, such as speech, language, or occupational skills, as needed.
• Provide for safety needs.
• Prevent self-injury. Be prepared to intervene if self-injury occurs.
• Teach about natural and normal feelings and emotions.
• Monitor for physical or emotional distress.
• Modify the behavior by teaching the child how to redirect energy.
• Keep communication brief, simple, and consistent.
• Teach caregivers to be patient, hopeful teachers as they work with the child to develop skills for as much independence as possible.

Self-care and support

• Teach the child adaptive skills, such as eating, dressing, grooming, and toileting.
• Demonstrate and help practice self-care skills.
• Work to increase compliance with conventional social norms and behaviors.
• Maintain a consistent and supervised environment.
• Maintain adequate environmental stimulation.
• Set supportive limits on activities.
• Work to establish satisfactory communication and social interaction patterns.
• Work to maintain and enhance positive feelings about self and daily accomplishments.

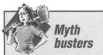

Myth busters

Settings for those with ID

It is often assumed that people with ID have to live in institutions.
Myth: Most people with ID live in institutional settings.
Reality: Since the advocacy movement of the 1970s, only persons with the most severe and profound ID less than 1% are institutionalized (National Council on Disability, 2009).

References

American Psychiatric Association. (2013). *Diagnostic and statistical manual of mental disorders* (5th ed.). Arlington, VA: Author.

Autism Speaks. (2014). *DSM-5 diagnostic criteria*. Retrieved from http://www.autismspeaks .org/what-autism/diagnosis/dsm-5-diagnostic-criteria

Barkley, R. (2013). *Taking charge of ADHD* (3rd ed.). New York, NY: Guilford Press.

Barry, C., Frick, P. J., Kamphaus, R. W., Geisinger, K. F., Bracken, B. A., Carlson, J. F., & Rodriguez, M. C. (Eds.). (2013). *APA handbook of testing and assessment in psychology, Vol. 2: Testing and assessment in clinical and counseling psychology.* Washington, DC: American Psychological Association.

Bernstein, B. (2014). *Conduct disorder*. Retrieved from http://emedicine.medscape.com/ article/918213-overview#a1

Carnevale, T. (2011). An integrative review of adolescent depression screening instruments: Applicability for use by school nurses. *Journal of Child & Adolescent Psychiatric Nursing, 24*(1), 51–57.

Centers for Disease Control and Prevention. (2013). *Attention deficit/hyperactivity disorder*. Retrieved from http://www.cdc.gov/ncbddd/adhd/data.html?mobile=nocontent

Centers for Disease Control and Prevention. (2014). *Adolescent health*. Retrieved from http:// www.cdc.gov/nchs/fastats/adolescent-health.htm

Clark, M. S., Jansen, K. L., & Cloy, J. A. (2012). Treatment of childhood and adolescent depression. *American Family Physician, 86*(5), 442–448.

Eapen, V., & Crncec, R. (2012). Strategies and challenges in the management of adolescent depression. *Current Opinion in Psychiatry, 25*(1), 7–13.

Harvard Medical School. (2011). Options for managing conduct disorder. *Harvard Mental Health Letter, 27*(9), 1–3.

Kieling, C., Baker-Henningham, H., Belfer, M., Conti, G., Ertem, I. Omigbodun, O., . . . Rahman, A. (2011). Child and adolescent mental health worldwide: Evidence for action. *The Lancet, 378*(9801), 1515–1525.

Loy, J. H., Merry, S. N., Hetricks, S. E., & Stasiak, K. (2012). *Atypical antipsychotics for disruptive behavior disorders in children and youths: The Cochrane Collaboration.* Somerset, NJ: John Wiley & Sons.

Mayo Clinic. (2012). *Oppositional defiant disorder*. Retrieved from http://www.mayoclinic .org/diseases-conditions/oppositional-defiant-disorder/basics/causes/con-20024559

Mayo Clinic. (2014). *Attention deficit/hyperactivity disorder (ADHD) in children.* Retrieved from http://www.mayoclinic.org/diseases-conditions/adhd/basics/risk-factors/ con-20023647

Merikangas, K. R., He, J., Burstein, M., Swanson, S. A., Avenevoli, S., Cui, L., . . . Swendsen, J. (2010). Lifetime prevalence of mental disorders in U.S. adolescents: Results from the National Comorbidity Study-Adolescent Supplement (NCS-A). *Journal of the American Academy of Child and Adolescent Psychiatry, 49*(10), 980–989.

Moreland, C., & Bonin, L. (2014). *Effects of antidepressants on suicide risk in children and adolescents*. Retrieved from http://www.uptodate.com/contents/effect-of-antidepressants-on-suicide-risk-in-children-and-adolescents

National Alliance on Mental Illness. (2014). *Depression in children and teens.* Retrieved from http://www.nami.org/Template.cfm?Section=By_Illness&template=/ContentManagement/ContentDisplay.cfm&ContentID=88551

National Council on Disability. (2009). *Institutions in brief.* Retrieved from http://www.ncd.gov/publications/2012/DIToolkit/Institutions/inBrief/

National Institute of Mental Health. (2011). *What is autism spectrum disorder? A parent's guide to autism spectrum disorder.* Retrieved from http://www.nimh.nih.gov/health/publications/a-parents-guide-to-autism-spectrum-disorder/index.shtml

National Institute of Neurological Disorders and Stroke. (2014). *Autism fact sheet.* Retrieved from http://www.ninds.nih.gov/disorders/autism/detail_autism.htm

O'Driscoll, C., Heary, C., Hennessy, E., & McKeague, L. (2012). Explicit and implicit stigma towards peers with mental health problems in childhood and adolescence. *Journal of Child Psychology and Psychiatry, 53,* 1054–1062.

Oppositional defiant disorder. (n.d.). In *A.D.A.M. medical encyclopedia.* Retrieved from http://www.ncbi.nlm.nih.gov/pubmedhealth/PMH0002504/

Turner, H. A., Finkelhor, D., & Ormrod, R. (2010). Child mental health problems as risk factors for victimization. *Child Maltreatment, 15*(2), 132–143.

WebMD. (2014). *Attention deficit hyperactivity disorder: ADHD in adults.* Retrieved from http://www.m.webmd.com/a-to-z-guides/adhd-adults

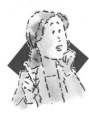

Quick quiz

1. What information should the nurse teach the parents of a child who's receiving methylphenidate (Concerta)?
  A. Obtain the child's blood glucose level yearly.
  B. Monitor the child's physical growth closely.
  C. Have the child's IQ tested every 2 years.
  D. Test the child's hearing and vision periodically.

Answer: B. The child's physical growth should be monitored because methylphenidate (Concerta) may cause weight loss and temporary interference with growth and development.

2. In a child with conduct disorder, what is aggressive behavior linked to?
  A. Severe anxiety
  B. Low self-esteem
  C. Relationship changes
  D. Genetic factors

Answer: B. A child with conduct disorder struggles with low self-esteem and a low tolerance for frustration, even though he or she may attempt to portray an aggressive image.

3. A child with depression has limited interaction with classmates. What is the nurse's top priority when working with this child?

    A.   Developing strengths and improving low self-esteem

    B.   Addressing problem solving and ways to complete tasks

    C.   Determining strategies for handling fears and failures

    D.   Developing peer communication and social networking skills

Answer: A. A depressed child needs assistance with learning how to feel good about self.

4. The nurse is teaching the parents of a child with a possible diagnosis of ODD. What major symptom of ODD would the nurse include in the teaching session?

    A.   Hurting siblings

    B.   Compulsive behavior

    C.   Testing limits

    D.   Repetitive movements

Answer: C. Children with ODD engage in persistent testing of limits, bully others to get what they want, and try to win no matter what the consequences may be.

5. The nurse is educating the caregiver of a high-functioning child who was recently diagnosed with autism. Which caregiver statement indicates that teaching has been effective?

    A.   "My child will get well soon."

    B.   "I will try to hug my child more."

    C.   "I have caused my child to be this way."

    D.   "I will create a daily schedule for our family to use."

Answer: D. Children with ASD respond more favorably to a predictable schedule.

Scoring

✰✰✰ If you answered all five items correctly, congrats! Your commitment to understanding kids is commendable!

  ✰✰ If you answered three or four items correctly, pat yourself on the back! We're proud of your pediatric proficiency!

    ✰ If you answered fewer than three items correctly, don't get depressed! Review the chapter—only this time, stop fidgeting and pay more attention!

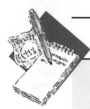

3

Disorders of the elderly

Just the facts

In this chapter, you'll learn:

♦ mental status changes associated with older adulthood

♦ roles and responsibilities of geropsychiatric nurses

♦ care settings for older adults with psychiatric conditions

♦ diagnosis, treatment, and nursing interventions for older adults with age-related cognitive decline, Alzheimer dementia, and vascular dementia.

A look at psychiatric disorders in older adults

Americans are living longer than ever before, with the vast majority surviving beyond the age of 65. Likewise, the elderly population is increasing. The U.S. population older than age 65 is expected to double from approximately 35 million in 2000 (13% of the total population) to 72 million in 2030 (20% of the population) (Administration on Aging, 2013).

A significant number of older adults are affected—sometimes severely—by psychiatric disorders, such as depression, anxiety, and dementia. As the life expectancy of Americans continues to rise, the number of older adults experiencing mental disorders will keep growing. Health care professionals must be educated to identify these disorders, whose symptoms may mimic those of other medical conditions. (See *Barriers to treatment*, page 98.)

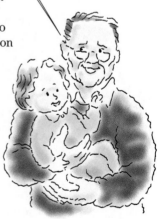

My granddaughter keeps me happy and alert. Sadly, some of my friends don't have family or friends to keep them company.

Barriers to treatment (Hatfield, 1999)

Many older adults need—but don't get—treatment for psychiatric disorders. Here are some reasons for this unmet need:

• Many people (elderly and otherwise) believe that senility, depression, and hopelessness are natural conditions of aging that can't or don't need to be treated.

• Many older adults are reluctant to discuss psychological symptoms, dwelling instead on their physical problems.

• Some older adults prefer primary care—yet many primary care providers lack the training to diagnose and treat psychiatric disorders in the elderly.

• Treatment of mental disorders in older adults can be complex even for properly trained professionals. Multiple prescriptions increase the risk for drug interactions.

• Some health care providers are reluctant to inform elderly patients that they have a mental disorder.

• Health care delivery systems may impose time pressures or fail to reimburse the costs of treating mental disorders.

• Stigma associated with mental health issues

• Lack of support systems

A depressing thought . . .

Approximately 15 of every 100 adults aged 65 or older in the United States experience some type of symptom of depression (Geriatric Mental Health Foundation [GMHF], 2014). Older adults have the highest suicide rate in the United States, accounting for 25% of suicides (GMHF, 2014).

Beyond recognition?

Despite the substantial need for mental health services, older adults may not seek or readily use available resources. Some elderly patients deny that they have mental disorders, and many health care providers fail to identify the characteristic signs and symptoms.

Even among older adults who acknowledge their mental disorders, not all seek or receive treatment from any health care provider, and only a fraction of those receive specialty mental health services (GMHF, 2014).

> I wanted to enjoy my "golden years" . . . I wonder why I am not happy?

Geropsychiatric nursing

Geropsychiatric nursing addresses the unique mental health care needs of elderly patients. It blends expertise from four specialties:

• gerontologic nursing
• psychiatric nursing
• medical-surgical nursing
• community health nursing.

The geropsychiatric nurse works as part of the mental health care team—typically as a case manager—and provides the bulk of direct patient care. Besides having a strong background in behavioral and social sciences, he or she must have a thorough knowledge of pathophysiology, psychopharmacology, and the normal aging process (Beck, Buckwater, Dudzik, & Evans, 2011).

The geropsychiatric nurse must also be familiar with the community resources in the local demographic area that exist to help older adults maintain the highest possible wellness level.

Geriatric and geropsychiatric advanced practice nurses

Geriatric and geropsychiatric advanced practice nurses (APNs) provide various specialty services to older adults with physical and mental health needs. These APNs have a master's or doctoral degree in nursing and advanced certification in a specialty area, such as clinical nurse specialist (CNS) or nurse practitioner (NP). In many states, APNs have some type of prescriptive authority and work in group or independent practices, or hospitals.

Geriatric APNs

Geriatric APNs serve as resources for the care of elderly adults, including those with mental health problems. They can see patients on site and intervene as needed with evidence-based, advanced clinical nursing skills.

Geropsychiatric APNs

Geropsychiatric APNs combine a strong background in medical-surgical and psychiatric nursing with patient education. Depending on the state in which they practice, they may be certified to provide psychotherapy and may have the authority to prescribe medications.

The accessible APN

Because of their accessibility, APNs are highly qualified to meet the special mental health care needs of older adults. They may be more geographically accessible than other providers of care, and older adults may feel more comfortable seeing the APN than the psychiatrist because of perceived negative preconceptions.

Community services for older adults

Community services for older adults with mental health care needs vary from one location to another. They may include:
• dementia evaluation centers
• geropsychiatric outpatient clinics
• group homes
• nutrition services
• transportation services
• home maintenance services.

Where to get information

To find out about community resources, referral sources, retirement campuses, and other support groups in your area, visit the public library; call the local department, council, or agency on aging; or contact the nearest chapter of the National Alliance on Mental Illness at 1-800-950-6264 (National Alliance on Mental Illness, 2014).

Other geriatric mental health care team members

Treatment by a geropsychologist or geropsychiatrist is one option for older adults with mental health needs.

Geropsychologists

Geropsychologists provide behavioral health care for older adults with mental health needs or behavioral concerns that diminish quality of life. Through programs that improve treatment adherence, stress management skills, and access to social support, they help older adults and their families maintain well-being, overcome problems, achieve maximum potential, manage disease, and prevent excessive disability.

Geropsychologists teach family caregivers about safe, effective caregiving techniques and help them locate resources to strengthen their coping skills. They also advise on safe, effective alternatives when medications are ineffective, when patients can't tolerate adverse effects, or when they are at risk for drug interactions.

Geropsychiatrists

Geropsychiatrists are physicians with advanced training in assessment and treatment of mental health needs and related medical problems of older adults. They are required to have a thorough understanding of psychopharmacology, the biological determinants of mental impairment, and age- and gender-related changes in physiology.

Their expertise also includes:
• understanding the stresses associated with hospitalization
• diagnosing atypical disease presentations
• detecting the presence of multiple medical conditions.

Mental status changes of older adulthood

Throughout life, a person continues to develop and change. The brain continuously interacts with and responds to multiple influences. At any given time, the expression of mental health needs can be subtle or pronounced.

Vulnerability to the various types of mental disorders changes throughout life. In children, this vulnerability is assumed, but in older adults, it is commonly overlooked, which means that mental health needs of this population can go undetected or undertreated.

As the brain ages . . .

During late adulthood, health changes may grow more pronounced and the ability to compensate for deficits may decrease. With age, the brain's capacity for certain mental tasks tends to diminish (Lu et al., 2011).

Other mental abilities normally remain intact. Well into late adulthood, cognitive skills training and problem-solving strategies can be used to enhance a person's ability to solve problems.

Neurobiological changes of normal aging

Normal aging brings certain changes in mental functioning. Most older adults experience slight declines in vocabulary, learning ability, short-term memory, and recall time. This may be related to changes in the hippocampal functioning (Besdine, 2013). These declines grow more significant by about age 70.

Physical changes of the brain

With age come certain physical changes in the brain (National Institute on Aging, 2014). These include:
- Certain parts of the brain shrink, especially the prefrontal cortex and the hippocampus.
- Communication between neurons decreases because white matter is degraded or lost.
- Blood flow decreases as arteries narrow.

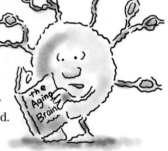

It says here that neurons shrink with age. Maybe that's why I am having trouble remembering things.

Cognitive changes

Cognition involves intelligence, language, learning, and memory. With advancing years, cognitive capacity declines somewhat, but important functions are spared. Age-related cognitive changes vary significantly among individuals (Persson et al., 2011).

Myth busters

Shaking off "old people" stereotypes

Does the brain grow brittle and inflexible with age, much the way bones do? Don't bet on it.

Myth: Older adults are slow-thinking, inflexible, and unproductive.

Reality: With normal aging, intellectual functioning remains stable, as does the capacity for change and productive engagement with life. People have the capacity for constructive change in later life—even in the face of mental health conditions, adversity, and chronic mental health problems. Many older adults remain flexible in both behavior and attitude and are able to grow intellectually and emotionally.

Cognitive research

Cognitive neuroscientists and cognitive aging psychologists continue to conduct research to determine:
- what happens to the mind as we age
- how changes in cognitive behaviors (such as remembering and problem solving) relate to brain function
- whether brains of younger people are more specialized
than those of older people
- whether brains of older people are able to reorganize so
that decreased functioning in one area is compensated for
by another area.

    Researchers are also investigating the aging mind
through brain-imaging techniques (Lu et al., 2011).

Cognitive disorders

Marked by disruption of cognitive functioning, cognitive
disorders manifest clinically as mental deficits in patients
who previously didn't seem to have problems. A cognitive
deficit is a prominent feature of many mental and physical conditions seen in older adults. Health care providers
must explore all possible causes for the underlying problem.

    A cognitive disorder can result from any condition that
alters or destroys brain tissue and, in turn, impairs cerebral
functioning.

Vocabulary, fluid intelligence, and processing capacity

A person's vocabulary increases slightly until about age 70
and then starts to decline (Besdine, 2013). Mental processing
capacity—the ability to understand text, make inferences,
and pay attention—also decreases with age. Likewise, fluid
intelligence—the ability to solve problems—also declines
over time. Research shows that fluid intelligence can be
enhanced through training in cognitive skills and problem-
solving strategies (National Institute on Aging, 2014).

Cognitive processes minimally affected by aging

In the normal brain, certain cognitive processes show little or no
decline with age. These include:
- implicit memory (information that can't be
brought to mind but that can affect behavior)
- prospective memory (remembering things you
need to do)
- highly practiced expert skills, such as typing or
playing bridge or chess
- picture recognition. (See *Using pictures and
words.*)

Memory jogger

To help re-
member the
possible causes of
cognitive disorders,
think of the three Ds:

- Disease—primary
brain disease

- Disturbance—the
brain's response to
a systemic distur-
bance, such as a
medical condition

- Drugs—the brain's
reaction to a toxic
substance, as in
substance abuse.

Highly
practiced skills
like typing and
playing bridge
rarely decline
with age.

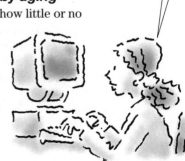

Advice from the experts

Using pictures and words

Aging doesn't seem to affect a person's ability to recognize pictures, so you can use pictures to help jog the memory of older adults with memory impairments.

Here are some other ways to aid memory retention:

• Choose text instructions that explicitly represent material rather than those that force the patient to make subtle inferences or draw conclusions.

• Avoid irrelevant details, which can be distracting and require more mental processing.

Working memory and long-term memory

It is not unusual for older adults to report subjective memory concerns associated with working memory or long-term memory. *Working* memory is used for tasks such as keeping a phone number in mind just long enough to write it down as well as in planning, organizing, and rehearsing. *Long-term* memory is responsible for storing information on a relatively permanent basis.

Haven't I seen you somewhere before?

Researchers have found that aging affects recall (the process of bringing an experience back into consciousness) more than it affects recognition (the ability to recognize someone or something through remembering).

Implications for teaching

Because age-related cognitive changes lead to slower learning, the nurse might need to repeat new information frequently when teaching older adults. Also, to reduce the memory load of new information, older patients should practice new skills and habits until these become automatic. When practiced sufficiently, a skill can become automatic—and isn't as likely to be completely lost at a later time.

Depression in older adults

Late-life depression can have serious consequences, including increased illness and death from suicide. Physical disorders can contribute to depression in older adults. Depression may be underestimated because its symptoms often mimic those associated with physical disorders. Depression may result from such losses as:

- deaths of friends and loved ones
- loss of physical capacities
- loss of social status and self-esteem.

Bereavement and depression

Bereavement—the natural response to a loved one's death—causes sorrow, anxiety, crying, agitation, insomnia, and appetite loss. Although these symptoms may coincide with major depression, they don't in themselves constitute a mental condition.

Woeful widows

Bereavement is an important risk factor for depression. Approximately 10% to 20% of widows and widowers develop clinically significant depression during the first year of bereavement (Townsend, 2014).

Without treatment, this depression may persist and become chronic, leading to further disability and health impairment (possibly including altered endocrine and immune function).

If bereavement symptoms last 2 months or more, the older adult is at risk for adjustment disorder or major depressive disorder. Even when it lasts less than 2 months, bereavement should receive clinical attention because it is a highly stressful condition that increases the likelihood of mental and somatic (physical) disorders.

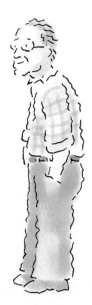

Bereavement red flags

Bereavement is common among older adults who survive family members and friends. Sometimes, though, bereavement can turn into a major depressive disorder. The nurse should suspect this may be happening if the patient experiences:

- frequent thoughts of death
- sense of worthlessness
- guilt about things other than the actions he or she took, or failed to take, at the time of the loved one's death
- pronounced slowing of psychomotor functions
- prolonged, marked functional impairment.

Not-so-harmless hallucinations

Some bereaved people hallucinate, thinking they've heard the dead loved one's voice or seen that person's face. Some report that they've seen their deceased spouses in a crowd or heard them call their name while drifting off to sleep. These hallucinations are common among bereaved people.

A patient who has other types of hallucinations may have a mental condition and needs to be evaluated by a health care provider.

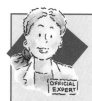

Advice from the experts

Guiding patients through grief

To help elderly patients most effectively, the nurse must recognize the signs and symptoms of grief and its phases. Grief refers to a sequence of mood changes that occur in response to an actual or perceived loss, such as a loved one's death or a change in family role, residence, or body image caused by illness or injury (Townsend, 2014).

Acute grief typically lasts 1 to 2 years. Prolonged grieving may persist for up to 12 years.

Grieving stages

Usually, successful adaptation requires progressing through grieving stages. Discrete stages of grieving are listed below. But patients don't necessarily move through the stages in an orderly way. They may experience several stages at once or may even regress.

- *Disequilibrium.* The patient has feelings of shock and disbelief, followed by a numbed sensation. He or she may cry and feel anger and guilt.
- *Disorganization.* Restlessness and the inability to organize and complete tasks are common. The patient typically experiences loss of self-esteem; profound feelings of loneliness, fear, and helplessness; preoccupation with the image of the lost person or object; feelings of unreality; and emotional distance from others.
- *Reorganization.* The patient establishes new goals and interpersonal relationships. He or she begins to test new behaviors and expand his or her sense of identity.

Pathologic grief

The patient who can't cope with change risks developing a maladaptive or pathologic grief reaction (Townsend, 2014). Stay alert for such warning signs as:

- prolonged, excessive activity with no sense of loss
- physical symptoms similar to those that the deceased person experienced
- psychosomatic illness
- progressive social isolation
- extreme hostility
- wooden or formal conduct
- activity detrimental to social or economic well-being
- manic episodes
- depression
- substance abuse or other self-destructive behavior.

Coping with grief

To help the patient cope with grief in a healthy manner, the nurse should:

- establish rapport and build trust
- explain the normal stages of grieving, emphasizing that a wide range of feelings and behaviors may occur
- convey a caring attitude to encourage the patient to express feelings
- discuss the patient's loss and the concrete changes that have resulted
- encourage the patient to express sadness, guilt, or anger. If he or she becomes angry with you, don't get defensive.
- help the patient to determine what realistic changes may need to be made
- suggest the use of more adaptive ways of coping and making concrete plans for the future
- urge the patient to review and share both good and bad memories.

Traumatic grief

Bereavement-related depression commonly coexists with traumatic grief. Signs and symptoms of traumatic grief include those exhibited in pathologic grief (extreme decline in functioning, harming oneself or others, changes in interpersonal relationships) and posttraumatic stress disorder (insomnia, an exaggerated startle response, angry outbursts, hypervigilance). Extremely disabling, these symptoms are associated with health and functional impairments as well as persistent thoughts of suicide (Townsend, 2014).

Preventing depression

With early recognition of symptoms, depression and suicidal behavior may be averted through grief counseling (Townsend, 2014). Suicide prevention strategies are essential for all residents of long-term facilities, especially those who are new—one-half of newly admitted patients are at increased risk for depression.

Assessment

Assessing and diagnosing psychiatric conditions in elderly patients can be challenging. These disorders may present differently in older adults than in younger ones. Additionally, older adults are more likely to report physical symptoms of depression than psychological ones; however, such somatic complaints may not meet the full criteria for depressive disorders.

History lessons

Obtaining an accurate patient history is crucial. If the patient's cognitive status is poor, you may need to gather history information from family members or caregivers.

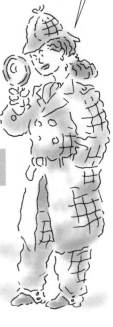

Shifting into detective mode can help you assess mental health needs for the older adult.

Treatment

Depending on the cause of the psychiatric condition, treatment may include medication, psychotherapy, support groups, and sociocultural supports. Ideally, a multidisciplinary team approach is used, with the patient (when able) and his or her family helping to set goals and make decisions about treatment options.

The team typically includes a nurse, physician, psychologist or psychiatrist, pharmacist, dietitian, social worker, and other professionals (such as a physical therapist or chemical dependency counselor) as needed. For optimal results, referrals should be made early in the treatment process.

Keep it confidential

All patients, including older adults, have a right to confidentiality in matters related to health care. Be sure to obtain a signed informed consent from the patient (or a family member, if the patient is incapacitated) before sharing information with loved ones, other health care professionals, and facilities. Never disclose the patient's identity to the public.

Outpatient therapy

Outpatient therapy is provided by experienced mental health professionals, such as psychiatrists, psychologists, psychotherapists, social workers, or psychiatric or geropsychiatric APNs. A multidisciplinary team approach helps to ensure comprehensive care.

Therapy can be provided to individuals, couples, families, or groups. Insurance may cover a portion of short-term outpatient psychotherapy costs.

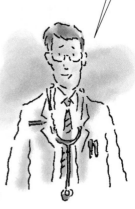

Some older adults see psychiatrists or other mental health professionals on an outpatient basis.

Support groups

Support groups give older adults a chance to discuss how their conditions affect their lives and to help each other by sharing workable solutions. The support group usually consists of patients (and family members) with a common problem. A mental health professional facilitates the group, monitoring and focusing the discussion.

Support groups commonly meet in churches, senior centers, hospitals, schools, and other public meeting places. The groups may be free or may charge a nominal fee.

Care settings

Nurses must be prepared to meet older adults' psychiatric needs in such settings as hospitals, patients' homes, outpatient clinics, partial hospitalization programs, short-term rehabilitation, adult day care, and long-term care facilities. (See *Providing psychiatric care for hospitalized older adults*, page 108.)

Home care

The home is one of the most common delivery settings for geropsychiatric nursing care. An older patient may be returning home after being discharged from the hospital, a partial hospitalization program, a rehabilitation center, or a group home. Or, he or she may simply need psychiatric nursing care to remain in the home. In-home services can involve many aspects of nursing care such as medication management, psychotherapy, detoxification, and dementia care.

Providing psychiatric care for hospitalized older adults

Health care professionals who provide psychiatric care for older adults in general hospitals must be knowledgeable in all aspects of geriatric health needs—not just the problem presenting at the time of admission.

Touting teamwork

Many hospitals have established multidisciplinary liaison-psychiatric intervention teams to aid in rapid expert assessment and interventions. These teams can de-escalate crisis situations, teach hospital staff specific interventions, counsel families, and make referrals for postdischarge specialty care.

Dealing with behavioral problems

Behavioral problems in hospitalized geriatric patients can lead to serious complications, so the staff must be trained to recognize these problems early.

Anxious, agitated elderly patients are at high risk for falls. Monitor the patient carefully, and remember that physical restraints should be used only in emergency situations after other interventions have failed.

Be aware that the use of physical restraints and side rails in elderly patients may lead to pressure ulcers, infections, incontinence, functional impairment, cardiac stress, altered nutrition, and agitation. Strangulation, accidental death, and serious injuries also have been reported.

Flex your mind

The geropsychiatric nurse must be prepared to draw on medical-surgical, community health, and psychiatric nursing expertise to meet home care patients' needs (Aine et al., 2011). Staying current in evidence-based information is crucial.

It's also important for the nurse to be able to professionally communicate frequently with other treatment team members and to respect the patient's right to choose his or her own lifestyle.

De-escalate and coordinate

When providing psychiatric care in a patient's home, the nurse must be thoroughly familiar with:
- physical assessment techniques
- commonly prescribed medications and their interactions
- crisis de-escalation
- community services for older adults.

The nurse may also serve as the care coordinator if the patient is receiving simultaneous services from a community mental health clinic, case management agency, and community support program.

Cutting down on crime

Older adults may be vulnerable to crime and abuse. If you learn of crimes against your patient, threats of crime, or other unusual situations, report these to the police. Remember, even if the patient has a mental condition, his or her descriptions of threatening situations may be reality-based and must not be ignored.

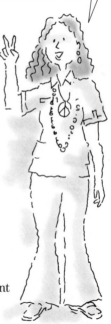

Peace and love, people! When caring for a patient at home, you may have to de-escalate a crisis.

Long-term care facilities

Admission to a nursing home or other long-term care facility can cause situational depression. Help the patient adjust to the change of environment and monitor for signs of depression.

If the patient was admitted for a short-term rehabilitation program, remind him or her that the stay is only temporary and that the goal is to return home.

Some older adults with chronic mental health conditions such as Alzheimer disease may need to be placed in specialized units in long-term care facilities. These units provide a low-stimulus environment with trained staff who assist in activities of daily living (ADLs), nutrition, and maintenance of safety.

Obeying OBRA

Psychiatric services provided to older adults in long-term care facilities are regulated by the Omnibus Budget Reconciliation Act (OBRA) of 1987. This act and its subsequent updates mandate the monitoring of physical restraints and chemical restraints (psychotropic drugs) in skilled nursing facilities.

OBRA guidelines require that older nursing home residents who have been diagnosed with a primary psychiatric disorder be treated for that disorder by a mental health professional. New residents in skilled nursing facilities must be screened for mental health conditions before admission. OBRA also requires that skilled nursing facilities have professional mental health consultants available to monitor patient behavior, work with the staff, and manage psychotropic medications (Yue, 2010).

Clinical nurse specialist consultants

An increasing number of geropsychiatric CNSs are working as consultants for long-term care facilities. They share their expertise with attending physicians, nursing staff, and families.

They are educationally prepared to successfully manage behavior problems in the facility and will consult a psychiatrist if needed.

Hospital emergency departments

An older adult may be taken to a hospital emergency department (ED) for a medical emergency, a suicide attempt, or an episode of violent or threatening behavior. A geriatric patient with a history of acting-out behavior should undergo a thorough physical assessment with baseline diagnostic tests, including electrocardiography, complete blood count with differential, chemistry panel, and urinalysis (Beauchet et al., 2012).

Intervention is targeted to:
- keep the patient from harming self or others
- provide calming treatment
- avoid overmedication and toxicity.

The linking liaison

To address the problems of caring for those with psychiatric conditions in the ED, some hospitals have community liaison nurses. Working collaboratively with other staff, these nurses act as the links among crisis intervention, outreach, and continuity of care staff. They can provide valuable information to the intervention team and expedite rapid referrals.

Inpatient geropsychiatric units

Inpatient geropsychiatric units are used to evaluate patients for suspected dementia and to stabilize aggressive or suicidal patients. Intervention focuses on rapid evaluation to rule out physical illness, stabilize mood, and design a treatment plan for the future. Stays on these units typically are brief, reflecting the trend toward community-based health care.

Partial hospitalization

Psychiatric partial hospitalization provides intense, structured, multidisciplinary therapy for patients who have more acute needs than outpatients do. Usually, patients are driven to the partial hospitalization site in the morning and returned to the home later that day. Many of these programs are associated with specialty psychiatric and chemical dependency programs.

Back to the real world

In a partial hospitalization program, nursing care focuses on:
• stabilizing lifestyle changes to help the patient stay well
• preparing the patient and family to manage the patient's mental condition
• providing the patient and family with tools for effective coping.

The patient receives education in methods of medication, stress, and ADL management.

Adult day care

In some locations, adult day care centers are available for patients with chronic mental conditions. These programs provide structured activities, personal care, recreation, socialization, nutrition support, and health care. They may also include social services and caregiver support.

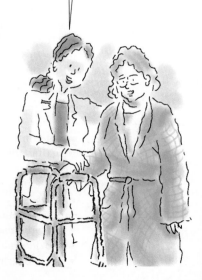

Teaching patients coping techniques is one of the things I love most about my job.

Adult day care offers respite for family members and other caregivers. It may also help to postpone or avoid institutionalizing the older adult.

Community education programs

In many communities, senior centers, hospitals, and churches sponsor public education programs on mental conditions. Often, these programs are free. Depression and anxiety screening programs encourage older adults and their families to learn more about mental health and help connect them with skilled practitioners for treatment.

Drug therapy

When a patient takes medication for a psychiatric condition, be aware of the increased possibility of adverse effects and drug interactions. Many older adults take concurrent multiple medications for coexisting illnesses—a practice called *polypharmacy*. This puts them at high risk for drug interactions and adverse effects (Beauchet et al., 2012).

A slowed metabolic rate in older adults increases the risk of drugs even further. Elderly patients are more vulnerable to adverse reactions, including tardive dyskinesia—a motor disorder causing involuntary jerky movements of the face, tongue, jaws, trunk, and limbs. Some prescribed drugs may worsen a coexisting medical disorder. Be sure to communicate with the health care provider who can adjust dosage and administration schedules appropriately.

Curbing prescriber chaos

Older adults may see a variety of health care providers for different medical conditions and thus have multiple drug prescribers. These prescribers may not be aware that the patient is seeing other practitioners.

To help ensure safe and effective drug administration, keep the patient's medication list up-to-date and monitor for adverse effects and drug interactions. Ask if the patient is taking nonprescription medications or nutritional or herbal supplements. Some of these may pose dangers to elderly patients (Akhondzadeh, Gerbarg, & Brown, 2013; Bottiglieri, 2013; Sarris, 2013).

Start low, titrate slow

Dosages for older adults may start lower than the amount used for younger adults; the health care provider may gradually increase the dose based on the patient's tolerance and report of therapeutic benefit. Blood or urine drug levels may be monitored to ensure that the patient isn't getting a toxic dose.

Meds matters

Using St. John's wort to treat depression

St. John's wort *(Hypericum perforatum)* is a wild-growing, yellow-flowered herb sometimes promoted for the treatment of mild to moderate depression and anxiety (Sarris, 2013). It's available as a capsule, tea, tincture (alcoholic or nonalcoholic), oil extract for topical use, and bulk dried leaves. Because St. John's wort can be obtained without a prescription, patients may feel that it is safe to take and not understand that it can interfere with prescribed medications.

Teach patients to talk with all of their health care providers before taking this herbal supplement.

Cautionary notes
• Be aware that St. John's wort shouldn't be taken concomitantly with other antidepressants.
• Teach the patient (and family members) to watch for adverse effects of St. John's wort, including dry mouth, dizziness, gastrointestinal symptoms, fatigue, and confusion.
• Advise the patient to follow sun exposure precautions to help prevent photosensitivity symptoms, such as dermatitis, severe burning, and blisters.

Compliance complaints

Compliance with drug treatment can be a challenge for older adults, especially those with moderate to severe cognitive deficits. Patients with poor vision may misread instructions or mistake one drug for another. Those with cognitive impairment may not remember whether they have taken all of their doses.

Other compliance challenges include impaired relationships with health care providers, inadequate patient teaching about the necessity or procedure for taking drugs, a large number of daily dosages, and multiple drugs taken at the same time.

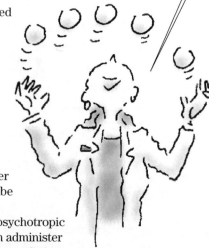

For many older patients, managing medications is a challenging juggling act.

Administering psychotropic drugs

Psychotropic drugs (such as antidepressants, sedatives, tranquilizers, or lithium) may cause oversedation in an older adult. Because of slower kidney and liver functions, drugs take longer to be metabolized and excreted in older people.

As a result, the patient may not respond to a psychotropic drug immediately. Misguided caregivers may then administer more of the medication, which can cause drug accumulation—with adverse effects that may range from light sedation to death.

Toxicology screening

If a patient is taking drugs to treat a psychiatric condition, the nurse will monitor laboratory results to detect toxicity. It is important to remember that diagnostic tests can also detect alcohol and illicit substances in the blood and/or urine as well. Use the list below to identify where toxic levels of these substances are detected.

Blood
- Alcohol (ethyl, isopropyl, and methyl)
- Ethchlorvynol (Placidyl)

Urine
- Chlorpromazine (Thorazine)
- Cocaine
- Cyanide
- Desmethyldoxepin (metabolite of doxepin)
- Heroin (metabolized to and detected as morphine)
- Imipramine (Tofranil)
- Lysergic acid diethylamide (LSD)
- Marijuana
- Methadone

- Morphine
- Phencyclidine (PCP)

Both blood and urine
- Acetaminophen
- Amitriptyline (Elavil)
- Amobarbital (Amytal)
- Butabarbital (Butisol)
- Butalbital (Fiorinal)
- Caffeine
- Carisoprodol (Soma)
- Chlordiazepoxide (Librium)
- Codeine
- Desipramine (Norpramin)
- Desmethyldiazepam (metabolite of diazepam)
- Diazepam (Valium)

- Diphenhydramine (Benadryl)
- Doxepin (Sinequan)
- Flurazepam (Dalmane)
- Glutethimide (Doriden)
- Ibuprofen (Advil, Motrin)
- Meperidine (Demerol)
- Mephobarbital (Mebaral)
- Meprobamate (Equanil, Miltown)
- Methapyrilene
- Methaqualone (Quaalude)
- Nortriptyline (Aventyl, Pamelor)
- Oxazepam (Serax)
- Phenobarbital (Luminal)
- Salicylates and their conjugates
- Secobarbital (Seconal)

Neurocognitive disorders and cognitive impairment

Neurocognitive disorders (NCD) can be identified based on changes in cognitive functioning. "NCDs are unique among *Diagnostic and Statistical Manual of Mental Disorders,* 5th Edition (*DSM-5*) categories in that these are syndromes for which the underlying pathology, and frequently the etiology as well, can potentially be determined" (American Psychiatric Association [APA], 2013, p. 591). Patients with NCDs experience some level of cognitive impairment, the severity of which is often based on the causative agent.

Causes

NCDs may stem from many different causes, not all of which are age-related. NCDs can develop from, or be associated with, medical conditions, cognitive disorders, vascular concerns, trauma, infections, and/or use of substances or medications.

The health care provider may also diagnose an NCD of unspecified or unknown etiology. Symptoms can range from mild problems with memory to complete cognitive impairment.

Signs and symptoms

Depending on the etiology of the NCD, patients with cognitive impairment may exhibit only a few, or many, symptoms. Suspect NCD if the following symptoms are noticed during assessment:
- poor hygiene
- inappropriate dress for climate or occasion
- general sense of confusion
- impairment in short- and/or long-term memory
- lack of ability to solve simple or complex problems
- decreased alertness and/or orientation to person, place, and/or time.

Treatment

Treatment will be based on whether the etiology of NCD is known. Various drugs, vitamins, herbs, and dietary therapies are being researched as treatments for cognitive impairment.

Interdisciplinary management should include psychiatrists, medical physicians, social workers, therapists (e.g., physical, occupational, and/or speech), and community resources.

Nursing interventions

These nursing interventions may be appropriate for a patient with cognitive impairment:

Cut through the confusion

- Reduce and eliminate factors that may worsen confusion associated with cognitive impairment, such as dehydration, malnutrition, and difficulty sleeping. Carefully monitor fluid and electrolyte status, and replace as needed. Promote adequate fluid intake. Provide a well-balanced diet.
- Promote normal sleep-rest activities. Avoid giving sedative-hypnotic drugs when possible.

Optimize senses and stimuli

- Promote optimal vision and hearing by keeping rooms well lit, cleaning cerumen out of ears, promoting frequent eye and ear examinations, and ensuring that hearing aids are in good working order and positioned properly in the ear.
- Reduce unnecessary stimulation and make the environment as stable as possible. Avoid changing rooms and moving furniture or possessions around.

Memory jogger

Use the acronym PILE to help patients with cognitive impairment maintain their maximum level of functioning.

P Promote "here and now" interactions.

I Interact briefly but frequently.

L Link conversations to meaningful topics.

E Encourage self-expression.

Orient—always

• Provide frequent meaningful sensory input and reorientation. Place a large clock and calendar in every room. Provide outdoor activities or a bed by the window.

• Add orienting material to every conversation. Frequently tell the patient your name and what you're going to do while you are with him or her.

• Encourage the patient to participate in therapeutic groups, such as those centered on reality orientation, remotivation, reminiscence, recreational therapy, pet therapy, music therapy, and sensory training.

• Frequently assess the patient's need for medications, appropriateness of dosage, and adverse effects. Be aware of possible drug interactions.

Avert injury

• Check the patient frequently to decrease the chance of falls, wandering, and self-poisoning.

• Take extra safety measures regarding bath water and food temperature to avoid accidental burns.

Major or mild neurocognitive disorder due to Alzheimer disease

Alzheimer disease is marked by global, progressive impairment of cognitive functioning, memory, and personality. The condition is irreversible and progressive which differs from symptoms that can be reversed with treatment (Alzheimer's Association, 2014a). The average duration of illness from symptom onset to death is 8 to 10 years, although patients may live up to 20 years following diagnosis (Alzheimer's Association, 2014a).

No safety in these numbers

Alzheimer disease affects an estimated 5.2 million Americans (Alzheimer's Association, 2014a). It affects more women than men and is the sixth leading cause of death in the United States (Alzheimer's Association, 2014a). As Americans live longer, the incidence of Alzheimer disease will likely continue to grow, unless a cure or effective means of prevention is discovered.

There goes the memory

Typically, memory loss is the earliest symptom of Alzheimer disease. As the disease progresses, symptoms progressively interfere with the patient's social and occupational functioning. (See *Debunking dementia myths*, page 116.)

Myth busters

Debunking dementia myths

Misunderstandings about dementia can lead to unrealistic expectations.

Myth: Dementia is reversible if diagnosed early.

Reality: Dementia takes a progressive, deteriorating, irreversible course.

Myth: Vascular dementia isn't as serious a health problem as Alzheimer disease.

Reality: Vascular dementia, which is characterized by a marked disruption in cerebral blood flow with destruction of brain cells, reduces life expectancy to a greater degree than does Alzheimer disease.

Myth: Dementia causes rapid loss of language skills.

Reality: Only the most severe forms of dementia result in aphasia and the inability to speak. As dementia progresses, though, most patients struggle to name objects and express themselves.

Causes

No one knows exactly what causes Alzheimer disease. Researchers suspect it's linked to specific biological factors, which may be triggered by various environmental and genetic factors (Alzheimer's Association, 2014d; Lu et al., 2011). When oxidants are overproduced, they can cause severe damage to cells and tissue. Oxidation is known to play a part in such diseases as coronary artery disease and cancer, and some experts believe it may contribute to Alzheimer disease. Researchers continue to explore whether environmental factors such as infection, metals, and toxins may trigger oxidation, inflammation, and the Alzheimer disease process (especially in people with genetic susceptibility). Other studies have explored such wide-ranging possibilities as vitamin deficiencies, depression, head injury, and lower educational levels as causative agents.

Genetic factors

Certain genetic factors are thought to play a role in the beta amyloid buildup found in the brain of patients with Alzheimer disease. A major focus of research is on the "risk gene" called *apolipoprotein E* (APOE-e4), which aids cholesterol transport and nerve cell repair.

Biological factors in the brain

In patients with Alzheimer disease, brain-imaging techniques have found a significant loss of neurons and volume in the brain regions devoted to memory and higher mental functioning (Alzheimer's Association, 2014d). Abnormalities found on biopsy include neurofibrillary tangles (twisted nerve cell fibers) and a buildup of beta amyloid (a sticky protein).

> Tangles and sticky proteins—two more things that are dangerous to my brain health!

Signs and symptoms

Decreased intellectual function, personality changes, impaired judgment, and changes in affect are common manifestations of Alzheimer disease, which has seven stages (Alzheimer's Association, 2014b). These stages may overlap, making it difficult to categorize a patient into a specific stage (Alzheimer's Association, 2014b).

Stage 1—no impairment

In stage 1, signs and symptoms typically include:
• no memory problems
• an interview with the health care provider does not reveal any evidence of symptoms.

Stage 2—very mild cognitive decline (may be mistaken for normal age-related changes)

In stage 2, expect to find:
• "memory lapses"
• forgetfulness of familiar words or the location of objects
• no symptoms upon medication examination by a health care provider.

> Signs and symptoms of Alzheimer disease occur in seven stages, matching the progression of the disease.

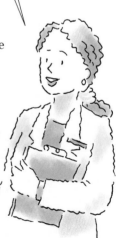

Stage 3—mild cognitive decline (early-stage Alzheimer disease can be diagnosed in some individuals)

In stage 3, look for:
• noticeable problems finding the right word or name
• trouble remembering people who are new to the patient
• difficulty performing tasks in social and/or work settings
• forgetfulness of material just read
• increased frequency of losing or missing familiar objects
• difficulty planning or organizing
• friends and family members who begin to notice difficulties
• problems with memory or concentration noted by the health care provider.

Stage 4—moderate cognitive decline (mild or early-stage Alzheimer disease)

In stage 4, expect:
- forgetfulness of recent happenings
- impaired cognitive ability to perform challenging mental math (e.g., counting backward from 100 by 7s)
- difficulty performing complex tasks (e.g., paying bills)
- forgetfulness of personal history
- moodiness or withdrawn behaviors, especially in situations where social engagement takes place
- identification of symptoms by a health care provider.

Stage 5—moderately severe cognitive decline (moderate or mid-stage Alzheimer disease)

In stage 5, anticipate:
- noticeable gaps in memory or thinking
- the patient begins to need minimal help with ADLs but still can dress, eat, and eliminate by self
- inability to recall personal facts (e.g., address, phone number)
- impaired cognitive ability to perform less challenging mental math (e.g., counting backward from 20 by 2s).

Stage 6—severe cognitive decline (moderately severe or mid-stage Alzheimer disease)

In stage 6, know that:
- memory continues to worsen
- personality and behavioral changes may take place (e.g., suspiciousness, delusions, repetitive behaviors like shredding tissue)
- the patient needs extensive help with ADLs
- the name of a spouse or caregiver may be forgotten
- sleep patterns may change
- incontinence may develop
- the patient may begin to wander or get lost.

Stage 7—very severe cognitive decline (severe or late-stage Alzheimer disease)

In stage 7, the patient:
- loses the ability to respond to their environment
- is unlikely to engage in a coherent conversation yet may still speak words or phrases
- may not be able to control movement
- need help with all ADLs
- may develop abnormal reflexes, demonstrate muscle rigidity, lose the ability to smile, and/or experience impaired swallowing.

Diagnosis

Because it's hard to obtain direct pathologic evidence of Alzheimer disease, diagnosis in a living patient is made by ruling out other possible causes of dementia and is based on the criteria set forth in the *DSM-5* (APA, 2013).

The full workup

Diagnostic tests that aid a health care provider in making a diagnosis include:

- cognitive assessment evaluation, which typically shows cognitive impairment in Alzheimer disease
- functional dementia scale, which may indicate the degree of dementia
- magnetic resonance imaging (MRI) of the brain, which typically shows structural and neurologic changes
- mini-mental status examination, which reveals disorientation and cognitive impairment
- spinal fluid analysis, which may show increased beta amyloid deposits.

Treatment

Although no cure exists for Alzheimer disease, certain drugs may be prescribed in an attempt to stabilize the symptoms and slow the progression of the disease. Likewise, care strategies and activities may minimize or prevent behavioral problems. Researchers continue to look for new treatments to alter the course of the disease and improve quality of life.

It's usually best for the patient to live at home as long as possible.

Native habitat preferred

In most cases, institutional placement should be delayed until absolutely necessary. Changes in living environment can contribute to increased confusion.

Drug therapy

Drugs used to treat Alzheimer disease (Shan, 2013) include:

- anticholinesterase agents, such as tacrine (Cognex), donepezil (Aricept), and rivastigmine (Exelon), to improve cognitive functioning
- antipsychotic agents, such as haloperidol (Haldol) and risperidone (Risperdal), to calm agitated behavior
- benzodiazepines, such as alprazolam (Xanax), to ease anxiety.

Agents under investigation for Alzheimer disease include estrogen, nonsteroidal anti-inflammatory agents, vitamin E, selegiline (Carbex, Eldepryl), and ginkgo biloba.

Psychotherapy

Brief psychotherapy techniques, such as reality orientation and memory retraining, may aid patients during certain stages of Alzheimer disease.

Preventive strategies

Alzheimer disease prevention might target individuals at increased genetic risk. Specific measures may involve prophylactic nutritional agents (such as vitamin E) or cholinergic- or amyloid-targeting interventions. A vaccine is also being studied in mice.

Nursing interventions

Nursing interventions for patients with NCDs are also appropriate for a patient with Alzheimer disease:

Memory jogger

How can you help keep a patient with Alzheimer disease safe? Just think of the word SAFE.

S Secure the area if the patient wanders.

A Arrange the room and furniture to accommodate the patient's needs.

F Frequently orient the patient to time, place, and situation.

E Easy access to self-care items is crucial.

Strive for safety

- Protect the patient from injury. Remove hazardous items or potential obstacles to help maintain a safe environment.
- Monitor the patient's food and fluid intake to decrease the risk for poor nutrition.

Recommend routines

- To the extent possible, have the patient follow a regular exercise routine, maintain normal social contacts with family and friends, and continue intellectual activities.
- Encourage the patient to see a health care provider every 3 to 6 months.

Soften your speech

- Speak to the patient calmly, using a soft, low-pitched voice.
- State expectations simply and completely.
- Minimize confusion by maintaining consistent, structured verbal and nonverbal communication.

Affirm emotions

- If the patient discusses an event that isn't happening or people who are no longer alive, affirm his or her emotions without adding to or refuting the fantasy. For example, if he or she talks about a dead spouse coming to a birthday party, you might say, "Birthdays are fun."

Orient often

- Add orienting material to every conversation. Frequently tell the patient your name and what you're going to do.
- Place a large clock and calendar in every room.
- Provide outdoor activities or a bed by the window.
- Redirect appropriate activities when behavior problems occur.

Stimulate to some extent

- Decrease environmental stimuli, such as noise, excessive artificial light, and television use.
- Provide frequent meaningful sensory input.
- Increase the patient's social interaction in reasonable amounts to encourage stimuli. Avoid placing the patient in large rooms with many people, such as dining rooms or group activity rooms.

Monitor medications

- Check the patient for adverse drug effects and drug interactions.
- Instruct the family to always check with the doctor before the patient begins nonprescription agents, especially if he or she has heart or liver problems or is taking a drug for heart problems, hypertension, diabetes, or another mental condition.

Offer information

- Educate the patient and family information about community resources, support groups, and placement in a long-term care facility (if necessary).
- Refer the patient to health care professionals skilled in caring for patients with Alzheimer disease.

Subdue stress

- Teach stress management techniques to the patient and caregivers.
- Provide support and education to home caregivers. Refer them to respite services as needed.
- If appropriate, refer to resources who specialize in helping the family with caregiver stress, financial pressures, and related issues.

Vascular dementia

Also called *vascular cognitive impairment* (VCI), vascular dementia can occur suddenly after blockage of a major brain blood vessel (Alzheimer's Association, 2014c). Initial symptoms may include confusion, disorientation, trouble speaking or understanding speech, and/or vision loss (Alzheimer's Association, 2014c). Memory loss may, or may not, be present.

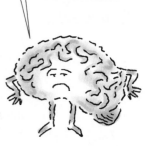

In vascular dementia, blockage of blood vessels leads to brain damage and cognitive impairment.

Think local, not global

Cerebral problems affect localized parts of the brain, sparing other brain function. Brain damage may be so slight that symptoms are barely noticeable. Over time, though, as more small vessels are blocked, the mental decline becomes more apparent.

Causes

Vascular dementia occurs when small focal deficits, typically caused by a series of small strokes, accumulate. The condition tends to progress in stages and causes patchy distribution of cognitive problems.

Besides advanced age, contributing factors include:
- cerebral emboli or thrombosis
- diabetes
- heart disease
- high blood cholesterol level
- hypertension (leading to stroke)
- transient ischemic attacks.

Signs and symptoms

Signs and symptoms of vascular dementia often develop progressively. They include:
- confusion or disorientation
- problems with recent memory
- wandering or getting lost in familiar places
- inappropriate emotional reactions, such as laughing or crying inappropriately
- difficulty following instructions
- problems handling money
- depression
- dizziness
- neurologic symptoms lasting only a few days
- slurred speech
- leg or arm weakness.

Diagnosis

Diagnostic test results may include:
- cognitive assessment scale showing deterioration in cognitive ability
- global deterioration scale indicating degenerative dementia
- mini-mental status examination revealing disorientation and difficulty with recall
- MRI or computed tomography scan showing structural, vascular, and neurologic changes in the brain.

Test time

An abbreviated mental examination can detect memory problems and aid differential diagnosis, treatment, and rehabilitation. To be most useful, the examination should be repeated periodically. (Be aware, though, that depressed patients may do poorly on these tests even if they don't have a memory problem.)

In a typical mental exam, the patient is asked to provide the following information:

- name
- date of birth
- age
- date and time of day
- address
- name of the president
- current location
- counting backward from 100 by 7s
- three objects that were told to him or her 5 minutes earlier (e.g., car, ball, umbrella).

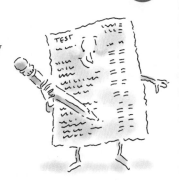

Assessing the patient's ability to count backward can help to diagnose vascular dementia.

Treatment

Treatment for vascular dementia may include:

- treatment for an underlying condition (such as hypertension, high cholesterol, or diabetes), including dietary interventions, medications, and smoking cessation
- carotid endarterectomy to remove blockages in the carotid artery
- drug therapy—for example, aspirin to decrease platelet aggregation and prevent clots.

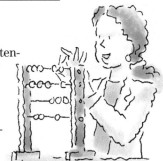

Nursing interventions

The same interventions you would use for a patient with NCD or Alzheimer disease apply to a patient with vascular dementia. The goal of interventions is to keep the patient safe and oriented.

Sweeten the surroundings

- Monitor the environment to prevent overstimulation.
- Reduce unnecessary stimulation and make the environment as stable as possible. Avoid changing rooms and moving furniture or possessions around.
- Minimize factors that may contribute to confusion, such as dehydration, malnutrition, and difficulty sleeping.

Orient at all times

- Orient the patient to surroundings to ease his or her anxiety.
- Provide frequent meaningful sensory input.

- Place a large clock and calendar in every room.
- Include orienting material in every conversation.
- Frequently tell the patient your name and what you're going to do.

Avert injury

- Check the patient often because he or she may be prone to falls, wandering, and self-poisoning.
- Take extra safety measures regarding food and bath water temperature to avoid accidental burns.
- Teach the patient and family members about proper diet, weight control, smoking cessation, limitation of alcohol consumption, and exercise to reduce cardiovascular risk factors.
- Frequently assess the patient's need for medications, appropriateness of the dosage, and adverse effects. Also, monitor for drug interactions.

References

Administration on Aging (2013). *Aging statistics*. Retreived from http://www.aoa.gov/AoARoot/Aging_Statistics/index.aspx

Aine, C. J., Sanfratello, L., Adair, J. C., Knoefel, J. E., Caprihan, A., & Stephen, J. M. (2011). Development and decline of memory functions in normal, pathological and healthy successful aging. *Brain Topography*, *24*(3–4), 323–339. doi:10.1007/s10548-011-0178-x

Akhondzadeh, S., Gerbarg, P. L., & Brown, R. P. (2013). Nutrients for prevention and treatment of mental health disorders. *The Psychiatric Clinics of North America*, *36*(1), 25–36.

Alzheimer's Association. (2014a). *2012 Alzheimer's disease facts and figures*. Retrieved from http://www.alz.org/alzheimers_disease_facts_and_figures.asp

Alzheimer's Association. (2014b). *Seven stages of Alzheimer's*. Retrieved from http://www.alz.org/alzheimers_disease_stages_of_alzheimers.asp

Alzheimer's Association. (2014c). *Vascular dementia*. Retrieved from http://www.alz.org/dementia/vascular-dementia-symptoms.asp

Alzheimer's Association. (2014d). *What is Alzheimer's?* Retrieved from http://www.alz.org/alzheimers_disease_what_is_alzheimers.asp

American Psychiatric Association. (2013). *Diagnostic and statistical manual of mental disorders* (5th ed.). Arlington, VA: Author.

Beauchet, O., Launay, C. P., Fantino, B., Lerolle, N., Maunoury, F., & Annweiler, C. (2012). Screening for elderly patients admitted to the emergency department requiring specialized geriatric care. *Journal of Emergency Medicine*, *45*(5), 739–745. doi:10.1016/j.jemermed.2012.11.110

Beck, C., Buckwalter, K. C., Dudzik, P. M., & Evans, L. K. (2011). Filling the void in geriatric mental health: The Geropsychiatric Nursing Collaborative as a model for change. *Nursing Outlook*, *59*, 236–242.

Besdine, R. (2013). *Changes in the body with aging. Merck Manual.* Retrieved from http://www.merckmanuals.com/home/older_peoples_health_issues/the_aging_body/changes_in_the_body_with_aging.html

Bottiglieri, T. (2013). Folate, vitamin B12 and S-adenosylmethionine. *The Psychiatric Clinics of North America, 36*(1), 1–13.

Geriatric Mental Health Foundation. (2014). *Depression in late life: Not a normal part of aging.* Retrieved from http://www.gmhfonline.org/gmhf/consumer/factsheets/depression_latelife.html

*Hatfield, A. B. (1999). Barriers to serving older adults with a psychiatric disability. *Psychiatric Rehabilitation Journal, 22*, 270–276.

Lu, P. H., Lee, G. J., Raven, E. P., Tingus, K., Khoo, T., Thompson, P. M., & Bartzokis, G. (2011). Age-related slowing in cognitive processing speed is associated with myelin integrity in a very healthy elderly sample. *Journal of Clinical and Experimental Neuropsychology, 33*(10), 1059–1068.

National Alliance on Mental Illness. (2014). Retrieved from www.nami.org

National Institute on Aging. (2014). *The changing brain in healthy aging.* Retrieved from http://www.nia.nih.gov/alzheimers/publication/part-1-basics-healthy-brain/changing-brain-healthy-aging

Persson, J., Pudas, S., Lind, J., Kauppi, K., Nilsson, L., & Nyberg, L. (2011). Longitudinal structure-function correlated in elderly reveal MTL dysfunction with cognitive decline. *Cerebral Cortex, 22*, 2297–2304.

Sarris, J. (2013). St. John's wort for the treatment of psychiatric disorders. *The Psychiatric Clinics of North America, 36*(1), 65–72.

Shan, Y. (2013). Treatment of alzhemier's disease. *Primary Health Care, 23*(6), 32–38.

Townsend, M. C. (2014). The bereaved individual. In M. C. Townsend (Ed.), *Essentials of psychiatric mental health nursing: Concepts of care in evidenced-based practice* (pp. 786–808). Philadelphia, PA: F. A. Davis.

Yue, L. (2010). Provision of mental health services in U.S. nursing homes, 1995–2004. *Psychiatric Services, 61*(4), 349–355.

*Asterisk indicates a classic or definitive work on this subject.

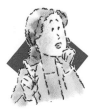

Quick quiz

1.   A patient with gradually occurring global impairments of cognitive functioning, memory, and personality is most likely to have:
   A.   delirium.
   B.   Alzheimer-type dementia.
   C.   vascular dementia.
   D.   dyskinesia.

Answer: B. A patient with Alzheimer-type dementia suffers global impairment of cognitive functioning, memory, and personality. The dementia occurs gradually but with a continuous decline.

2. Age-related declines in intelligence, learning ability, short-term memory, and reaction time may grow more significant after age:
    A.   60.
    B.   65.
    C.   70.
    D.   75.

Answer: C. After age 70, declines in intelligence, learning ability, short-term memory, and reaction time may become more significant.

3. An appropriate way to teach an elderly patient is to use:
    A.   audiotapes.
    B.   pictures and simple wording.
    C.   television programs.
    D.   musical recordings.

Answer: B. Because picture recognition doesn't seem to be affected by aging, using pictures can help older adults with memory.

4. OBRA requires that nursing home residents who have been diagnosed with a primary psychiatric disorder receive treatment for that disorder by a:
    A.   neurologist.
    B.   physical therapist.
    C.   mental health professional.
    D.   social worker.

Answer: C. Nursing home residents with primary psychiatric disorders must receive treatment from a mental health professional (who might be a neurologist, geropsychiatric CNS, psychiatrist, or other qualified person).

5. A drug used to treat Alzheimer disease is:
    A.   aripiprazole (Abilify).
    B.   valproic acid (Depakote).
    C.   donepezil (Aricept).
    D.   sertraline (Zoloft).

Answer: C. Donepezil (Aricept) is a cholinesterase inhibitor used to treat Alzheimer disease.

Scoring

☆☆☆ If you answered all five items correctly, marvy! Your mastery of older adults' mental conditions is magnificent!

☆☆ If you answered three or four items correctly, mazel tov! Your knowledge of mental disorders is maturing quite nicely.

☆ If you answered fewer than three items correctly, don't be melancholic! Just read the chapter again—your working memory is bound to improve.

4

Schizophrenia

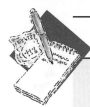

Just the facts

In this chapter, you'll learn:

♦ symptoms of schizophrenia

♦ theories on the cause of schizophrenia

♦ assessment, diagnosis, and treatment of patients with schizophrenia

♦ nursing interventions for patients with schizophrenia.

A look at schizophrenia

Schizophrenia refers to a group of severe, chronic, and disabling psychiatric disorders marked by withdrawal from reality, illogical thinking, possible delusions and hallucinations, and other emotional, behavioral, or intellectual disturbances. These disturbances may affect everything from speech, affect, and perception to psychomotor behavior, interpersonal relationships, and sense of self.

Patients with schizophrenia may have trouble distinguishing reality from fantasy. Their speech and behavior may frighten or mystify those around them.

Statistically speaking . . .

In any given year, approximately 2.5 million Americans experience schizophrenia. Approximately 1% of Americans—1 in every 100 persons—develops schizophrenia during their lifetime (National Institute of Mental Health, 2009).

Schizophrenia is a debilitating and chronic disease and is one of the most economically and emotionally costly of all mental disorders, not only on the individuals and their families but also on society.

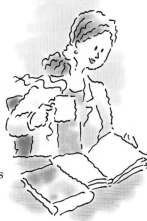

It says here that patients with schizophrenia have trouble distinguishing reality from fantasy.

Functional fade-out

The patient's overall disability depends mainly on the severity of cognitive impairment. Symptoms may impair the individual's ability to hold a job, stay in school, maintain relationships, and even perform self-care. Unfortunately, it is not uncommon for the patient with schizophrenia to be found unemployable, socially isolated, and estranged from family and friends.

Life interrupted

Many people with schizophrenia neglect personal hygiene and ignore their health needs. As a result, their life expectancy is about 10 years shorter than that of the general population. Approximately 20% to 40% of people with schizophrenia attempt suicide more than once, with 5% to 13% of people with schizophrenia dying by suicide (WebMD, 2013). Risk of suicide is high among young male people with schizophrenia who have comorbid substance use. Risk of suicidal behavior is also high among those who have been newly diagnosed after a psychotic break, which is associated with feelings of hopelessness and depression.

Symptom start-up

Although sudden onset of full-blown schizophrenia symptoms may occur, the majority of people with schizophrenia develop signs and symptoms in a more gradual and insidious fashion. Many individuals begin by experiencing prodromal symptoms such as development of depressive symptoms, gradual isolation from friends and family, cognitive alteration, and personality changes in late adolescent years. The first psychotic episode for males usually occurs by their early to mid-twenties, whereas females tend to have a later peak age by their mid- or late 20s.

Prognosis

The prognosis for patients with schizophrenia worsens with the occurrence of each acute episode. Few of these patients experience just a single psychotic episode. Some individuals suffer through periods of exacerbations and remissions. Between periods of exacerbation, some patients may have no disability, whereas others need continuous institutional care. Unfortunately, a number of patients with schizophrenia continue to suffer from a progressive course of increasingly debilitating and deteriorating symptoms.

Progress and promise

Although schizophrenia was previously thought as a disorder from which a patient never recovered, more recent studies demonstrate that management, and potential recovery, is more possible than previously thought (Glynn, 2014). Research has brought forth safer and promising treatments. New discoveries into possible causes and cutting-edge brain-imaging techniques hold the promise of further insights and therapeutic advances. (See *Prognosis and probability.*)

Psychosocial and economic issues

Schizophrenia is a devastating illness—and the afflicted person isn't the only one who suffers. Family, friends, clinical caregivers, and the entire community feel the effects. (See *The truth about schizophrenia and violence,* page 130.)

Denial

People with schizophrenia do not often seek initial treatment on their own. Because of impaired thought processes and perceptual problems, they may deny that they need help and resist seeking health care.

Economic and social consequences

Schizophrenia is more prevalent among lower socioeconomic groups in urban areas—perhaps because its disabling effects often lead to unemployment and poverty.

It is also more common among single persons. This may reflect the effects of the illness or its precursors on the person's social functioning.

Prognosis and probability

Overall, about one-third of patients with schizophrenia achieve significant and lasting improvement. Another third improve somewhat but have intermittent relapses and residual disability. The remaining third are severely and permanently incapacitated.

However, during any given 1-year period, the prognosis depends largely on the patient's compliance with the prescribed drug regimen.

Good omens

Besides treatment compliance, other factors that contribute to a good prognosis include:
• late or sudden disease onset
• female sex

• relatively good pre-illness functioning
• minimal cognitive impairment
• paranoid schizophrenia subtype or many positive symptoms
• family history of mood disorders rather than schizophrenia.

Unfavorable outlook

Factors linked to a poor prognosis include:
• early age at onset
• poor pre-illness functioning
• family history of schizophrenia
• disorganized schizophrenia subtype with many negative symptoms.

Myth busters

The truth about schizophrenia and violence

Are people with schizophrenia harmless victims of mental illness or unpredictable perpetrators of violence?

Myth: People with schizophrenia are more violent than other people.

Reality: People with schizophrenia pose a relatively modest risk for violent behavior. Although some threaten violence and have minor aggressive outbursts, few commit violent acts. In fact, people with schizophrenia are 14 times more likely to become victims of violence than being arrested as perpetrators of violence (Wehring & Carpenter, 2011). They are far less likely to behave violently than substance abusers.

Nonetheless, a patient with schizophrenia who obeys hallucinatory voices telling him or her to attack someone poses a real danger. In rare cases, a depressed, isolated, paranoid patient with schizophrenia attacks or kills someone he or she views as the cause of his or her problems.

Impact on the family

Schizophrenia profoundly affects the patient's family. Although the patient needs the understanding and support of family members, his or her behavior may frighten and frustrate loved ones.

Family ferment

Family members may be uninformed about schizophrenia and its management. Few families are adequately prepared to deal with the stressors caused by chronic schizophrenia, which include personality decompensation, hospitalizations, and medication noncompliance.

> Unfortunately, many people with schizophrenia also abuse substances—which certainly doesn't aid recovery.

Substance abuse

People with schizophrenia are more likely than the general population to abuse alcohol and substances (National Institute of Mental Health, 2009). People with schizophrenia who abuse drugs (other than tobacco) are associated with poorer outcomes and functioning. Substance abuse may contribute to noncompliance with prescribed medication, increased psychotic symptoms, repeated illness relapses, frequent hospitalizations, declining function, and loss of social support.

Possible causes of schizophrenia

Schizophrenia is a complex illness whose precise cause is unknown. It is thought that genetics, environment, and brain chemistry and structure may contribute to this condition (National Institute of Mental Health, 2009).

Genetic factors

Experts have long known that schizophrenia runs in families. Persons who have a first-degree relative with the disease stand a 10% chance of developing it themselves— compared to a 1% chance among the general population (National Institute of Mental Health, 2009).

> If one of us develops schizophrenia, the other one stands a 50% chance of getting it.

Double jeopardy

Those at highest risk are the identical twins of people with schizophrenia and the children of two parents with schizophrenia—roughly 50% will develop this condition.

However, nearly two-thirds of diagnosed people with schizophrenia have no family history of the disease.

Predictable—not!

Most likely, multiple genes are involved in creating a predisposition to schizophrenia. Other factors (such as prenatal infections, perinatal complications, and certain stressors) seem to influence disease development.

Researchers don't understand how the genetic predisposition is transmitted and can't predict whether a given person will develop the disease. (See *Vulnerability-stress theory*.)

Vulnerability-stress theory

Some experts believe schizophrenia occurs when a biologically susceptible person experiences an environmental stressor. According to the vulnerability-stress theory, a stressful event (such as the death of a loved one, job loss, or divorce) can trigger symptom onset in a vulnerable person.

Fetal forebodings

What causes this vulnerability in the first place? Some researchers blame such factors as:
- genetic predisposition
- viral infections of the central nervous system
- illness or complications during pregnancy, delivery, or the neonatal period.

Scientists have found a connection between pregnant mothers' exposure to influenza and their children that eventually develop schizophrenia. A study by Parboosing et al. identified that there was a fourfold increased risk for schizophrenia that could be linked back to a maternal influenza infection at any time during pregnancy (National Institute of Mental Health, 2013).

Genome jumble

Scientists are investigating several regions of the human genome to identify the genes involved in schizophrenia. A 2014 study revealed that schizophrenia is not just one disease but eight disorders with genetically distinct causes (Arnedo et al., 2014).

Continued genetic research will yield significant information about schizophrenia. This knowledge will guide the development of better treatments.

Biochemical theories

Scientists strongly suspect that people with schizophrenia have abnormalities in the chemical brain messengers called *neurotransmitters*—particularly dopamine, serotonin, and glutamate.

Dopamine theory

Studies exploring the role of neurotransmitters in schizophrenia have focused on the dopamine neurotransmitter. According to the dopamine hypothesis of schizophrenia, the disease results when the dopamine system in the brain is disturbed. Hyperactivity of dopaminergic activity in the limbic regions of the brain results in positive symptoms such as hallucinations, agitation, delusional thinking, and grandiosity. Hypoactivity of dopaminergic activity in the frontal region results in negative symptoms such as flattened affect, anhedonia, and defects in executive functions (Tusaie & Fitzpatrick, 2013). Despite strong evidence supporting the dopamine theory, not all the data support it. Some people with schizophrenia don't show high levels of this neurotransmitter. This suggests that other factors are involved in their disease process.

Serotonin theory

Serotonin has been identified to play a role in the causation of schizophrenic symptoms, and its significance is reflected in the development of a newer generation of drugs for schizophrenia that targets both dopamine and serotonin receptors in the brain (Tusaie & Fitzpatrick, 2013).

Glutamate theory

Some cognitive symptoms of schizophrenia may be associated with abnormalities of glutamate—a neurotransmitter involved in dopamine breakdown as well as learning and memory impairment. The glutamate theory posits that excessive glutamate activity leads to a neurotoxic effect that results in schizophrenic symptoms (Tusaie & Fitzpatrick, 2013).

Other brain chemicals

Schizophrenia may involve abnormalities of endorphins (peptide hormones that bind to opiate receptors in the brain) or other neurotransmitters, such as norepinephrine, acetylcholine, and gamma-aminobutyric acid.

Structural brain abnormalities

Postmortem examinations of brains of people with schizophrenia have found small changes in the distribution or number of brain cells. Scientists have studied the brains of people living with schizophrenia using neuroimaging techniques and have discovered:
• lateral and third ventricle enlargement
• cortical gray matter deficits
• reductions in the sizes of certain brain regions
• abnormalities in specific brain functions, including decreased metabolic activity in some brain regions.

However, these abnormalities weren't found in all people with schizophrenia—and *were* found in some people without the disease.

Developmental factors

Developmental neurobiologists suspect that schizophrenia results from faulty connections formed by neurons during fetal development. These errors may lie dormant until puberty, when the brain changes that occur normally at this time may interact adversely with the faulty connections. Researchers are trying to identify any and all prenatal factors that may influence the apparent abnormality.

Vulnerability markers

Proposed vulnerability markers for schizophrenia include psychophysiologic deficits in eye tracking, information processing, attention, and sensory inhibition. (See *Psychophysiologic markers of schizophrenia*, page 134.)

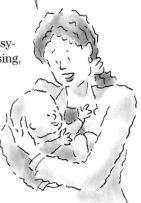

An infant whose mother had the flu during the second trimester of pregnancy has an increased risk for developing schizophrenia.

Other possible causes

Many additional physical conditions have been linked to schizophrenia, including:
• viral infection
• birth trauma

Psychophysiologic markers of schizophrenia

Schizophrenia is known to affect eye movements.

Not so smooth pursuit

When tracking a moving object, such as a baseball in flight, the human eye uses a movement called *smooth pursuit*. The neuromuscular system produces pursuit movement by adjusting the moving eyeball's velocity to that of the object being viewed. This allows a stable image to be reflected onto the retina.

In people with schizophrenia, smooth pursuit eye movements are interrupted inappropriately by rapid eye movements, such as those used to read or look around. Although this genetically driven abnormality doesn't directly relate to the cause or effects of schizophrenia, it may serve as a genetic marker and a predictor of possible disease development.

Other abnormalities

Studies also show that people with schizophrenia are more likely to have abnormal results on cognition and attention tests as well as deficient sensory gating (blocking of an incoming sensory message when other stimuli are occupying the person's attention). These markers, also found in first-degree relatives of people with schizophrenia, may signal vulnerability before the overt onset of illness.

- head injury
- epilepsy (especially of the temporal lobe)
- Huntington chorea
- cerebral tumor
- stroke
- systemic lupus erythematosus
- myxedema
- parkinsonism
- Wilson disease (a rare inherited disorder of poor copper metabolism)
- alcohol abuse.

Assessment

Although behaviors and functional deficiencies may vary widely among patients—and even in the same patient at different times—some characteristic signs and symptoms usually are detectable during the assessment.

To assess a patient for schizophrenia, a comprehensive history is gathered and a physical examination is conducted. It is often necessary to obtain information from family, friends, teachers, and others who know the patient well, as many people with schizophrenia may suffer from cognitive alterations that prevent insight on their illness, perceptions, emotions, and behavior. Keep in mind that assessment findings will depend partly on the disease subtype, prevailing symptom type, and illness phase. (See *Recognizing schizophrenia.*)

Advice from the experts

Recognizing schizophrenia

During the assessment interview, you may note characteristic signs and symptoms in a patient with schizophrenia.

Speech abnormalities
The patient's speech may include:
• clang associations—words that rhyme or sound alike, used in an illogical, nonsensical manner (e.g., "It's the rain, train, pain")
• echolalia—meaningless repetition of words or phrases
• flight of ideas—rapid succession of incomplete ideas that aren't connected by logic or rationality
• word salad—illogical or random word groupings (e.g., "She had a star, barn, plant")
• neologisms—bizarre words that have meaning only for the patient.

Thought distortions
Stay alert for evidence of:
• overly concrete thinking—inability to form or understand abstract thoughts
• delusions—false ideas or beliefs accepted as real by the patient

• hallucinations—false sensory perceptions with no basis in reality
• thought blocking—sudden interruption in the train of thought
• magical thinking—a belief that thoughts or wishes can control other people or events.

Social interactions
Note whether the patient exhibits:
• poor interpersonal relationships
• withdrawal and apathy—disinterest in objects, people, or surroundings.

Other findings
In some people with schizophrenia, you also may assess:
• regression—return to an earlier developmental stage
• ambivalence—coexisting strong positive and negative feelings, leading to emotional conflict
• echopraxia—involuntary repetition of movements observed in others.

Symptom categories

Many clinicians refer to positive, negative, and disorganized symptoms of schizophrenia. In most patients, one of these symptom clusters predominates. (See *Tall tales about schizophrenia*, page 136.)

Positive symptoms

Positive symptoms are symptoms that are not present in most individuals but are found in patients with schizophrenia. They include primarily delusions, hallucinations, and disordered speech and thoughts.

Keep in mind that in this context, "positive" does not mean "good." Quite the contrary—positive symptoms are psychotic and show that there is a disconnection between actual reality and the patient's perception of reality.

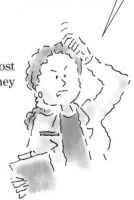

How odd . . . they're called positive symptoms but that doesn't mean they are "good."

Myth busters

Tall tales about schizophrenia

The behavior of people with schizophrenia can be frightening and puzzling to individuals who are not familiar with this condition. This can lead to misconceptions about the disease. Two of these misconceptions are addressed below.

Myth: The agitated psychomotor behavior of some patients with schizophrenia reflects excessive energy, which causes them to engage in violent acts.

Reality: People with schizophrenia frequently show a lack of energy and have difficulty performing activities of daily living and interacting with other people.

Myth: A person with schizophrenia may experience either hallucinations or delusions but not both.

Reality: Individuals who experience positive symptoms of schizophrenia may experience both hallucinations and delusions—especially delusions of paranoia or persecution.

Hallucinations

The most common feature of schizophrenia is hallucinations, which involve hearing, seeing, smelling, tasting, or touching things that aren't actually there. For instance, the patient may "hear" voices commenting on his or her behavior, conversing with one another, or making critical and abusive comments.

Delusions

Delusions are erroneous beliefs that usually grow out of misinterpretations of experience. They may cause the patient to think that someone is reading his or her thoughts, involved in a conspiracy against him or her, or monitoring him or her—or that he or she can control the minds of other people.

Delusional distinctions

Delusions fall into several categories. A patient with a *persecutory* delusion thinks he or she is being tormented, followed, tricked, or spied on.

A patient with a *reference* delusion may think that passages in books, newspapers, television shows, song lyrics, or other environmental cues are directed at him or her.

In delusions of *thought withdrawal* or *thought insertion*, the patient believes others can read his or her mind, that his or her thoughts are being transmitted to others, or that outside forces are imposing thoughts or impulses on him or her.

Negative symptoms

Negative (deficit) symptoms reflect the absence of normal characteristics. They include apathy, lack of motivation, blunted affect, poverty of speech, anhedonia, and asociality.
- *Apathy* refers to a lack of interest in people, things, and activities.
- *Lack of motivation* impairs the ability of the person to start and follow through with activities.
- *Blunted affect* refers to flattening of the emotions. The person's face may appear immobile and inexpressive. As schizophrenia progresses, blunted affect may grow more pronounced. (Keep in mind that inability to *show* emotions does not mean inability to *feel* emotions.)
- *Poverty of speech* refers to speech that is brief and lacks content. The person may give terse replies to questions, creating the impression of inner emptiness.
- *Anhedonia* is diminished capacity to experience pleasure.
- *Asociality* refers to avoidance of relationships. A person with schizophrenia may withdraw socially because of depression. He or she may feel relatively safe when alone, or may be completely caught up in personal feelings and fears, or it may be difficult to manage the company of others.

Disorganized symptoms

Disorganized symptoms include thought disorder, speech abnormalities, and bizarre behavior.
- *Thought disorder* refers to confused thinking and speech, ranging from mildly disorganized speech to incoherent ramblings. The person may make loose associations, jumping from one idea to another, and wander further and further from the original topic. He or she may have trouble carrying on conversations with others.
- Speech abnormalities may include incoherent speech and frequent derailment from the topic at hand.
- *Bizarre behavior* may include childlike silliness; agitation; and inappropriate appearance, hygiene, or conduct. The patient may move slowly, repeat rhythmic gestures, or walk in circles. It may be difficult or impossible to make sense of everyday sights, sounds, and feelings.

Disease phases

Schizophrenia usually progresses in three distinct phases—prodromal, active, and residual.

Prodromal phase

During the *prodromal phase*, which may arise a year or so before the first hospitalization, the person shows a clear decline from his or her previous level of functioning.

A low profile

The person may withdraw from friends, hobbies, and other interests and may exhibit peculiar behavior, neglect personal hygiene and grooming, and lack energy and initiative. Work or school performance may deteriorate.

Active phase

During the *active phase* (commonly triggered by a stressful event), the person has acute psychotic symptoms, such as hallucinations, delusions, incoherence, or catatonic behavior. (See *What is catatonia, as in* DSM-5?) Functional deficits worsen.

Symptomatic periods may occur episodically (with identifiable exacerbations and remissions) or continuously (with no identifiable remissions).

Number of acute episodes

Up to one-third of people with schizophrenia have just one acute episode and no more. Others have repeated, acute exacerbations of the active phase. With each acute episode, the prognosis worsens.

Residual phase

During the *residual phase*, which follows the active phase, symptoms resemble those of the prodromal phase. However, blunted affect and impaired role functioning may be more pronounced. Some psychotic symptoms, such as hallucinations, may persist but without strong affect.

What is catatonia, as in *DSM-5*?

Catatonia refers to abnormal and bizarre psychomotor disturbance that may involve decreased motor activity such as immobility or increased motor activity such as agitation or echopraxia.

The clinical picture of catatonia as in *DSM-5* is defined by the presence of three or more of the following symptoms:

1. Stupor (i.e., no psychomotor activity; not actively relating to environment)
2. Catalepsy (i.e., passive induction of a posture held against gravity)
3. Wavy flexibility (i.e., slight, even resistance to positioning by examiner)
4. Mutism (i.e., no, or very little, verbal response; exclude if known aphasia)
5. Negativism (i.e., opposition or no response to instructions or external stimuli)
6. Posturing (i.e., spontaneous and active maintenance of a posture against gravity)
7. Mannerism (i.e., odd, circumstantial caricature of normal actions)
8. Stereotypy (i.e., repetitive, abnormally frequent, non-goal-directed movements)
9. Agitation, not influenced by external stimuli
10. Grimacing
11. Echolalia (i.e., mimicking another's speech)
12. Echopraxia (i.e., mimicking another's movements)

During the residual phase, the illness pattern may become established, disability levels may stabilize, or late improvements may appear.

Remissions

Although few people with schizophrenia return to their full pre-illness functioning level, some full remissions have occurred.

Disease course

The course of schizophrenia varies among patients and depends largely on compliance with prescribed antipsychotic drug regimen.

Mild course

The person with a mild disease course is usually stable. This person always complies with drug treatment, has just one or two major relapses by age 45, and experiences only a few mild symptoms.

Moderate course

Typically, the person with a moderate disease course takes drugs as prescribed most of the time but isn't fully compliant. The person has several major relapses by age 45 and has experienced increased symptoms during stressful periods. Between relapses, symptoms persist.

Severe, unstable course

The person with a severe disease course doesn't com-ply with the prescribed drug regimen—or discontinues it entirely. He or she has frequent relapses and is stable only for brief periods between relapses. The person experi-ences bothersome symptoms and needs help with activities of daily living. There is also the likeli-hood of coexisting other problems (such as substance abuse) that make recovery more difficult.

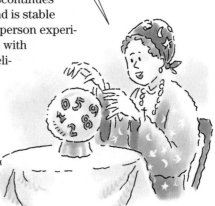

Symptoms over time

During the first 5 years of the illness, the person's level of functioning may deteriorate. Social and work skills may decline, cognitive deficits grow more pronounced, and self-care neglect may worsen progressively. Also, negative symptoms may grow more severe.

In the most common disease course, acute episodes are followed by residual impairment. During the first few years of schizophrenia, impairment between episodes commonly increases.

Respite and relief

After the first 5 years, the disability level tends to plateau. Some evidence suggests that illness severity may lessen later in life, particularly among women.

Diagnosis

A mental status examination, psychiatric history, and careful clinical observation form the basis for diagnosing schizophrenia.

For a thorough evaluation, the patient should undergo physical and psychiatric examinations to rule out other possible causes of symptoms—including physical disorders, substance-induced psychosis, and primary mood disorders with psychotic features.

The stamp of authority

Official diagnosis, determined by a provider of care, is based on the criteria in the *Diagnostic and Statistical Manual of Mental Disorders*, 5th Edition (*DSM-5*).

Diagnostic test results

There are no diagnostic tests that definitively confirm schizophrenia. To support a diagnosis, the provider of care may order a dexamethasone suppression test, which fails to show suppression in some people with schizophrenia. (However, some clinicians question the test's accuracy.) Because other disorders such as vitamin deficiencies, uremia, thyrotoxicosis, and electrolyte imbalances can cause symptoms that mimic schizophrenia, other tests may be done to rule out these types of conditions.

Computed tomography (CT) scans and a ventricular-brain ratio (VBR) analysis may show structural brain abnormalities that suggest schizophrenia.

Views of the ventricles

In approximately half of the people diagnosed with schizophrenia, CT scans show structural brain abnormalities, such as:
- lateral ventricular enlargement (common in males but not females)
- enlargement of the sulci or fissures on the cerebral surface
- atrophy of the cerebellum.

Magnetic resonance imaging has found certain abnormalities in the brain's amygdala, limbic system, frontal cortex, temporal lobes, hippocampus, basal ganglia, and thalamus. It may also show decreased blood flow to the thalamus, which may cause a flood of sensory information.

General treatment

Antipsychotic drugs (sometimes called *neuroleptics*) are the mainstay of treatment. Continuous prophylactic antipsychotic drug therapy can reduce the 1-year relapse rate to about 30%. Without prophylactic drugs, 70% to 80% of patients who have had one schizophrenia episode experience a subsequent one within the next 12 months.

Value of early treatment

People with schizophrenia who develop psychotic symptoms may wait months to years before they present for medical care. The interval between symptom onset and the first treatment correlates with the speed and quality of the initial treatment response and severity of negative symptoms. Patients treated soon after being diagnosed are more likely to respond more quickly and fully than those who do not begin drug therapy until later in the disease course.

> The sooner a patient with schizophrenia begins treatment, the faster and more fully he or she is likely to respond.

Mixed modalities

Although psychopharmacology remains the foundation of treatment of schizophrenia, a more holistic and comprehensive treatment plan requires the integration of other treatment modalities such as:
- psychosocial treatment and rehabilitation
- compliance promotion programs
- vocational counseling
- psychotherapy
- appropriate use of community resources.

Certain people with schizophrenia also may be candidates for electroconvulsive therapy (ECT).

Treatment goals

Treatment goals for the patient with schizophrenia include:
- reducing the severity of psychotic symptoms
- preventing recurrences of acute episodes and associated functional decline

Myth buster

Myths about dependence

People may think that individuals with schizophrenia are unable to manage everyday life.
Myth: People with schizophrenia are incapable of making life decisions and need the help of a legal guardian.
Reality: Although some people with schizophrenia need guidance through certain periods, only a small minority must depend on others to fully make decisions and care for them. Most handle their own affairs successfully.

Memory jogger

The word PRESSURE can help you remember the treatment goals for a patient with schizophrenia.

P Psychiatric medications administered properly and monitored

R Realistic perceptions and self-expectations developed

E Environmental situations managed effectively

S Safety needs addressed

S Self-care performed adequately

U Use of community resources on an ongoing basis

R Relationships developed and sustained

E Establishment and maintenance of family involvement in care

• meeting the patient's physical, psychosocial, developmental, cultural, and spiritual needs
• helping the patient function at the highest level possible. (See *Myths about dependence.*)

Drug therapy

Antipsychotic drugs control symptoms adequately in most people with schizophrenia. The wide choice of drug treatment options available today has improved patients' chances for remission and recovery.

Just say no to dopamine

Antipsychotic drugs appear to work at least in part by blocking postsynaptic dopamine receptors. These drugs have multiple benefits, including:
• reducing positive symptoms, such as hallucinations and delusions
• easing thought disorders
• relieving anxiety and agitation
• maximizing the patient's level of functioning.

Antipsychotic drug categories

Two categories of antipsychotics are available—conventional antipsychotics and newer atypical antipsychotics.

Conventional antipsychotics

In the past, conventional antipsychotics were traditionally used to treat patients with schizophrenia. Because of their potential for adverse effects and the advent of newer atypical antipsychotics, they are no longer the first-line treatment of choice.

(See *Adverse effects of antipsychotic drugs.*) However, patients who do well on them without experiencing troublesome effects are usually advised to continue taking them.

Conventional antipsychotics include:

- fluphenazine (Prolixin)
- haloperidol (Haldol)
- perphenazine (Trilafon)
- thioridazine (Mellaril)
- thiothixene (Navane)
- trifluoperazine (Stelazine).

Adverse effects of antipsychotic drugs

Patients with schizophrenia must take antipsychotic drugs for a long time—usually for life. Unfortunately, some of these drugs may cause unpleasant side effects.

Sedative, anticholinergic, and extrapyramidal effects

High-potency conventional antipsychotics (such as haloperidol) can cause some sedation and anticholinergic effects, such as rapid pulse, dry mouth, inability to urinate, and constipation.

These drugs carry a high incidence of extrapyramidal (motor) effects. The most common motor effects are dystonia, parkinsonism, and akathisia.

- *Dystonia* refers to prolonged, repetitive muscle contractions that may cause twisting or jerking movements—especially of the neck, mouth, and tongue. It's most common in young males, usually appearing within the first few days of drug treatment.
- Drug-induced *parkinsonism* results in bradykinesia (abnormally slow movements), muscle rigidity, shuffling gait, stooped posture, flat facial affect, tremors, and drooling. It may emerge 1 week to several months after drug treatment begins.
- *Akathisia* causes restlessness, pacing, and an inability to rest or sit still.

Intermediate-potency conventional antipsychotics have a moderate incidence of extrapyramidal effects. Low-potency agents (such as chlorpromazine) are highly sedative and anticholinergic but cause few extrapyramidal effects.

Orthostatic hypotension

Low-potency antipsychotics may cause orthostatic hypotension (low blood pressure when standing).

Tardive dyskinesia

With prolonged use, antipsychotics may cause tardive dyskinesia—a disorder characterized by repetitive, involuntary, purposeless movements. Signs and symptoms include grimacing, rapid eye blinking, tongue protrusion and smacking, lip puckering or pursing, and rapid movements of the hands, arms, legs, and trunk.

Symptoms may persist long after the patient stops taking the antipsychotic drug. With careful management, though, some symptoms may eventually lessen or even disappear.

Neuroleptic malignant syndrome

Although infrequent, antipsychotic drugs can cause neuroleptic malignant syndrome. This life-threatening condition leads to fever, extremely rigid muscles, and altered consciousness. It may occur hours to months after drug therapy starts or the dosage is increased.

Atypical antipsychotics

The introduction of newer atypical antipsychotics has given new hope to many people with schizophrenia. These drugs are referred to as *atypical* because they work differently than conventional antipsychotics, and they are much less likely to cause tardive dyskinesia.

Clozapine

Introduced in 1990, clozapine was the first atypical antipsychotic. It has proven to be effective in many patients who do not respond to conventional antipsychotics. The drug controls a wider range of signs and symptoms (including negative symptoms) than conventional agents and causes few or no adverse motor effects.

Agranulocytosis and other adversities

Clozapine carries the risk of serious side effects such as agranulocytosis—a potentially fatal blood disorder marked by a low white blood cell count and pronounced neutrophil depletion. Patients receiving it should undergo routine blood monitoring to detect the disorder. When caught early, agranulocytosis can be reversible.

Cardiomyopathy and myocarditis are two other rare but potentially serious conditions that may result from using clozapine. Other adverse effects include drowsiness, sedation, hypotension, weight gain, excessive salivation, hyperglycemia, tachycardia, dizziness, and seizures.

Other atypical antipsychotics

The main atypical antipsychotics being used in the market include:

- olanzapine (Zyprexa)
- quetiapine (Seroquel)
- risperidone (Risperdal)
- ziprasidone (Geodon)
- aripiprazole (Abilify)
- lurasidone (Latuda)
- paliperidone (Invega)
- iloperidone (Fanapt)
- asenapine (Saphris)

Patients should take these drugs for a trial of at least 3 weeks and up to 9 weeks to assess their efficacy, with the exception of Clozaril that can take up to 3 months (Tusaie & Fitzpatrick, 2013). For acute treatment, rapid symptom resolution is the goal. For maintenance, patients should receive the lowest dose that is sufficient to prevent relapse.

Atypicals' advantages

Newer atypical antipsychotics offer many benefits. They:
• have a selective affinity for brain regions involved in schizophrenia symptoms
• relieve positive symptoms
• may improve negative symptoms more effectively than conventional antipsychotics
• enhance the brain's serotonin levels while stabilizing dopamine levels
• may improve neurocognitive deficits
• are more effective in treating refractory schizophrenia (in particular, clozapine)
• are less likely to cause motor adverse effects
• produce little or no prolactin elevation (a possible adverse effect of conventional antipsychotics).

Better symptom coverage, fewer adverse effects, higher serotonin levels—atypical antipsychotics offer many benefits.

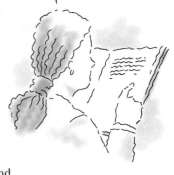

But . . .

The use of atypical antipsychotics has been associated with the development of metabolic syndrome, which includes dyslipidemia, obesity, hypertension, and non-insulin-dependent diabetes. Monitor metabolic parameters prior to and during treatment with antipsychotics to reduce the risk of other health issues.

Drug depots

Commonly referred to as *depot formulations*, a number of long-acting injectable antipsychotics are available. These are administered intramuscularly, and the drug then gradually releases over time. Depot antipsychotics may require administration on a biweekly or monthly basis. At time of writing, depot formulation is available for fluphenazine (Prolixin) and haloperidol (Haldol), risperidone (Risperdal Consta) and paliperidone (Invega Sustenna), and olanzapine (Zyprexa Relprevv) and aripiprazole (Abilify Maintena).

Depot formulation of antipsychotics can improve medication adherence, reduce relapse, and prevent hospitalization.

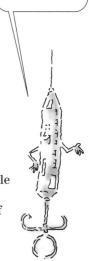

The key benefit of using drug depots is better medication adherence. People with schizophrenia who have difficulty remembering to take medication daily, or those who lack the insight to take their medication regularly, can benefit from receiving medication in this manner. Other benefits of depot formulations include maintenance of stable drug levels in the body, prevention or delay of relapse and subsequent acute hospitalizations, and better monitoring of patient compliance.

Other drugs

Antidepressants and anxiolytics may be used to control associated signs and symptoms in some patients. Mood-stabilizing agents, such as lithium, carbamazepine (Tegretol), and valproic acid (Depakote), may be given to manage negative symptoms.

Psychosocial treatment and rehabilitation

Besides antipsychotic drugs, most patients need support to manage their illness and the isolation, stigma, and fear that often accompany it. Psychosocial treatment, rehabilitation services, and special living arrangements to aid in the various stages of recovery can be helpful. (See *Home is where the help is.*)

Psychosocial treatment

Key components of psychosocial treatment for patients with schizophrenia include:
• patient and family teaching about the disease and its treatment
• collaborative decision making
• monitoring of drug therapy and symptoms
• social services assistance with obtaining prescribed drugs and resources
• supervision of financial resources, as needed
• training and assistance with activities of daily living
• peer support and self-help groups
• psychotherapy.

Psychotherapy

Used as a singular method of treatment, individual or group psychotherapy has little value in managing schizophrenia. However, adjunctive psychotherapy provides emotional support, reinforces health-promoting behaviors, aids adjustment to the illness, and helps patients make the most of their abilities. Typically, psychotherapy is used during the maintenance phase or during the stabilization phase that follows an acute episode.

Go it alone or hang with a gang?

The focus of individual therapy is reality-based and supportive. Group therapy helps patients to encourage socialization, develop coping skills, and resolve interpersonal conflicts.

Family psychotherapy and teaching

Because schizophrenia may be disruptive to the family, all family members may benefit from psychotherapy. This type of therapy can reduce guilt and disappointment, foster acceptance of the patient and behavior, and teach the family stress-management

Home is where the help is

A stable place to live is an important component of treating schizophrenia. Depending on the patient's geographic location, different types of residential options may be available.

Brief respite or crisis homes

Brief respite or crisis homes are intensive residential programs with on-site clinical staff who can provide 24-hour supervision and treatment. These homes may be a good choice for patients experiencing acute episodes or during the stabilization phase that follows an acute episode. For patients experiencing relapse, these homes may help them avoid the need for hospitalization.

Transitional group homes

Transitional group homes are structured programs that typically offer in-house daily training in living skills and 24-hour coverage by paraprofessionals. They help stabilize patients after acute episodes or after a stay in a hospital or brief respite home.

Foster or boarding homes

Foster or boarding homes are supportive group living situations run by laypersons. Usually, the staff provides supervision during the day, with one staff member sleeping over at night. These homes may be recommended for patients in long-term recovery and maintenance.

Supported or supervised apartments

Supported or supervised apartments usually have a specially trained on-site residential manager who provides support, assistance, and supervision. Alternatively, a mental health professional or family member may provide these services.

These apartments are useful for patients in long-term recovery and maintenance. They help the patient remain autonomous while providing sufficient care to minimize the chance of relapse and the need for inpatient hospitalization.

Family living

For some patients, living with family members may be an acceptable long-term arrangement. For others, it may be needed only during acute episodes. Support and advocacy groups can provide families with information and support.

Independent living

During long-term recovery and maintenance, independent living is recommended for most patients. Of course, this may be impossible during acute episodes and for patients with a more severe disease course.

skills. For patients who live with their families, psychoeducational family interventions can reduce the relapse rate.

Rehabilitation

Rehabilitation may be particularly important for patients who need to sharpen their job skills, want to work, and have only a few symptoms.

A range of rehab

During the long-term recovery and maintenance phases of the illness, three types of rehabilitation programs may be used.

Psychosocial rehabilitation programs help patients improve work skills so they can get and keep jobs.

Psychiatric rehabilitation teaches patients the skills needed to define and achieve their personal goals regarding education, work, socialization, and living arrangements.

Vocational rehabilitation involves work assessment and training to help patients prepare for full-time employment.

Electroconvulsive therapy

ECT may be used in the treatment of patients with acute schizophrenia and for those who cannot tolerate or do not respond to medication. It has been effective in reducing depressive and catatonic symptoms associated with schizophrenia.

Preserving the people's rights

Remember that patients with schizophrenia have the same rights as other hospitalized patients.

Schizophrenia in children

Although schizophrenia usually presents during adolescence, there are rare instances where symptoms begin during childhood. It is imperative that clinicians be mindful of other medical or organic conditions that may produce symptoms that mimic symptoms of schizophrenia. The social norm and the individual child's stage of development should be considered in the assessment of symptoms in ruling out other developmental disorders. Certain antipsychotics have been approved for use for children with schizophrenia who are aged 13 to 17: risperidone (Risperdal), aripiprazole (Abilify), olanzapine (Zyprexa), and quetiapine (Seroquel) (Mayo Clinic, 2014).

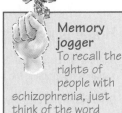

Memory jogger

To recall the rights of people with schizophrenia, just think of the word RIGHTS.

R Refusal of nonemergency treatment

I Individualized care

G Grievances addressed as they occur

H Health alternatives given

T Treatment obtained in the least restrictive setting

S Security of the patient's civil rights

Schizophrenia in elderly

Late-onset schizophrenia (LOS) is defined as onset of symptoms after age 40 and very-late-onset schizophrenia-like psychosis (VLOSLP) consists of onset after age 60 (Vannorsdall & Schretlin, 2013). Such phenomenon is more commonly seen among women and usually consists of paranoia and persecutory delusions. Risk of suicide in this population is high. Medication management for older people with schizophrenia may be more conservative to factor in the aging body's diminished ability to metabolize and excrete drugs. Dosage of medication is often adjusted lower to decrease incidence of fall, sedation, confusion, orthostatic hypotension, and toxicity.

References

Arnedo, J., Svrakic, D. M., del Val, C., Romero-Zaliz, R., Hernández-Cuervo, H., Fanous, A. H., . . . Zwir, I. (2014). Uncovering the hidden risk architecture of the schizophrenias: Confirmation in three independent genome-wide association studies. *The American Journal of Psychiatry*. Advance online publication. Retrieved from http://ajp .psychiatryonline.org/doi/abs/10.1176/appi.ajp.2014.14040435?journalCode=ajp

Glynn, S. (2014). Bridging psychiatric rehabilitation and recovery in schizophrenia: A life's work. *American Journal of Psychiatric Rehabilitation, 17*(3), 214–224.

Mayo Clinic. (2014). *Childhood schizophrenia: Treatment and drugs*. Retrieved from http:// www.mayoclinic.org/diseases-conditions/childhood-schizophrenia/basics/treatment/ con-20029260

National Institute of Mental Health. (2009). *What is schizophrenia?* Retrieved from http:// www.nimh.nih.gov/health/topics/schizophrenia/index.shtml

National Institute of Mental Health. (2013). *NIH-funded study adds to evidence of overlap with schizophrenia*. Retrieved from http://www.nimh.nih.gov/news/science-news/2013/ flu-in-pregnancy-may-quadruple-childs-risk-for-bipolar-disorder.shtml

Tusaie, K., & Fitzpatrick, J. (2013). *Advanced practice psychiatric nursing*. New York, NY: Springer.

Vannorsdall, T., & Schretlin, D. (2013). Late-onset schizophrenia. In L. D. Ravdin & H. L. Katzen (Eds.), *Handbook on the neuropsychology of aging and dementia: Clinical handbooks in neuropsychology* (pp. 487–500). New York, NY: Springer.

WebMD (2013). *Schizophrenia and suicide*. Retrieved from http://www.webmd.com/ schizophrenia/guide/schizophrenia-and-suicide

Wehring, H., & Carpenter, W. (2011). Violence and schizophrenia. *Schizophrenia Bulletin, 37*(5), 877–878.

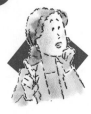

Quick quiz

1. Flattening of emotions refers to:
   A.   anhedonia.
   B.   asociality.
   C.   blunted affect.
   D.   regression.

Answer: C. Blunted affect is the flattening of emotions. The person's face may be immobile and inexpressive, with poor eye contact.

2. False ideas or beliefs that the person accepts as real are called:
   A.   delusions.
   B.   hallucinations.
   C.   illusions.
   D.   magical thinking.

Answer: A. Delusions are false ideas or beliefs accepted as real by the patient. Among people with schizophrenia, delusions of grandeur, persecution, and reference are common.

3. A newly admitted patient is presenting with psychomotor rigidity with arms folded in unnatural angle. The patient is resisting efforts by the nurse to assume a more comfortable position. This form of catatonia is best described as:
   A.   echopraxia.
   B.   echolalia.
   C.   wavy flexibility.
   D.   mutism.

Answer: C. Wavy flexibility is a rigid maintenance of body position seen in people with schizophrenia with catatonia features.

4. A patient with schizophrenia who began taking haloperidol (Haldol) 1 week ago now exhibits jerking movements of the neck and mouth. These are signs of:
   A.   dystonia.
   B.   psychosis.
   C.   akathisia.
   D.   parkinsonism.

Answer: A. Haloperidol and other high-potency conventional antipsychotics cause a high incidence of dystonia and other extrapyramidal adverse effects. Dystonia is marked by prolonged, repetitive muscle contractions that cause twisting or jerking movements—especially of the neck, mouth, and tongue.

5. A positive symptom of schizophrenia is:
A.   hallucination.
B.   blunted affect.
C.   anhedonia.
D.   asociality.

Answer: A. Characterized by an excess or distortion of normal functions, positive symptoms of schizophrenia include hallucinations and delusions.

Scoring

☆☆☆   If you answered all five items correctly, spectacular! We hereby declare you the Grand Sage of understanding schizophrenia!

☆☆   If you answered three or four items correctly, good show! You're exhibiting superior savvy in understanding schizophrenia.

☆   If you answered fewer than three items correctly, don't get paranoid! We'll just chalk it up to a few faulty dopamine receptors.

5

Mood disorders

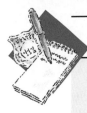

Just the facts

In this chapter, you'll learn:

♦ effects of mood disorders on functioning

♦ proposed causes of mood disorders

♦ how to assess a patient's suicide risk

♦ types of bipolar and depressive disorders

♦ assessment and interventions for patients with mood disorders.

A look at mood disorders

Mood disorders are disturbances in the regulation of mood, behavior, and affect that go beyond the normal fluctuations that most people experience. In the United States, more than 20 million people suffer from mood disorders (World Health Organization, 2013). Throughout the world, mood disorders are the leading cause of disability.

This chapter discusses bipolar disorders and depressive disorders. These potentially disabling mood disorders can affect every aspect of a person's life—thought processes, emotions, behaviors, and even physical health. Many people with mood disorders have coexisting mental and physical disorders.

Mood and affect

Mood refers to a pervading feeling. With a mood disorder, a person's mood becomes so intense and persistent that it interferes with social and psychological functioning. Mood is one element of the mental status examination that is historical and not typically able to be observed.

Special affects

Affect refers to the outward expression of emotion attached to ideas—including but not limited to facial expression and vocal modulation. Variations in affect are termed the *range of emotional expression.*

Patients with mood disorders may exhibit various abnormalities in affect, such as:

• blunted affect—severe reduction in the intensity of outward emotional expression

• flat affect—complete or almost complete absence of outward expressional expression

• restricted affect constricted (not restricted)—reduction in the intensity of outward emotional expression

• inappropriate affect—affect that doesn't match the situation or the content of the verbalized message (for instance, laughter when describing a loved one's death)

• labile affect—rapid and easily changing affective expression unrelated to external events or stimuli.

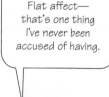

Flat affect— that's one thing I've never been accused of having.

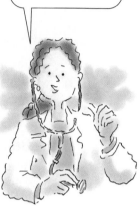

Causes

Theories regarding the causes of mood disorders center on genetic, biological, and psychological factors.

Genetic factors

Genetics appear to play a major role in mood disorders. Major depressive disorder and bipolar disorders occur much more often in first-degree relatives than in the general population. (Singh et al., 2010).

Double the displeasure

Also, studies of identical twins show that when one twin is diagnosed with major depression, the other twin has more than a 70% chance of developing depression. Research is underway to pinpoint the specific genetic underpinnings of the various mood disorders.

Biological factors

Biological research into the roots of mood disorder focuses on deficiencies or abnormalities in the brain's chemical messengers—neurotransmitters such as norepinephrine, serotonin, dopamine, and acetylcholine. The success of drugs that affect neurotransmitter levels in treating mood disorders supports the theory that these illnesses have biological roots.

Psychological theories

Cognitive, behavioral, and psychoanalytic theories also offer explanations for mood disorders.

Cognitive theory

Cognitive theory suggests that people who suffer from depression process information in a characteristically negative way. They view themselves and the world in a negative light and believe these negative perceptions will continue in the future (Beck, 1995).

Behavioral theory

According to the learned helplessness theory, people may become depressed after a negative event, such as a loved one's death or loss of a job, if the event makes them feel helpless. The perceived lack of control over life events dampens motivation, self-esteem, and initiative. Lack of social support and ineffective stress management and problem-solving skills increase the risk of depression after stressful events.

Psychoanalytic theory

According to psychoanalytic theory, depression results from a harsh superego (the "conscience" of the unconscious mind) and feelings of loss and aggression. Loss—especially at an early age—makes a child more susceptible to depression later in life.

Anger turned inward

The child interprets the loss as rejection and a sign that he or she's unworthy of love. He may feel aggressive toward those who have rejected him or her but realizes that these aggressive feelings could lead to further rejection, so he or she pushes those feelings out of awareness and turns them against himself or herself—and becomes depressed.

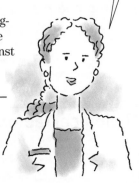

A child who feels rejected may ultimately turn his or her anger inward.

Signs and symptoms

Mood and affect

Mood refers to a pervading feeling. Mood must be assessed by patient report, as it is a subjective symptom (Mohr, 2013).

With a mood disorder, a person's mood becomes so intense and persistent that it interferes with social and psychological functioning. Mood is the only element of the mental status examination that is historical and not observed.

Challenges in caring for patients with mood disorders

Caring for patients with mood disorders poses numerous challenges.

• Mood disorders may cause primarily somatic (physical) symptoms, so they may be mistaken for physical illnesses.

• The patient may neglect self-care because of lowered motivation and energy levels.

• Mood disorders may alter family and social relationships and lead to frustration, anger, and guilt. As a result, the patient may be the victim or perpetrator of abuse.

• If the patient is unable to work because of the mood disorder, financial hardship may occur.

• A seriously depressed patient may be at increased risk for suicide.

Bipolar disorders

Bipolar disorders (previously called *manic-depressive disorders*) are mood disorders marked by severe, pathologic mood swings. Typically, the patient experiences extreme highs (mania or hypomania) with alternating extreme lows (depression). Interspersed between the highs and lows are periods of normal mood.

Variations in the pattern of highs and lows can occur. For instance, some people experience only acute episodes of mania.

Millions of moody people

An estimated 3 million people in the United States have bipolar disorders. Men and women are affected equally. Women, however, are likely to have more depressive episodes, whereas men experience more manic episodes. (See *Bipolar disorder and psychotic symptoms*.)

Onset usually occurs between ages 20 and 30 years, although symptoms sometimes arise in late childhood or early adolescence. Many patients with bipolar disorder have difficulties in work performance and psychosocial functioning.

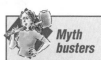

Myth busters

Bipolar disorder and psychotic symptoms

Many people are confused about the potential for psychotic symptoms in patients with bipolar disorder.

Myth: Patients with bipolar disorder never experience psychotic symptoms.

Reality: Some patients with bipolar disorder have rapidly alternating moods, severe impairment in functioning, and psychotic features that necessitate hospitalization.

Episodes and residuals

Most patients with bipolar disorder have recurring episodes of
mania and depression across the life span, with symptom-free
periods between episodes. Many patients experience residual
symptoms and some have chronic, unremitting symptoms despite
treatment.

Mania and hypomania

The highs of bipolar disorder may involve either mania
or hypomania. *Mania* is characterized by:

- elation
- euphoria
- agitation or irritability
- hyperexcitability
- hyperactivity
- rapid thought and speech
- exaggerated sexuality
- decreased sleep.

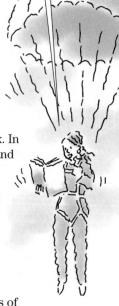

I may be high
right now, but I'm
not manic.

Not quite so manic

Hypomania refers to an expansive, elevated, or
agitated mood that resembles mania but is less intense
and lacks psychotic symptoms. For some patients, hypomania doesn't cause problems in social activities or work. In
fact, it may feel good, bringing high energy, confidence, and
enhanced social functioning and productivity.

You call that progress?

For others, however, hypomanic episodes can be
troublesome. Without proper treatment, these episodes
may progress to severe mania or switch to depression.

Psychotic symptoms

Some patients with bipolar disorder have severe episodes of
mania or depression that involve psychotic symptoms, such as
hallucinations (hearing, seeing, touching, smelling, or tasting
things that aren't actually there) or delusions (false beliefs not
influenced by logical reasoning or explained by a person's usual
cultural concepts). These patients may be misdiagnosed with
schizophrenia. (For information on schizophrenia, see Chapter 4.)

Implications

The impulsive behavior of a manic episode may have far-reaching
emotional and social consequences—divorce, child abuse, job-
lessness, bankruptcy, and promiscuity, to name a few.

STDs and suicide

People with bipolar disorders have an increased incidence of sexually transmitted diseases and unwanted pregnancies. Hyperactivity and sleep disturbances may lead to exhaustion and poor nutrition.

Bipolar disorder also increases the suicide risk. A suicide attempt may occur impulsively during a manic episode or after a depressive episode resolves. Lifetime rates of completed suicide for people with bipolar disorder are as high as 10% to 15% (American Psychiatric Association, 2006).

Classification

Bipolar disorder occurs in three major types.
• *Bipolar I disorder* is the classic and most severe disease form. The patient has manic episodes or mixed episodes (with symptoms of both mania and depression) that alternate with major depressive episodes. The depressive phase may immediately precede or follow a manic phase, or it may be separated from the manic phase by months or years.
• In *bipolar II disorder*, the patient doesn't experience severe mania but instead has milder episodes of hypomania that alternate with depressive episodes.
• In *cyclothymic disorder*, the patient has a history of numerous hypomanic episodes intermingled with numerous depressive episodes that don't meet the criteria for major depressive episodes.

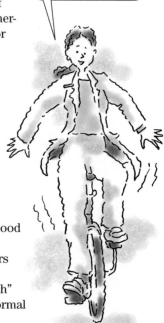

For someone with rapid-cycling bipolar disorder, mood swings come fast and furious.

Rapid cycling

Some patients who have bipolar disorder have rapid cycling. In this variant, four or more distinct periods of depression, mania, hypomania, or mixed states occur within a 12-month period. Periods of normal mood may be brief or even absent. Rapid cycling tends to develop later in the course of illness.

Pedaling as fast as they can

The more rapid the cycling, the more numerous the mood swings. Some sufferers experience multiple illness episodes within a single week. Some ultra-rapid cyclers have several mood swings in a single day.

Experts believe that any bipolar patient can "switch" to a rapid cycling pattern—but most return to their normal bipolar pattern in time.

Causes

The precise cause of bipolar disorder isn't known. However, genetic, biochemical, and psychological factors probably play a role.

Genetic factors

Twin, family, and adoption studies strongly suggest that bipolar disorder has a genetic component. First-degree relatives of a person with bipolar disorder are more likely than the general population to develop the disorder. In affected families, researchers have found autosomal dominant inheritance.

Biochemical factors

Experts think bipolar disorder stems at least in part from neurotransmitter abnormalities or imbalances. Some studies suggest the illness involves sensitivity of receptors on nerve cells.

Precipitating events

Stressful life events, such as a serious loss, chronic illness, or financial problems, may trigger a bipolar episode in persons who are predisposed to the disorder. Other possible triggers include:
• treatment of depression with an antidepressant drug, which may cause a switch to mania
• sleep deprivation
• hypothyroidism.
     However, bipolar episodes can occur with no obvious trigger.

Signs and symptoms

Bipolar disorder can be difficult to diagnose. Assessment findings vary with the illness phase.

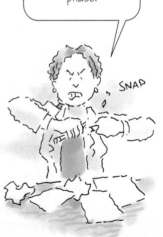

Some people get super irritable during the manic phase.

SNAP

During the manic phase

Signs and symptoms that may appear during the manic phase include:
• expansive, grandiose, or hyperirritable mood
• increased psychomotor activity, such as agitation, pacing, or hand wringing
• excessive social extroversion
• short attention span
• rapid speech with frequent topic changes (flight of ideas)
• decreased need for sleep and food
• impulsivity

- impaired judgment
- easy distractibility
- rapid response to external stimuli, such as background noise or a ringing telephone.

Maximal mania

With severe mania, the patient may have delusions, paranoid thinking, and an inflated sense of self-esteem ranging from uncritical self-confidence to marked grandiosity.

During the depressive phase

During a depressive episode, the patient may report or exhibit:
- low self-esteem
- overwhelming inertia
- social withdrawal
- feelings of hopelessness, apathy, or self-reproach
- difficulty concentrating or thinking clearly (without obvious disorientation or intellectual impairment)
- psychomotor retardation (sluggish physical movements and activity)
- slowing of speech and responses
- sexual dysfunction
- sleep disturbances (such as difficulty falling or staying asleep or early morning awakening)
- decreased muscle tone
- weight loss
- slow gait
- constipation.

Diagnosis

The diagnosis of bipolar disorder is confirmed if the patient meets the criteria in the *Diagnostic and Statistical Manual of Mental Disorders*, 5th Edition, (*DSM-5*). (See *Diagnostic criteria: Bipolar disorder*, pages 160–162.)

Treatment

Treatment of bipolar disorder requires drug therapy. Lithium is highly effective in both preventing and relieving manic episodes. It curbs accelerated thought processes and hyperactive behavior without the sedating effect of antipsychotic drugs. Lithium also may prevent the recurrence of depressive episodes (although it's ineffective in treating acute depression).

(Text continues on page 162.)

Diagnostic criteria: Bipolar disorder from *DSM-5*

Diagnostic criteria: Bipolar I disorder from *DSM-5*

For a diagnosis of bipolar I disorder, it is necessary to meet the following criteria for a manic episode. The manic episode may have been preceded by and may be followed by hypomanic or major depressive episodes.

Manic episode

A. A distinct period of abnormally and persistently elevated, expansive, or irritable mood and abnormally and persistently increased goal-directed activity or energy, lasting at least 1 week and present most of the day, nearly every day (or any duration if hospitalization is necessary).

B. During the period of mood disturbance and increased energy or activity, three (or more) of the following symptoms (four if the mood is only irritable) are present to a significant degree and represent a noticeable change from usual behavior:

1. Inflated self-esteem or grandiosity.
2. Decreased need for sleep (e.g., feels rested after only 3 hours of sleep).
3. More talkative than usual or pressure to keep talking.
4. Flight of ideas or subjective experience that thoughts are racing.
5. Distractibility (i.e., attention too easily drawn to unimportant or irrelevant external stimuli), as reported or observed.
6. Increase in goal-directed activity (either socially, at work or school, or sexually) or psychomotor agitation (i.e., purposeless non-goal-directed activity).
7. Excessive involvement in activities that have a high potential for painful consequences (e.g., engaging in unrestrained buying sprees, sexual indiscretions, or foolish business investments).

C. The mood disturbance is sufficiently severe to cause marked impairment in social or occupational functioning or to necessitate hospitalization to prevent harm to self or others, or there are psychotic features.

D. The episode is not attributable to the physiological effects of a substance (e.g., a drug of abuse, a medication, other treatment) or to another medical condition.

Note: A full manic episode that emerges during antidepressant treatment (e.g., medication, electroconvulsive therapy) but persists at a fully syndromal level beyond the physiological effect of that treatment is sufficient evidence for a manic episode and, therefore, a bipolar I diagnosis.

Note: Criteria A–D constitute a manic episode. At least one lifetime manic episode is required for the diagnosis of bipolar I disorder.

Hypomanic episode

A. A distinct period of abnormally and persistently elevated, expansive, or irritable mood and abnormally and persistently increased activity or energy, lasting at least 4 consecutive days and present most of the day, nearly every day.

B. During the period of mood disturbance and increased energy and activity, three (or more) of the following symptoms (four if the mood is only irritable) have persisted, represent a noticeable change from usual behavior, and have been present to a significant degree:

1. Inflated self-esteem or grandiosity.
2. Decreased need for sleep (e.g., feels rested after only 3 hours of sleep).
3. More talkative than usual or pressure to keep talking.
4. Flight of ideas or subjective experience that thoughts are racing.
5. Distractibility (i.e., attention too easily drawn to unimportant or irrelevant external stimuli), as reported or observed.
6. Increase in goal-directed activity (either socially, at work or school, or sexually) or psychomotor agitation.
7. Excessive involvement in activities that have a high potential for painful consequences (e.g., engaging in unrestrained buying sprees, sexual indiscretions, or foolish business investments).

C. The episode is associated with an unequivocal change in functioning that is uncharacteristic of the individual when not symptomatic.

Diagnostic criteria: Bipolar disorder from *DSM-5* (continued)

D. The disturbance in mood and the change in functioning are observable by others.

E. The episode is not severe enough to cause marked impairment in social or occupational functioning or to necessitate hospitalization. If there are psychotic features, the episode is, by definition, manic.

F. The episode is not attributable to the physiological effects of a substance (e.g., a drug of abuse, a medication, other treatment).

Note: A full hypomanic episode that emerges during antidepressant treatment (e.g., medication, electroconvulsive therapy) but persists at a fully syndromal level beyond the physiological effect of that treatment is sufficient evidence for a hypomanic episode diagnosis. However, caution is indicated so that one or two symptoms (particularly increased irritability, edginess, or agitation following antidepressant use) are not taken as sufficient for diagnosis of a hypomanic episode, nor necessarily indicative of a bipolar diathesis.

Note: Criteria A–F constitute a hypomanic episode. Hypomanic episodes are common in bipolar I disorder but are not required for the diagnosis of bipolar I disorder.

For bipolar II disorder

• The patient currently has, or his history includes, one or more major depressive episodes.

• He currently has, or his history includes, at least one hypomanic episode.

• He has never had a manic or a mixed episode.

• The first two exacerbations of the mood episode described previously aren't better explained by schizoaffective disorder and aren't superimposed on schizophrenia, schizophreniform disorder, delusional disorder, or psychotic disorder not otherwise specified.

• Symptoms cause clinically significant distress or impairment in social, occupational, or other important areas of functioning.

Diagnostic criteria: Bipolar II disorder from *DSM-5*

For a diagnosis of bipolar II disorder, it is necessary to meet the following criteria for a current or past hypomanic episode and the following criteria for a current or past major depressive episode:

Hypomanic episode

A. A distinct period of abnormally and persistently elevated, expansive, or irritable mood and abnormally and persistently increased activity or energy, lasting at least 4 consecutive days and present most of the day, nearly every day.

B. During the period of mood disturbance and increased energy and activity, three (or more) of the following symptoms have persisted (four if the mood is only irritable), represent a noticeable change from usual behavior, and have been present to a significant degree:

1. Inflated self-esteem or grandiosity.
2. Decreased need for sleep (e.g., feels rested after only 3 hours of sleep).
3. More talkative than usual or pressure to keep talking.
4. Flight of ideas or subjective experience that thoughts are racing.
5. Distractibility (i.e., attention too easily drawn to unimportant or irrelevant external stimuli), as reported or observed.
6. Increase in goal-directed activity (either socially, at work or school, or sexually) or psychomotor agitation.
7. Excessive involvement in activities that have a high potential for painful consequences (e.g., engaging in unrestrained buying sprees, sexual indiscretions, or foolish business investments).

C. The episode is associated with an unequivocal change in functioning that is uncharacteristic of the individual when not symptomatic.

D. The disturbance in mood and the change in functioning are observable by others.

E. The episode is not severe enough to cause marked impairment in social or occupational functioning or to necessitate hospitalization. If there are psychotic features, the episode is, by definition, manic.

(continued)

Not much wiggle room

Lithium has a narrow margin of safety and can easily cause toxicity. Treatment must begin cautiously with a low dose, which is adjusted slowly as needed. The patient must maintain therapeutic blood levels for 7 to 10 days before the desired effects appear, so the doctor may prescribe antipsychotic drugs in the interim for sedation and symptomatic relief. (See *Lithium alert.*)

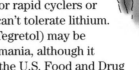

Lithium can be tricky because of its narrow margin of safety.

Other drugs

The doctor may prescribe valproic acid (Depakote) for rapid cyclers or for patients who can't tolerate lithium. Carbamazepine (Tegretol) may be useful in treating mania, although it isn't approved by the U.S. Food and Drug Administration for bipolar disorder.

Flip-flop effect

Antidepressants occasionally are prescribed to treat depressive symptoms. They must be used cautiously, however, because they may trigger a manic episode in patients with bipolar disorders.

Nursing interventions

Appropriate nursing interventions vary with the phase of bipolar disorder.

Advice from the experts

Lithium alert

For a patient who's receiving lithium, blood level monitoring is crucial because of the medication's narrow therapeutic margin. In fact, lithium shouldn't be used if the patient can't have regular blood tests. In addition, because lithium is excreted by the kidneys, it shouldn't be given to patients with renal impairment.

Blood levels should be checked 8 to 12 hours after the first dose, two or three times weekly for the first month, and then weekly to monthly during maintenance therapy.

Patient teaching

• Instruct the patient to maintain a fluid intake of 2,500 to 3,000 ml/day to promote adequate lithium excretion.

• Teach the patient that the lithium may cause sodium depletion, especially during initial therapy until consistent blood levels are achieved. Instruct the patient not to make dietary changes that might alter sodium intake because this might reduce lithium elimination and increase the toxicity risk.

• Inform the patient that raising salt intake may increase lithium excretion—which could lead to the return of mood symptoms. So stress the need to maintain adequate salt and water intake and to eat a normal, well-balanced diet. Remind the patient that sodium loss (which can result from diarrhea, illness, extreme sweating, or other conditions) may alter lithium levels.

• Teach the patient and family to watch for evidence of toxicity—diarrhea, vomiting, tremors, drowsiness, muscle weakness, and ataxia. Instruct patients to withhold one dose and call the doctor if toxic symptoms occur—but not to stop taking the drug abruptly.

During a manic episode

• Provide for the patient's physical needs. Involve the patient in activities that require safe gross motor movements.

• Encourage the patient to eat. He or she may be permitted to jump up and walk around the room after every mouthful but will sit down again if you remind him or her. If the patient can't sit still long enough to finish a meal, offer high-calorie finger foods, sandwiches, and cheese and crackers to supplement his or her diet.

• Suggest short daytime naps and help with personal hygiene. As symptoms subside, encourage the patient to assume responsibility for personal care.

• Provide diversionary activities suited to a short attention span. Firmly discourage the patient if he or she tries to overextend himself or herself.

Mission: Harmony

• Maintain a calm environment and protect the patient from overstimulation, such as from large groups, loud noises, and bright colors.

• Provide emotional support and set realistic goals for behavior.

- Tactfully divert the conversation if it becomes intimately involved with other patients or staff.
- Avoid reinforcing socially inappropriate or suggestive comments.

Limit-setting and listening

- In a calm, clear, self-confident manner, set limits for the patient's demanding, hyperactive, manipulative, and acting-out behaviors. Don't leave an opening for testing or argumentative behaviors.
- Listen to requests attentively and with a neutral attitude, but avoid power struggles if the patient pressures you for an immediate answer. Explain that you'll seriously consider the request and respond later.
- Collaborate with other staff members to provide consistent responses to the patient's manipulations or acting out.
- Anticipate the need for excessive verbalization.

> Listen to the patient's requests with a neutral attitude.

No Oscars for acting out

- Watch for early signs of frustration—when the patient's anger escalates from verbal threats to hitting an object.
- Tell the patient firmly that threats and hitting are unacceptable and indicate that help may be needed to control behavior. Inform the patient that the staff will help with movement to a quiet area and help with control of behavior so the patient won't hurt himself or herself or others. Staff members who have practiced as a team can work effectively to prevent acting-out behavior or to remove and confine the patient.
- Alert the care team promptly when acting-out behavior escalates. It's safer to have help available before you need it than to try controlling an anxious or frightened patient by yourself.
- When the acting-out incident ends and the patient is calm and in control, discuss feelings with the patient and offer suggestions to prevent recurrence.

Minding medications

- Advise the patient to take lithium with food or after meals to avoid stomach upset.
- Because lithium may impair mental and physical function, caution the patient against driving or operating dangerous equipment.
- Encourage to stay well hydrated because lithium is excreted via the kidneys.

During a depressive episode

- Provide for the patient's physical needs. If too depressed to provide self-care, help with personal hygiene.

• Encourage eating, or feed the patient if necessary. If constipated, add high-fiber foods to the diet; offer small, frequent meals; and encourage physical activity.
• To help the patient sleep, give back rubs or warm milk at bedtime.

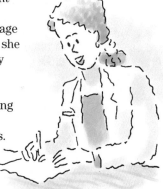

Be sure to assess and document the severity, duration, and other features of the patient's pain.

Provide pick-me-ups

• Keep in mind that a depressed patient needs continual positive reinforcement to improve self-esteem. Provide a structured routine, including activities to boost confidence and promote interaction with others (for instance, group therapy). Keep reassuring the patient that the depression will lift.
• Assume an active role in communicating. Encourage the patient to talk or to write down feelings if he or she is having trouble expressing them. Listen attentively and respectfully. If the patient seems sluggish, give adequate time to formulate thoughts. Record your observations and conversations to assist in evaluating the patient's condition.
• Avoid overwhelming the patient with expectations.

Injury aversion

• To prevent self-injury or suicide, remove harmful objects (such as glass, belts, rope, shoe laces, paper clips, and bobby pins) from the patient's environment.
• Institute suicide precautions as dictated by facility policy.
• Observe the patient closely and strictly supervise medications.

Medication teaching

• If the patient is taking lithium, instruct the patient to maintain a normal diet with normal salt and water intake. Inform the patient that restricting sodium intake increases lithium toxicity.
• Teach the patient the importance of continuing medication regimen even if he or she does not feel a need for it.
• If the patient is taking an antidepressant, watch for signs and symptoms of mania.

Cyclothymic disorder

In cyclothymic disorder, short periods of mild depression alternate with short periods of hypomania. Between the depressive and manic episodes, brief periods of normal mood occur. The person never goes more than 2 months without symptoms of depression or hypomania.

In many persons with cyclothymic disorder, manic episodes emerge over a few days to weeks—although onset within hours is possible.

Cyclothymic disorder affects men and women equally. Typically, onset occurs in the teens or early 20s.

Mood indigo

Both the depressive and hypomanic periods of cyclothymic disorder are shorter and less severe than in bipolar I or II disorder. Also, delusions don't occur, and few patients required hospitalization.

Nonetheless, mood swings may impair social and occupational functioning. Also, many patients progress to a more severe form of bipolar illness. Many experience a full-blown manic episode or major depression, with a consequent change in diagnosis to bipolar I or II disorder.

Damage and instability

Hypomanic periods of cyclothymic disorder may enhance a person's achievement in business and artistic endeavors—but also may damage interpersonal and social relationships. The patient's instability may lead to an uneven work and academic history, impulsive and frequent changes of residence, repeated romantic or marital breakups, and an episodic pattern of alcohol and drug abuse. Many cyclothymic patients self-medicate with alcohol or illegal drugs.

Signs and symptoms

General features of cyclothymia include:
• an odd, eccentric, or suspicious personality
• dramatic, erratic, or antisocial personality features
• inability to maintain enthusiasm for new projects
• a pattern of pulling close and then pushing away in interpersonal relationships
• abrupt changes in personality from cheerful, confident, and energetic to sad, blue, or mean.

Other signs and symptoms vary with the illness phase.

During the hypomanic phase

The patient experiencing the hypomanic phase may report or exhibit:
• insomnia
• hyperactivity
• inflated self-esteem

- increased productivity and creativity
- overinvolvement in pleasurable activities, including sex
- physical restlessness
- rapid speech.

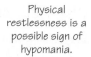

Physical restlessness is a possible sign of hypomania.

During the depressive phase

Signs and symptoms during the depressive phase may include:
- insomnia or hypersomnia
- feelings of inadequacy
- decreased productivity
- social withdrawal
- loss of libido
- loss of interest in pleasurable activities
- lethargy
- depressed speech
- crying.

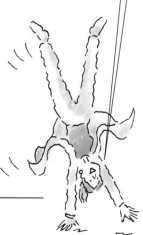

Causes

Most likely, genetic factors influence the development of cyclothymic disorder. Many patients have a family history of bipolar disorder, major depression, substance abuse, or suicide.

Diagnosis

The doctor must rule out various disorders to accurately diagnose cyclothymia. Medical disorders that can mimic cyclothymia include:
- acquired immunodeficiency syndrome
- Cushing disease
- epilepsy
- Huntington disease
- hyperthyroidism
- premenstrual dysphoric syndrome
- migraines
- multiple sclerosis
- neoplasm
- postpartum depression
- stroke
- systemic lupus erythematosus
- uremia
- vitamin deficiency
- Wilson disease.

Diagnostic criteria: Cyclothymic disorder

Diagnostic criteria: Cyclothymia from *DSM-5*

A. For at least 2 years (at least 1 year in children and adolescents) there have been numerous periods with hypomanic symptoms that do not meet criteria for a hypomanic episode and numerous periods with depressive symptoms that do not meet criteria for a major depressive episode.

B. During the above 2-year period (1 year in children and adolescents), the hypomanic and depressive periods have been present for at least half the time and the individual has not been without the symptoms for more than 2 months at a time.

C. Criteria for a major depressive, manic, or hypomanic episode have never been met.

D. The symptoms in Criterion A are not better explained by schizoaffective disorder, schizophrenia, schizophreniform disorder, delusional disorder, or other specified or unspecified schizophrenia spectrum and other psychotic disorder.

E. The symptoms are not attributable to the physiological effects of a substance (e.g., a drug of abuse, a medication) or another medical condition (e.g., hyperthyroidism).

F. The symptoms cause clinically significant distress or impairment in social, occupational, or other important areas of functioning.

Specify if:

• With anxious distress

Copycat conditions

Psychiatric disorders that can mimic cyclothymic disorder include:
• mood disorder caused by substance abuse or a general medical condition
• bipolar I or II disorder with rapid cycling
• borderline personality disorder.

The diagnosis is confirmed if the patient meets the criteria in the *DSM 5*. (See *Diagnostic criteria: Cyclothymic disorder*.)

Treatment

Pharmacologic options for cyclothymic disorder include:
• lithium
• carbamazepine (Tegretol)
• valproic acid (Depakote)
• verapamil (Calan).

Other therapies may include individual psychotherapy and couple or family therapy, which can help patients deal with relationship problems associated with the disorder.

Nursing interventions

These nursing interventions may be appropriate for patients with cyclothymic disorder.
- Explore ways to help the patient cope with frequent mood changes.
- Encourage vocational opportunities that allow flexible work hours.
- Urge a patient with artistic ability to pursue a career in the arts, where mood changes may be better tolerated.

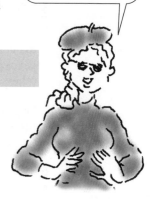

Some roses are red, dude. And violets are blue. If you're cyclothymic, the art world's calling you.

Major depressive disorder

Major depressive disorder (also called *unipolar major depression*) is a syndrome of a persistent sad mood lasting 2 weeks or longer. The feeling of sadness is accompanied by:
- feelings of guilt, helplessness, or hopelessness
- poor concentration
- sleep disturbances
- lethargy
- appetite loss
- anhedonia (inability to feel pleasure)
- loss of mood reactivity (failure to feel a mood uplift in response to something positive)
- thoughts of death.

Major depression often goes undiagnosed, and those who have it commonly receive inadequate treatment.

Beyond sad to bad

In major depressive disorder, sad feelings go beyond—and last longer than—"normal" sadness or grief. Also, some symptoms of severe depression (such as disinterest in pleasurable activities, hopelessness, and loss of mood reactivity) rarely accompany "normal" sadness.

In harm's way

Major depression can profoundly alter a person's social, family, and occupational functioning. Suicide—the most serious complication—can occur if feelings of worthlessness, guilt, and hopelessness are so overwhelming that the person no longer considers life worth living.

Nearly 15% of patients with untreated depression commit suicide. Most of them sought help from a doctor within 1 month of death.

What a bummer

At some time in their lives, about 22% of women and 16% of men in the United States experience major depressive disorder. In health care settings, an estimated 6% to 8% of patients meet the diagnostic criteria for this disorder.

The incidence of major depression rises with age. Onset usually occurs in early adulthood, with recurrences throughout the patient's lifetime.

It's baaaaack!

Recurrences may follow a prolonged symptom-free period or may occur sporadically. For some people, they come in clusters. For others, recurrences grow more frequent with age.

About 50% of those affected have their first episode of depression at about age 40—but this may be shifting downward to the 30s. More than 50% of patients who have one episode go on to have at least two more. An untreated episode can last from 1 month to a year—or even longer.

Causes

Genetic, biochemical, physical, psychological, and social factors have been implicated in major depression. The relationship between psychological stress, stressful life events, and depression onset is unclear. However, the patient history often reveals a specific personal loss or severe stress. According to one theory, the stressor interacts with the person's predisposition to provoke major depression.

SISTER-IN-LAW/ BROTHER-IN-LAW
MOTHER-IN-LAW / FATHER-IN-LAW
GREAT GRANDMOTHER/ GREAT GRANDFATHER
COUSINS
AUNT/ UNCLE
GRANDSON/ GRANDDAUGHTER
GRANDMOTHER/ GRANDFATHER
MOTHER/ FATHER
DAUGHTER/SON
SISTER/ BROTHER
NIECE/NEPHEW
FAMILY TREE

Genetic basis

Depression is more common in people with first-degree relatives with the disorder, indicating a genetic vulnerability. Although some researchers believe a single depression gene exists, mounting evidence suggests several genes may be involved in depression (Sullivan & Kendler, 2001).

Biochemical defects

The neural networks of the brain's prefrontal cortex and basal ganglia may be the primary defect sites in major depressive disorder.

The serotonin, neuroendocrine, and hypothalamic-pituitary-adrenal regulation systems may also be involved in development of depression. Differences in biological rhythms may also play a role, as seen by changes in circadian rhythms and various neurochemical and neurohormonal factors.

Finally, some researchers are homing in on abnormal cortisol levels as a factor in depression. In the dexamethasone suppression test, about 50% of patients with depression fail to suppress cortisol levels.

Organic causes

Health care professionals must distinguish major depression from depression caused by a specific event or a recognizable organic condition. Secondary depression can result from a wide range of physical disorders, including:
- metabolic disturbances, such as hypoxia and hypercalcemia
- endocrine disorders, such as diabetes and Cushing's disease
- neurologic diseases, such as Parkinson disease and Alzheimer disease
- cancer (especially of the pancreas)
- viral and bacterial infections, such as influenza and pneumonia
- cardiovascular disorders, such as heart failure
- pulmonary disorders, such as chronic obstructive lung disease
- musculoskeletal disorders, such as degenerative arthritis
- gastrointestinal disorders, such as irritable bowel syndrome
- genitourinary problems, such as incontinence
- collagen vascular diseases, such as lupus
- anemias.

Medications that can cause depression

Drugs prescribed for certain medical and psychiatric conditions can cause depression; examples include:
- antihypertensives
- psychotropics
- antiparkinsonian drugs
- opioids and nonnarcotic analgesics
- numerous cardiovascular medications
- oral antidiabetics
- antimicrobials
- steroids
- chemotherapeutic agents
- cimetidine.
  Alcohol use may also contribute to depression.

Signs and symptoms

During the assessment interview, a patient with major depression may seem unhappy or apathetic. The patient may report such changes as:
- feeling "down in the dumps"
- increased or decreased appetite
- sleep disturbances (e.g., insomnia or early awakening)
- disinterest in sex
- difficulty concentrating or thinking clearly
- easy distractibility
- indecisiveness
- low self-esteem
- poor coping
- constipation or diarrhea.

    The patient may report that symptoms are worse in the morning.

    During the physical examination, you may note agitation (such as hand wringing or restlessness) or psychomotor retardation (slow movements). With severe depression, the patient may have delusions of persecution or guilt, which can have an immobilizing effect.

Psychosocial clues

The psychosocial history may reveal life problems or losses that may explain or contribute to depression. Or, the medical history may implicate a physical disorder or use of a prescription drug or other substance that can cause depression.

A danger to oneself

Stay alert for clues to suicidal thoughts, a preoccupation with death, or previous suicide attempts. Many patients are reluctant to verbalize suicidal thoughts unless prompted, so you may need to assess the patient's suicide risk by asking direct questions.

    A patient who has specific suicide plans or significant risk factors (such as a history of a suicide attempt, profound hopelessness, concurrent medical illness, substance abuse, or social isolation) should be referred to a mental health specialist for immediate care. (See *Obstacles to detecting depression.*)

Memory jogger

Can't remember the things that may predispose a patient to suicide? The term RISK FACTORS can guide you.

R: Relationship difficulties

I: Intense feelings of hopelessness or helplessness

S: Sex differences (females make more suicide attempts; males succeed more often)

K: Kinship supports are weak or nonexistent

F: Family abuse or other types of abuse

A: Age extremes (those younger than age 19 and older than age 65 are at highest risk)

C: Chronic or debilitating health problems

T: Thinking is distorted

O: Overreacts to stress

R: Revenge or rage present

S: Substance abuse

Diagnosis

The doctor may administer psychological tests, such as the Beck Depression Inventory, to determine symptom onset, severity, duration, and progression.

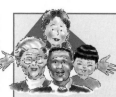

Bridging the gap

Obstacles to detecting depression

Always consider the patient's cultural background and values when assessing for signs and symptoms of depression. In most parts of world, depression and other mood disorders are viewed as social or moral problems—not as mental health problems appropriate to discuss with health care providers.

Even in the United States, many people from both mainstream and immigrant cultures feel that depression implies a moral weakness. As a result, they're likely to deny or minimize their emotional distress and express it instead as more socially acceptable somatic (physical) symptoms.

African American attitudes

Among African Americans, depression often has been misdiagnosed as some other condition because of mistrust of health care professionals (based in part on historical higher-than-average institutionalization rates for African Americans with mental illness). Also, during periods of emotional distress, African Americans tend to rely more on the support of family and the religious community rather than mental health professionals.

Memory jogger

For a depressed patient, positive OUTCOMES include:

O: Overwhelming feelings of grief and loss are processed

U: Uses problem-solving and reasoning skills to handle stressors

T: Talks with others willingly and appropriately

C: Cognitive distortions are decreased or eliminated

O: Overcomes thoughts of physically harming self

M: Maintains a positive sense of self

E: Eats nutritionally balanced meals and snacks

S: Sleeps 6 to 8 hours each night

The dexamethasone suppression test may show failure to suppress cortisol secretion in depressed patients (although this test has a high false-negative rate). Toxicology screening may suggest drug-induced depression.

The diagnosis is confirmed if the patient meets the criteria in the *DSM-5* (See *Diagnostic criteria: Major depressive disorder*, pages 174 and 175.)

Treatment

The primary treatments for major depressive disorder are pharmacologic therapy, electroconvulsive therapy, and psychotherapy.

Evidence-based treatment of mild to moderate depression includes:
• treatment of coexisting anxiety
• advice on sleep hygiene
• active monitoring
• low-intensity psychosocial interventions (cognitive-behavioral therapy [CBT], computerized cognitive-behavioral therapy [CCBT])
• group CBT
• antidepressant medication treatment in limited cases
• advice against using St. John's wort

Diagnostic criteria: Major depressive disorder

Diagnostic criteria for major depression from *DSM-5*

A. Five (or more) of the following symptoms have been present during the same 2-week period and represent a change from previous functioning; at least one of the symptoms is either (1) depressed mood or (2) loss of interest or pleasure.

Note: Do not include symptoms that are clearly attributable to another medical condition.

1. Depressed mood most of the day, nearly every day, as indicated by either subjective report (e.g., feels sad, empty, hopelessness) or observation made by others (e.g., appears tearful). (Note: In children and adolescents, can be irritable mood.)

2. Markedly diminished interest or pleasure in all, or almost all, activities most of the day, nearly every day (as indicated by either subjective account or observation).

3. Significant weight loss when not dieting or weight gain (e.g., a change of more than 5% of body weight in a month), or decrease or increase in appetite nearly every day. (Note: In children, consider failure to make expected weight gain.)

4. Insomnia or hypersomnia nearly every day.

5. Psychomotor agitation or retardation nearly every day (observable by others, not merely subjective feelings of restlessness or being slowed down).

6. Fatigue or loss of energy nearly every day.

7. Feelings of worthlessness or excessive or inappropriate guilt (which may be delusional) nearly every day (not merely self-reproach or guilt about being sick).

8. Diminished ability to think or concentrate, or indecisiveness, nearly every day (either by subjective account or as observed by others).

9. Recurrent thoughts of death (not just fear of dying), recurrent suicidal ideation without a specific plan, or a suicide attempt or a specific plan for committing suicide.

B. The symptoms cause clinically significant distress or impairment in social, occupational, or other important areas of functioning.

C. The episode is not attributable to the physiological effects of a substance or to another medical condition.

Note: Criteria A–C represent a major depressive episode.

Note: Responses to a significant loss (e.g., bereavement, financial ruin, losses from a natural disaster, a serious medical illness or disability) may include the feelings of intense sadness, rumination about the loss, insomnia, poor appetite, and weight loss noted in Criterion A, which may resemble a depressive episode. Although such symptoms may be understandable or considered appropriate to the loss, the presence of a major depressive episode in addition to the normal response to a significant loss should also be carefully considered. This decision inevitably requires the exercise of clinical judgment based on the individual's history and the cultural norms for the expression of distress in the context of loss.

In distinguishing grief from a major depressive episode (MDE), it is useful to consider that in grief the predominant affect is feelings of emptiness and loss, while in MDE it is persistent depressed mood and the inability to anticipate happiness or pleasure. The dysphoria in grief is likely to decrease in intensity over days to weeks and occurs in waves, the so-called pangs of grief. These waves tend to be associated with thoughts or reminders of the deceased. The depressed mood of MDE is more persistent and not tied to specific thoughts or preoccupations. The pain of grief may be accompanied by positive emotions and humor that are uncharacteristic of the pervasive unhappiness and misery characteristic of MDE. The thought content associated with grief generally features a preoccupation with thoughts and memories of the deceased, rather than the self-critical or pessimistic ruminations seen in MDE. In grief, self-esteem is generally preserved, whereas in MDE feelings of worthlessness and self-loathing are common. If self-derogatory ideation is present in grief, it typically involves perceived failings vis-à-vis the deceased (e.g., not visiting frequently enough, not telling the deceased how much he or she was loved). If a bereaved individual thinks about death and dying,

(continued)

Diagnostic criteria: Major depressive disorder (continued)

such thoughts are generally focused on the deceased and possibly about "joining" the deceased, whereas in MDE such thoughts are focused on ending one's own life because of feeling worthless, undeserving of life, or unable to cope with the pain of depression.

D. The occurrence of the major depressive episode is not better explained by schizoaffective disorder, schizophrenia, schizophreniform disorder, delusional disorder, or other specified and unspecified schizophrenia spectrum and other psychotic disorders.

E. There has never been a manic episode or a hypomanic episode.

Note: This exclusion does not apply if all of the manic-like or hypomanic-like episodes are substance-induced or are attributable to the physiological effects of another medical condition.

Coding and recording procedures

The diagnostic code for major depressive disorder is based on whether this is a single or recurrent episode, current severity, presence of psychotic features, and remission status. Current severity and psychotic features are only indicated if full criteria are currently met for a major depressive episode. Remission specifiers are only indicated if the full criteria are not currently met for a major depressive episode. Codes are as follows:

In recording the name of a diagnosis, terms should be listed in the following order: major depressive disorder, single or recurrent episode, severity/psychotic/remission specifiers, followed by as many of the following specifiers without codes that apply to the current episode. Specify:

With anxious distress
With mixed features
With melancholic features
With atypical features
With mood-congruent psychotic features
With mood-incongruent psychotic features
With catatonia. Coding note: Use additional code 293.89 (F06.1).
With peripartum onset
With seasonal pattern (recurrent episode only)

Evidence-based treatment of moderate and severe depression includes:

- antidepressant drug treatment (selective serotonin reuptake inhibitor [SSRI])
- high-intensity psychological intervention (CBT, interpersonal therapy, behavioral activation, behavioral couples therapy)
- combined antidepressant medication and high-intensity psychological intervention
- counseling
- short-term psychodynamic psychotherapy
- choice of antidepressant medication other than SSRI (e.g., venlafaxine, duloxetine, and tricyclic antidepressants [TCAs])
- assessing during the initial phase of medication treatment (e.g., suicide risk, side effects)
- treatment choice based on depression subtypes and personal characteristics
- enhanced care for depression: referral to specialist mental health services

- switching antidepressants
- combining and augmenting medications (e.g., addition of lithium, an antipsychotic, another antidepressant)
- continuation and relapse prevention.

Evidence-based management of complex and severe depression includes:
- referral to specialist mental health services
- inpatient care
- crisis resolution
- home treatment teams
- pharmacologic management of depression with psychotic symptoms
- electroconvulsive therapy
- transcranial magnetic stimulation (not recommended outside of research studies) (National Collaborating Centre for Mental Health, 2009).

Pharmacologic therapy

Medication is the most effective means of achieving remission and preventing relapse. Combining medication with psychotherapy can improve the treatment outcome by helping the patient cope with low self-esteem and demoralization.

Types of antidepressants

Generally, antidepressant drugs work by modifying the activity of relevant neurotransmitter pathways. These agents fall into several categories:
- SSRIs
- serotonin and norepinephrine reuptake inhibitors (SNRIs)
- atypical antidepressants
- TCAs
- monoamine oxidase inhibitors (MAOIs)
- other antidepressants.

No ideal antidepressant exists for all patients. The doctor must consider the patient's metabolism, possible adverse effects, agents that have been effective with family members, and potential for toxicity (if suicidal overdose is a concern).

Whichever drug is prescribed, the patient's response should be reevaluated after the first 2 months of therapy, with dosage changes made as needed. After remission, drug therapy should continue for at least 6 to 9 months. (See *Matching the treatment to the culture*.)

Bridging the gap

Matching the treatment to the culture

No matter what the diagnosis, always consider your patient's cultural and religious background. Some patients, for instance, may have cultural or religious reasons for not complying with the prescribed medication regimen. Some Brazilians oppose taking medication for fear they'll become addicted. Cambodians may refuse medications in the belief that Western medicine is too strong for their bodies.

When this occurs, consider possible alternative treatments.

Selective serotonin reuptake inhibitors

SSRIs include citalopram (Celexa), fluoxetine (Prozac), fluvoxamine (Luvox), paroxetine (Paxil), escitalopram (Lexapro), and sertraline (Zoloft). These agents inhibit serotonin reuptake and may inhibit the reuptake of other neurotransmitters as well.

SSRIs have become the first-choice treatment for most patients. They lack most of the disturbing adverse effects associated with TCAs and MAOIs.

Serotonin/norepinephrine reuptake inhibitors

SNRIs, such as venlafaxine (Effexor), inhibit norepinephrine uptake. They're generally used as second-line agents for patients with major depressive disorder.

Atypical antidepressants

Atypical antidepressants include bupropion (Wellbutrin), nefazodone (Serzone), trazodone (Desyrel), and mirtazapine (Remeron). These medications' mechanisms of action aren't well understood. Buproprion is thought to inhibit reuptake of serotonin, norepinephrine, and dopamine to varying degrees. Nefazodone and trazodone inhibit serotonin and norepinephrine reuptake. Mirtazapine is thought to inhibit serotonin and norepinephrine reuptake while blocking two specific serotonin receptors.

Although effective in certain patients, atypical antidepressants generally are used as second-line agents.

Tricyclic antidepressants

An older class of antidepressants, TCAs inhibit the reuptake of norepinephrine, serotonin, and dopamine and cause a gradual decline in beta-adrenergic receptors.

Specific TCAs include:
- amitriptyline (Elavil)
- amoxapine (Asendin)
- clomipramine (Anafranil)
- desipramine (Norpramin)
- doxepin (Sinequan)
- imipramine (Tofranil)
- nortriptyline (Pamelor)
- trimipramine (Surmontil).

Although TCAs can be effective, they may cause intolerable adverse effects. TCA overdose can quickly be lethal. For this reason, most TCAs have a black box warning for prescribers indicating a high suicide risk for patients on TCA therapy (Chew, Hales, & Yudofsky, 2005).

Consequently, they generally aren't used as first-line agents.

Monoamine oxidase inhibitors

MAOIs, such as phenelzine (Nardil) and tranylcypromine (Parnate), increase norepinephrine, serotonin, and dopamine levels by inhibiting MAO, an enzyme that inactivates them. They may have additional actions that contribute to their antidepressant effect.

MAOIs may be prescribed for patients with atypical depression (e.g., depression marked by an increased appetite and increased sleep rather than anorexia and insomnia) or for patients who don't respond to TCAs.

Although often effective, MAOIs carry a high risk of adverse effects and dangerous interactions with various foods and medications. Consequently, they're rarely used today—although conservative doses may be combined with a TCA for patients refractory to either type of drug alone.

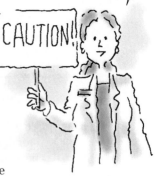

MAOIs can cause serious adverse effects and dangerous interactions with foods and other drugs.

CAUTION!

Other antidepressants

Other antidepressants, such as mirtazapine (Remeron) and nefazodone (Serzone), have varying mechanisms of action. They're generally used as second-line agents. (See *Pharmacologic therapy for mood disorders.*)

Electroconvulsive therapy

In electroconvulsive therapy (ECT), a tiny electrical current is applied to the patient's brain through electrodes. The current produces a seizure lasting from 30 seconds to 1 minute. ECT is indicated primarily for the treatment of severe major depression, in the context of either unipolar or bipolar disorders (Kellner et al., 2012).

A quicker picker-upper

Although controversial, ECT sometimes is used to treat severe depression when psychotherapy and medication aren't effective, when ECT poses a lower risk than other treatments, or when the patient is at immediate risk of suicide. ECT produces faster results than antidepressant drugs.

Get ready, get set . . .

The patient fasts for 6 to 8 hours before ECT. Just before the session, dentures, glasses, hearing aids, contact lenses, and hairpins are removed and the patient is asked to void. The patient may be given a variety of medications before the procedure, including:
• atropine or glycopyrrolate to reduce secretions, prevent aspiration, and reduce the risk of bradycardia
• a short-acting general anesthetic
• a muscle relaxant
• oxygen.

(Text continues on page 182.)

Meds matters

Pharmacologic therapy for mood disorders

This chart highlights several of the drugs used to treat mood disorders.

Drug	Adverse effects	Contraindications	Nursing considerations
Monoamine oxidase inhibitor (MAOI)			
Isocarboxazid (Marplan)	• Blurred vision • Constipation • Dry mouth • Drowsiness or insomnia • Fatigue • Hepatic dysfunction (jaundice, malaise, right upper abdominal quadrant pain, change in stool color or consistency) • Hypertensive crisis • Hypomania • Muscle twitching • Orthostatic hypotension • Skin rash • Vertigo • Weakness • Weight gain	• Cardiovascular or cerebrovascular disease • Confusion, uncooperativeness • Elderly or debilitated patients • Glaucoma • Heart failure • History of severe headaches • Impaired renal function • Liver disease • Paranoid schizophrenia • Pregnancy	• Monitor patient's blood pressure every 2 to 4 hours during initial therapy. Instruct patient to change positions slowly. • Assess for signs and symptoms of hypertensive crisis. • Monitor fluid intake and output. • Assess patient for suicidal risk. • Caution patient not to ingest foods and beverages containing tyramine, caffeine, or tryptophan. Warn the patient that ingesting tyramine can cause a hypertensive crisis. Give him or her a list of foods and beverages that contain such substances, which include aged cheeses, sour cream, beer, Chianti, aged sherry, pickled herring, liver, canned figs, raisins, bananas, avocados, chocolate, soy, smoked fish, sausage, liver, bologna, fava beans, yeast extracts, meat tenderizers, coffee, and colas. • Instruct patient to avoid meperidine (Demerol), epinephrine, local anesthetics, decongestants, cough medicines, diet pills, and most over-the-counter agents. • Teach patient to wear medical identification jewelry. • Advise patient to go to emergency department immediately if hypertensive crisis develops.
Tricyclic antidepressant			
Amitriptyline (Elavil) Imipramine (Tofranil)	• Agranulocytosis • Arrhythmias • Blurred vision • Bone marrow depression • Constipation	• Concomitant use of MAOIs • Recent myocardial infarction (MI) • Renal or hepatic disease	• Supervise patient's drug ingestion. • Monitor blood pressure and pulse for signs of orthostatic hypotension. • Monitor liver function and complete blood counts. • Institute suicide precautions as needed.

(continued)

Pharmacologic therapy for mood disorders *(continued)*

Drug	Adverse effects	Contraindications	Nursing considerations
Tricyclic antidepressant (continued)			
Amitriptyline (Elavil) Imipramine (Tofranil)	• Dry mouth • Esophageal reflux • Galactorrhea • Hallucinations • Heart failure • Increased or decreased libido • Jaundice and fatigue • Mania • MI • Orthostatic hypotension or hypertension • Palpitations • Shock • Slowed intracardiac conduction • Urinary hesitancy • Weight gain		• Know that special monitoring is required if patient poses a suicide risk or has a history of angle-closure glaucoma or seizure disorder. • Instruct patient to change positions slowly. • Tell patient to avoid driving or hazardous machinery if drowsiness occurs. • Instruct patient to avoid alcohol and over-the-counter agents unless the doctor approves. • Inform patient that the drug may take up to 4 weeks to become effective.
Selective serotonin reuptake inhibitor			
Fluoxetine (Prozac)	• Dry mouth • Insomnia • Nausea • Nervousness • Rash • Vertigo • Weight loss	• Within 14 days of taking an MAOI	• Know that drug medication is usually given in the morning with or without food. • Assess patient for weight loss if nausea occurs. • Know that patient should wait 5 weeks after stopping fluoxetine before starting an MAOI. • Tell patient to avoid alcoholic beverages. • Instruct patient to report adverse effects to the doctor, especially rash or itching.
Anticonvulsant (for treatment of bipolar disorder)			
Divalproex sodium (Depakote)	• Abdominal cramps • Diarrhea or constipation • Double vision or seeing "spots" • Increased urination • Indigestion • Nausea	• Liver disease	• Assess liver function tests and platelet counts. • Instruct patient to take drug with meals if stomach upset occurs. • Urge patient to report excessive bruising or unexplained bleeding. • Caution patient not to discontinue the drug abruptly.

Pharmacologic therapy for mood disorders *(continued)*

Drug	Adverse effects	Contraindications	Nursing considerations
Anticonvulsant (for treatment of bipolar disorder) (continued)			
Divalproex sodium (Depakote)	• Prolonged bleeding time • Sedation • Skin rashes • Vomiting		• Instruct patient not to crush tablets. • Caution patient to avoid alcohol while taking this drug.
Antimanic drug			
Lithium carbonate (Eskalith)	• Below 1.5 mEq/L: fine hand tremors, dry mouth, increased thirst, increased urination, nausea • 1.5 to 2.0 mEq/L: vomiting, diarrhea, muscle weakness, ataxia, dizziness, confusion, slurred speech • 2.0 to 2.5 mEq/L: persistent nausea and vomiting, blurred vision, muscle twitching, hyperactive deep tendon reflexes • 2.5 to 3.0 mEq/L: myoclonic twitches or movements of an entire limb, choreoathetoid movements, urinary and fecal incontinence • Above 3.0 mEq/L: seizures, cardiac arrhythmias, hypotension, peripheral vascular collapse, death	• Early pregnancy	• Assess serum drug levels. • Instruct patient not to chew extended-release preparations but to swallow them whole. • Supervise patient during administration to ensure that the medication is swallowed. • To relieve dry mouth or increased thirst, instruct patient to increase fluids or eat sugarless gum or hard candy. • If patient has increased urination, suggest limiting fluids after 8 p.m. Evaluate for diabetes insipidus, dilute urine, or low specific gravity. • For nausea, suggest patient take drug with food. • Instruct patient to maintain adequate sodium intake. • Inform patient that metallic taste may occur while taking this drug. • Teach patient to take drug even when feeling better and not to stop it abruptly. • Instruct patient to monitor weight weekly. • Caution the patient not to take drug with alcohol. • Instruct patient to notify doctor if severe vomiting or diarrhea occurs. • Instruct female patient to use a reliable form of birth control while on this drug. • Tell patient to get the doctor's approval before taking any new medications. • Instruct patient not to stop taking drug without discussing it with the doctor.

A bite block is inserted to prevent tongue-biting during the seizure, and the patient is connected to devices that monitor his or her brain waves, heart rhythm, and arterial oxygen saturation. Vital signs (heart rate, blood pressure, and temperature), blood oxygen saturation, end-tidal carbon dioxide levels, electrocardiogram, electroencephalogram, and electromyogram (to record the duration of the motor component of the seizure) are monitored during ECT (Kellner et al., 2012).

. . . Get zapped

Then a 1-second electrical current is applied to the brain through electrodes placed above the temples. The current produces a brief seizure.

In a typical course of treatment for major depression, the patient receives two or three ECT treatments a week, for a total of 6 to 12 treatments. Contraindications include recent myocardial infarction, a history of stroke, and intracranial lesions.

Psychotherapy

Short-term psychotherapy can aid in relieving major depression. Many psychiatrists believe the best results occur from combining individual, family, or group psychotherapy with medication.

After the acute episode of depression resolves, a patient with a history of recurrent depression may be maintained on a low dose of an antidepressant drug as a preventive measure.

Nursing interventions

These nursing interventions may be appropriate for a patient with major depression.

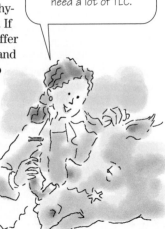

With this beastly mood you're in, you need a lot of TLC.

• Provide for the patient's physical needs. If the patient is too depressed to perform self-care, help with personal hygiene. Encourage the patient to eat or feed if necessary. If constipated, add high-fiber foods to the patient's diet; offer small, frequent meals; and encourage physical activity and fluid intake. Give warm milk or back rubs at bedtime to improve sleep.
• Record all observations and conversations with the patient. They're valuable in evaluating the response to treatment.
• Plan activities for times when the patient's energy level peaks.

Connection and communication

• Assume an active role in initiating communication.
• Share your observations of the patient's behavior. You might say, "You're sitting all by yourself, looking sad. Is that how you feel?"

• The patient may think and react sluggishly, so speak slowly and allow ample time for response.
• Avoid feigned cheerfulness, but don't hesitate to laugh and point out the value of humor.
• Encourage the patient to talk about and write down feelings. Show that the individual is important by listening attentively and respectfully, avoiding interruptions, and remaining nonjudgmental.

Structure and socialization

• Provide a structured routine, including noncompetitive activities, to build the patient's self-confidence and promote interaction with others. Urge socialization and joining group activities.
• Try to spend some time with the patient each day to decrease isolation. Avoid long periods of silence, which tend to increase anxiety.

Self-help suggestions

• Reassure the patient that expressing his or her feelings, engaging in pleasurable activities, and improving grooming and hygiene help to decrease depression.
• Teach the patient about depression. Emphasize that effective methods are available to relieve symptoms.
• Help with recognition of distorted perceptions and link them to depression. Once depressive thought patterns are recognized, the patient can begin to substitute self-affirming thoughts.

Inklings of suicide

• Ask the patient about having thoughts of death or suicide. Such thoughts signal an immediate need for consultation and assessment. Failure to detect suicidal thoughts early may encourage a suicide attempt.
• Be aware that the suicide risk rises as depression lifts. (See *Recognizing suicide potential*, page 184.)

Medication edification

• If the patient is taking an antidepressant, stress the need for compliance and review adverse reactions. For drugs that produce strong anticholinergic effects (such as amitriptyline and amoxapine), suggest using sugarless gum or hard candy to relieve dry mouth. For sedating antidepressants (such as amitriptyline and trazodone), warn the patient to avoid activities that require alertness, including driving and operating mechanical equipment.
• Some antidepressants lower the seizure threshold, so monitor the patient for seizures.
• Inform the patient that antidepressants may take several weeks to produce the desired effect.

Advice from the experts

Recognizing suicide potential

A patient with a mood disorder may be at risk for attempting suicide. Stay alert for:
• overwhelming anxiety (the most frequent trigger for a suicide attempt)
• withdrawal and social isolation
• saying farewell to friends and family
• putting affairs in order
• giving away prized possessions
• sending covert suicide messages and death wishes
• expressing obvious suicidal thoughts ("I'd be better off dead")
• describing a suicide plan
• hoarding medications
• talking about death and a feeling of futility
• behavior changes, especially as depression begins to subside.

Taking action
If you think your patient is at risk for suicide, take these steps:
• Keep communication lines open. Maintaining personal contact may help the suicidal patient feel less alone or without resources or hope. Continuity of care and consistency of primary nurses also can help the patient maintain emotional ties to others—the ultimate technique for preventing suicide.
• To ensure a safe environment, check for dangerous conditions, such as exposed pipes, windows without safety glass, and access to the roof or open balconies.
• Remove belts; sharp objects such as razors, knives, nail files, and clippers; suspenders; light cords; and glass from the patient's room.
• Make sure an acutely suicidal patient is observed around the clock. Stay alert when the patient uses a sharp object (as when shaving), takes medications, or uses the bathroom (to prevent hanging or other injury). Assign the patient a room near the nurses' station and with another patient.

• Caution the patient taking a TCA or an SSRI to avoid drinking alcoholic beverages or taking other central nervous system depressants during therapy.

FYI on MAOIs

• If the patient is taking an MAOI, emphasize that he or she must avoid foods that contain tyramine, caffeine, or tryptophan. Warn him or her that ingesting tyramine can cause a hypertensive crisis. Give him or her a list of foods and beverages that contain these substances, which include aged cheeses, sour cream, beer, Chianti, sherry, pickled herring, liver, canned figs, raisins, bananas, avocados, chocolate, soy sauce, fava beans, yeast extracts, meat tenderizers, coffee, and colas.

> Alcohol is a big no-no for a patient during TCA or SSRI therapy.

Dysthymic disorder

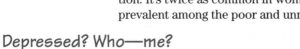

Dysthymic disorder, or dysthymia, refers to mild depression that lasts at least 2 years in adults or 1 year in children. The depression is relatively mild or moderate, and most patients aren't certain when they first became depressed.

Despite its relative mildness, dysthymic disorder may impair functioning at home, in school, or at work. However, hospitalization rarely is needed unless suicidal intent is present.

Dysthymic disorder may affect up to 3% of the population. It's twice as common in women as in men and more prevalent among the poor and unmarried.

Depressed? Who—me?

This disorder often goes unrecognized by those experiencing it, as well as by their family and friends. Dysthymic persons may not consider themselves depressed. Because of the mild symptoms—which may be physical rather than emotional—patients typically see a mental health professional only if dysthymia progresses to major depression.

Even when recognized, dysthymia is hard to treat. Recovery is slower if the condition becomes chronic and goes untreated.

> A patient who's under a lot of stress and lacks the skills to cope may be destined for dysthymia.

Additional agonies

Many patients with dysthymic disorder have a coexisting psychiatric or medical disorder, such as heart disease, cancer, diabetes, or another psychiatric disorder (e.g., substance abuse or an anxiety disorder).

Causes

Biological, psychological, and medical factors may play a role in dysthymic disorder. Patients with dysthymic disorder may have below-normal serotonin levels, so it's likely that serotonin is involved in development of this disorder.

As with many other psychiatric disorders, personality problems and multiple stressors, combined with inadequate coping skills, may increase a person's vulnerability to this disorder.

Signs and symptoms

Signs and symptoms of dysthymic disorder include:
- persistent sad, anxious, or empty mood
- loss of interest in activities previously enjoyed
- excessive crying
- increased feelings of guilt, helplessness, or hopelessness
- weight or appetite changes
- sleep difficulties
- poor school or work performance
- social withdrawal
- conflicts with family and friends
- increased restlessness and irritability
- poor concentration
- inability to make decisions
- reduced energy level
- thoughts of death or suicide or suicide attempts
- physical symptoms, such as headache or backache.

Diagnosis

The patient may be diagnosed with dysthymic disorder after a careful psychiatric examination and medical history are performed by a psychiatrist or other mental health professional. The diagnosis is confirmed if the patient meets the criteria in the *DSM-5*. (See *Diagnostic criteria: Dysthymic disorder.*)

Treatment

Short-term psychotherapy teaches the patient more constructive ways of communicating with family, friends, and coworkers. It also allows ongoing assessment of suicidal ideation and suicide risk.

Behavioral therapy may be used to reeducate the patient in social skills. Group therapy can help the patient to change maladaptive social functioning.

Pharmacologic treatment of dysthymic disorder may involve antidepressants, such as SSRIs or TCAs. Patients who exhibit pessimism, disinterest, and low self-esteem typically respond to antidepressant drugs.

Diagnostic criteria: Dysthymic disorder

Dysthymic disorder is diagnosed if the patient meets these criteria from the *DSM-5*.

Diagnostic criteria: Persistent depressive disorder (dysthymia) from *DSM-5*

This disorder represents a consolidation of *DSM-IV*–defined chronic major depressive disorder and dysthymic disorder.

A. Depressed mood for most of the day, for more days than not, as indicated by either subjective account or observation by others, for at least 2 years.

   Note: In children and adolescents, mood can be irritable and duration must be at least 1 year.

B. Presence, while depressed, of two (or more) of the following:
   1. Poor appetite or overeating.
   2. Insomnia or hypersomnia.
   3. Low energy or fatigue.
   4. Low self-esteem.
   5. Poor concentration or difficulty making decisions.
   6. Feelings of hopelessness.

C. During the 2-year period (1 year for children or adolescents) of the disturbance, the individual has never been without the symptoms in Criteria A and B for more than 2 months at a time.

D. Criteria for a major depressive disorder may be continuously present for 2 years.

E. There has never been a manic episode or a hypomanic episode, and criteria have never been met for cyclothymic disorder.

F. The disturbance is not better explained by a persistent schizoaffective disorder, schizophrenia, delusional disorder, or other specified or unspecified schizophrenia spectrum and other psychotic disorder.

G. The symptoms are not attributable to the physiological effects of a substance (e.g., a drug of abuse, a medication) or another medical condition (e.g., hypothyroidism).

H. The symptoms cause clinically significant distress or impairment in social, occupational, or other important areas of functioning.

   Note: Because the criteria for a major depressive episode include four symptoms that are absent from the symptom list for persistent depressive disorder (dysthymia), a very limited number of individuals will have depressive symptoms that have persisted longer than 2 years but will not meet criteria for persistent depressive disorder. If full criteria for a major depressive episode have been met at some point during the current episode of illness, they should be given a diagnosis of major depressive disorder. Otherwise, a diagnosis of other specified depressive disorder or unspecified depressive disorder is warranted.

Specify if:
   With anxious distress
   With mixed features
   With melancholic features
   With atypical features
   With mood-congruent psychotic features
   With mood-incongruent psychotic features
   With peripartum onset

Specify if:
   In partial remission
   In full remission

Specify if:
   Early onset: If onset is before age 21 years.
   Late onset: If onset is at age 21 years or older.

Specify if (for most recent 2 years of persistent depressive disorder):
   With pure dysthymic syndrome: Full criteria for a major depressive episode have not been met in at least the preceding 2 years.

   With persistent major depressive episode: Full criteria for a major depressive episode have been met throughout the preceding 2-year period.

   With intermittent major depressive episodes, with current episode: Full criteria for a major depressive episode are currently met, but there have been periods of at least 8 weeks in at least the preceding 2 years with symptoms below the threshold for a full major depressive episode.

   With intermittent major depressive episodes, without current episode: Full criteria for a major depressive episode are not currently met, but there has been one or more major depressive episodes in at least the preceding 2 years.

Specify current severity: Mild, Moderate, Severe

Nursing interventions

These nursing interventions may be appropriate for a patient with dysthymic disorder.

• Provide supportive measures, such as reassurance, warmth, availability, and acceptance—even if the patient becomes hostile.

• Teach the patient about the illness and prescribed antidepressant medication.

• Urge the patient to engage in activities that enhance his or her sense of accomplishment.

• Encourage positive health habits, such as eating well-balanced meals, avoiding drugs and alcohol (which can worsen depression), and getting physical exercise (which can lift his or her mood).

References

American Psychiatric Association. (2006). *Practice guidelines. Treating bipolar disorder: A quick reference guide.* Arlington, VA: American Psychiatric Publishing. doi:10.1176/appi.books.9780890423370.110108

American Psychiatric Association. (2013). *Diagnostic and statistical manual of mental disorders* (5th ed.). Arlington, VA: Author.

Beck, J. S. (1995). *Cognitive therapy: Basics and beyond.* New York, NY: Guilford.

Chew, R. H., Hales, R. E., & Yudofsky, S. C. (2005). *What your patients need to know about psychiatric medications* (2nd ed.). Arlington, VA: American Psychiatric Publishing. doi:10.1176/appi.books.9781585623877.228000

Kellner, C. H., Greenberg, R. M., Murrough, J. W., Bryson, E. O., Briggs, M. C., & Pasculi, R. (2012). ECT in treatment-resistant depression. *The American Journal of Psychiatry, 169*(12), 1238–1244. doi:10.1176/appi.ajp.2012.12050648

National Collaborating Centre for Mental Health. (2009). *Depression. The treatment and management of depression in adults.* London, United Kingdom: National Institute for Health and Clinical Excellence.

Singh, A. L., D'Onofrio, B. M., Slutseke, W. S., Turkheimer, E., Emery, R. E., Harden, K. P., . . . Martin, N. G. (2010). Parental depression and offspring psychopathology: A children of twins study. *Psychological Medicine, 41*(7), 1385–1395. doi:10.1017/S0033291710002059

Sullivan, P., & Kendler, K. (2001). Genetic case-control studies in neuropsychiatry. *Archives of General Psychiatry, 58*(11), 1015–1024.

World Health Organization. (2013). *Depression.* Retrieved from http://www.who.int/topics/depression/en/

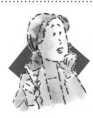

Quick quiz

1. A nurse is caring for a patient with a psychiatric disorder and understands that severe pathologic mood swings, from hyperactivity and euphoria to sadness and depression, occur in which of the following?

    A. dysthymic disorder.
    B. cyclothymic disorder.
    C. bipolar disorder.
    D. depressive disorder.

Answer: C. Severe pathologic mood swings occur in bipolar disorder. The mood swings of cyclothymic disorder are much milder.

2. The nurse understands that a bipolar episode may be triggered by which of the following physical causes?

    A. hypothyroidism.
    B. hyperthyroidism.
    C. antimanic drugs.
    D. antiseizure medications.

Answer: A. In a patient who's predisposed to bipolar disorder, hypothyroidism may trigger a disease episode.

3. The terminology of *rapid cycling* refers to bipolar disorder in a patient that exhibits which of the following patterns?

    A. one or more episodes of depression or mania in 1 year.
    B. two or more episodes of depression or mania in 1 year.
    C. four or more episodes of depression or mania in 1 year.
    D. no episodes of depression.

Answer: C. Rapid cycling is bipolar disorder in which four or more episodes of depression and mania occur within a 12-month period.

4. ECT may be used to treat which of the following psychiatric problem?

    A. dysthymic disorder.
    B. major depressive disorder.
    C. cyclothymic disorder.
    D. bipolar I disorder.

Answer: B. ECT sometimes is used to treat major depression as well as certain psychotic disorders.

5. A patient who has been prescribed lithium (Eskalith) should be taught to do which of the following with regard to maintaining best health while on the medication?

A. limit fluids to 1,500 ml daily.
B. maintain a high fluid intake.
C. restrict sodium intake.
D. exercise outside in hot weather.

Answer: B. A patient taking lithium must maintain a high fluid intake.

Scoring

☆☆☆ If you answered all five items correctly, you should be feeling elated! Your performance was grandiose!

☆☆ If you answered three or four items correctly, feel free to indulge in an episode of hypomania. Your insight into mood disorders is expansive.

☆ If you answered fewer than three items correctly, don't get depressed. By the end of the next chapter, your mood should stabilize.

6

Anxiety, anxiety-related, and obsessive disorders

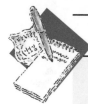

Just the facts

In this chapter, you'll learn:

♦ effects of anxiety

♦ neurobiological theories for anxiety disorders

♦ how anxiety disorders impair functioning

♦ risk factors and proposed causes of anxiety disorders

♦ risk for suicide for those with anxiety disorders

♦ assessment and intervention for patients with an anxiety disorder.

A look at anxiety disorders

Anxiety disorders are a group of conditions marked by extreme or pathologic anxiety or dread. Those with anxiety experience disturbances of thinking, mood, behavior, and physiologic activity. Many feel anxious most of the time, with no apparent reason.

The anxiety may be so uncomfortable that they stop doing certain everyday activities to avoid the feeling of dread. Some have terrifying bouts of intense anxiety that immobilize them. To relieve overwhelming feelings of anxiety, impending catastrophe, guilt, shame, helplessness, or worthlessness, sufferers may cling to maladaptive behaviors, which only make their symptoms worse. "The two core symptoms shared by all anxiety disorders are anxiety or fear coupled with some form of worry" (Stahl & Grady, 2010, p. 2).

> What? . . . Me worry?

The anatomy of anxiety

From time to time, everyone experiences worry, uncertainty, or apprehension—particularly when confronting a stressful event such as a job interview or a first date. Mild or moderate anxiety rarely threatens one's coping ability. In fact, it can motivate us to try new things and take risks. In that sense, it's useful and productive.

The degree of anxiety experienced and the ability to perceive it accurately and channel it appropriately determine if the anxiety will help or hinder the person's level of functioning. Someone who perceives anxiety as severe will feel threatened—and either avoid it or become overwhelmed by it.

Sure—this is risky and makes me a little anxious. But I thrive on that feeling.

Oodles of anxiety

"Anxiety disorders affect about 40 million American adults age 18 and older in a given year" (National Institute of Mental Health, 2014). Although the number of individuals officially diagnosed is high, it is suggested that the numbers of those who have undiagnosed anxiety may be even higher. Treatment for anxiety disorder is readily available and, in most cases, very successful in restoring a productive and fulfilling life to those with anxiety.

Over and above anxiety

Anxiety disorders are often accompanied by other psychiatric illnesses, especially mood disorders and substance abuse—as well as medical disorders. Health care providers must stay alert for this possibility. There is also quite a bit of overlap in symptoms with major depression. (See *Plain talk about anxiety disorders*.)

Causes

Anxiety disorders are thought to result from a combination of genetic, biochemical, neuroanatomic, and psychological factors—plus life experiences. Specific causes for each disorder will be discussed with that disorder.

Myth busters

Plain talk about anxiety disorders

Here's a reality check to help the nurse stay on course when caring for patients with anxiety disorders.

Myth: All anxiety disorders cause psychological symptoms, but only panic attacks cause physiologic symptoms.

Reality: Both physiologic and psychological symptoms accompany all levels of anxiety, from mild to severe.

Myth: With posttraumatic stress disorder, patients who frequently talk about their trauma tend to relive the traumatic experience.

Reality: Talking about the trauma with a mental health professional can help the patient acknowledge the traumatic event, learn coping strategies, and obtain support during the recovery process.

Genetic factors

Research shows that some anxiety disorders are inherited. Many of them—including panic disorder, obsessive-compulsive disorder (OCD), generalized anxiety disorder (GAD), and major phobias—run in families. Up to 50% of those with an anxiety disorder also have a first-degree relative with an anxiety disorder (Sadock & Sadock, 2007, p. 586).

Researchers are looking for specific genetic factors that might explain or contribute to an inherited risk. Some studies are focusing on defective genes that regulate specific chemical messengers in the brain (neurotransmitters), such as serotonin, dopamine, norepinephrine, glutamate, and gamma-aminobutyric acid (GABA).

Biochemical factors

Some experts believe that people with anxiety disorders have a biological vulnerability to stress, which makes them more susceptible to environmental stimuli. Neurotransmitter (see previous list) imbalances may also contribute to anxiety disorders.

Neuroanatomic factors

Scientists are using functional magnetic resonance imaging (fMRI), positron emission tomography, single photon emission computed tomography (SPECT), electroencephalography (EEG), and other functional brain imaging studies to locate the brain areas or abnormalities associated with anxiety responses. So far, they've identified brain atrophy, underdeveloped frontal and temporal lobes, and abnormalities involving the amygdala (which regulates fear, memory, and emotion) and the hippocampus (which plays a role in emotion and memory storage) (Stahl & Grady, 2010, p. 35). The hypothalamic-pituitary-adrenal axis is chronically activated in situations where there is chronic stress. With chronic stress, "excessive glucocorticoid release may lead to hippocampal atrophy . . . and increase the risk for an anxiety disorder" (Stahl & Grady, 2010, p. 8).

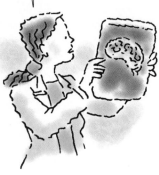

MRI scans have found brain abnormalities in some patients with anxiety disorders.

The other component of anxiety disorders is worry. This involves the cortico-striato-thalamo-cortical feedback loops from the prefrontal cortex (Stahl, 2013, p. 395).

Psychological factors

Some theories suggest that certain anxiety disorders arise when unconscious defense mechanisms become overwhelmed and dysfunctional. The ego can be in an imbalance where there are interpersonal and/or intrapsychic conflicts (Sadock & Sadock, 2007, p. 581).

Fear in the family

The family's role in phobias is also under investigation. Several studies show a strong correlation between a parent's fears and those of their children. In other words, a child "learns" fears by observing the parent's fearful reaction to an object or situation.

Traumatic life events

Traumatic events can trigger anxiety disorders; the most obvious example is posttraumatic stress disorder (PTSD). Panic disorders have also been associated with anxiety following separation and loss.

Some experts, however, believe that only someone who's vulnerable because of psychological, genetic, or biochemical factors will develop an anxiety disorder in response to trauma. Some people may even have a biological propensity for specific phobias (such as a fear of snakes) that's triggered by a single exposure.

Medical conditions

Some anxiety symptoms are associated with particular medical conditions. For example, someone who has a hyperthyroid condition or adrenal disorder may mimic an anxiety disorder. Withdrawal of certain medications as well as alcohol can promote symptoms of anxiety. Many health conditions can lead to feelings of anxiety such as vertigo, cardiac disease, gastrointestinal (GI) disorders, asthma, and cigarette smoking (Boyd, 2012). However, it is important to distinguish symptoms of anxiety as they relate to an underlying medical problem versus symptoms of anxiety as they relate to anxiety disorder. Anxiety disorder is diagnosed when the symptoms are not attributable to another medical condition or medication (American Psychiatric Association [APA], 2013).

Risk factors

- Female gender
- Physical comorbidity
- Depression or other psychiatric disorder

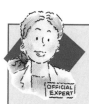

Advice from the experts

Differentiating fear, anxiety, worry, and panic

When assessing patients for anxiety disorders, keep in mind the key differences among fear, anxiety, worry, and panic:

- Fear is a response to external stimuli. "The emotional aspect of fear is regulated by connections between the amygdala and specific areas of the prefrontal cortex" (Stahl & Grady, 2010, p. 5). The amygdala is located near the hippocampus. The motor responses (i.e., fight, flight, or freeze) to fear are also regulated between a connection from the amygdala to a part of the brainstem (locus coeruleus) (Stahl, 2013, p. 392). Breathing output is affected in the fear response, which is regulated by the amygdala and another part of the brain stem (parabrachial nucleus). Symptoms such as shortness of breath, asthma attack, or the feeling of being smothered all stem from increases in respiratory rate in a panic attack (Stahl & Grady, 2010, p. 9).

- Anxiety is a response to internal conflict that may influence behavior even after the cause of the anxiety is removed. "Anxiety is a state that encompasses both an internal 'feeling' of fear and the physiologic expression of that fear" and the amygdala (limbic system), hippocampus, cortical regions, and locus coeruleus plays an important role in this (Stahl & Grady, 2010, pp. 3 and 6).
- Worry may include anxious misery, apprehensive expectation, catastrophic thinking, and obsessions (Stahl & Grady, 2010, p. 13). Worry is linked to a feedback loop in the prefrontal cortex (Stahl, 2013, p. 395).
- Panic is an extreme level of anxiety characterized by "a sudden overwhelming feeling of terror or impending doom" (Townsend, 2014, p. 531).

Panic disorder

Panic disorder represents anxiety in its most severe form. In this disorder, the person has recurrent, unexpected panic attacks that cause intense apprehension and feelings of impending doom. Between attacks, the patient persistently worries about having additional panic attacks and the consequences of the attacks and may change his or her behavior because of them. The frequency of panic attacks and the high level of anxiety may cause functional impairments. Panic attacks can occur in the context of other diagnoses and in and of itself is not a mental disorder (Katon & Ciechanowski, 2013).

Thirty minutes of terror: Panic attacks

Panic attacks occur suddenly, with no warning. They usually build to peak intensity within 10 to 15 minutes and rarely last longer than 30 minutes. However, repeated attacks may continue to recur for hours.

During the attack, the patient may fear he or she is dying, going crazy, or losing control of his or her emotions or behavior. The patient has a strong urge to escape or flee the place where the attack began. If the patient experiences chest pain or shortness of breath, he or she may go to a hospital emergency department or seek some other type of urgent assistance.

The frequency and severity of panic attacks vary from one person to the next. Attacks may arise once a week or in clusters separated by months. Because they occur spontaneously—without exposure to a known anxiety-producing situation—the patient worries about when the next one will occur and may restrict his or her lifestyle to avoid them.

Panic tally

Roughly 4.7% of the U.S. general population experiences panic disorder at some time in their lives. The disorder affects about twice as many women as men. The prevalence of panic disorder peaks in late adolescence and again at 35 to 50 years old (Katon & Ciechanowski, 2013). The earlier the onset, the greater the risk of coexisting illnesses, chronicity, and impairment. "Onset after the age of 45 is unusual but can occur" (APA, 2013, p. 210).

Affliction overlap

For many sufferers, panic disorder is complicated by major depressive disorder (10% to 65% lifetime comorbidity, [APA, 2013, p. 213]). The tendency to self-medicate with alcohol or antianxiety drugs may result in alcoholism and substance abuse disorders. Many patients with panic disorder also have additional anxiety disorders—including social phobia, GAD, specific phobia, and OCD.

Risk for suicide

According to the American Psychiatric Association (2013), panic attacks and a diagnosis of panic disorder are related to higher rates of suicide attempts and suicidal ideations. Katon and Ciechanowski (2013) state that "studies have shown a higher likelihood of suicide attempts among people with panic disorder than the general population." This risk increases in patients with a comorbid diagnosis of a mood disorder, personality disorders, or alcohol abuse.

Causes

Although intense stress or a sudden loss may trigger panic disorder, the underlying cause of the disorder involves a combination of genetic, biochemical, and other factors.

Genetic factors

Panic disorder tends to run in families. Eighteen percent to 41% of patients have first-degree relatives with the disorder. It also occurs to a much higher degree in identical twins, supporting the theory of a genetic basis (Katon & Ciechanowski, 2013). "A tendency to experience negative emotions, often labeled neuroticism or negative affect, is largely inherited and has been shown to be predictive of panic attacks" (Prenoveau & Craske, 2010, p. 79).

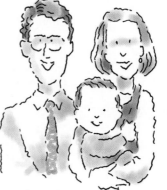

Biochemical abnormalities

Higher norepinephrine levels have been found in patients with panic attacks, suggesting a defect in the body's catecholamine system. The hypothalamic-pituitary-adrenal axis is involved in stress, which is related to the risk for anxiety disorders (Stahl & Grady, 2010, p. 8).

Some researchers believe that people with panic disorder may have a heightened sensitivity to somatic (physical) symptoms. This sensitivity, in turn, may trigger the autonomic system, which sets off a series of events leading to a panic attack (Sadock & Sadock, 2007, p. 588). Increases in respiratory rate, which is controlled partly by the amygdala, can cause shortness of breath, asthma, or a feeling of being smothered (Stahl & Grady, 2010, p. 9).

Cognitive and behavioral theory

Learning theory, which proposes that a person misinterprets symptoms, may explain some cases of panic disorder. The person fears that mild anxiety symptoms are the start of a major physical illness. The exaggerated fear triggers a panic attack. Behavioral theorists think "anxiety is a learned response either from parental behavior or through the process of classical conditioning" (Sadock & Sadock, 2007, p. 589).

Psychoanalytic theory

Some psychoanalysts think panic disorder results from failure to resolve the early childhood conflict of dependence versus independence. "Panic attacks [may] arise from an unsuccessful defense against anxiety-provoking impulses" (Sadock & Sadock, 2007, p. 589).

Medical conditions (Katon & Ciechanowski, 2013)

"Panic disorder is significantly comorbid with numerous medical symptoms and conditions, including, but not limited to, dizziness, cardiac arrhythmias, hyperthyroidism, asthma, chronic obstructive pulmonary disease, and irritable bowel syndrome" (APA, 2013, p. 214).

Life events

Intensely stressful life events or multiple stressors can contribute to panic disorder. Childhood adversity increases the risk of panic disorder developing as an adult. Childhood asthma and smoking also have been shown to increase this risk (Katon & Ciechanowski, 2013).

Temperament

"Anxious temperaments and anxiety sensitivity have also been shown to be risk factors for the development of panic disorder" (Katon & Ciechanowski, 2013).

Risk factors

Such physical illnesses as asthma, cardiovascular disease, and GI disorders may predispose a person to panic disorder by causing fear. The first experience of one of these conditions may be so frightening that it causes a panic attack.

Signs and symptoms of panic attack

- Extreme anxiety and fear
- Feelings of "impending doom" (term used when a person just "feels" like something bad is going to happen even when there is no evidence to support)
- Palpitations
- Breathing difficulty
- Chest pain
- Nausea
- Dizziness
- Chills or hot flashes.

"Typically, panic attacks come 'out of the blue' (i.e., suddenly and not in response to stress), are extremely intense, last a matter of minutes, and then subside" (Halter, 2014, p. 284). Patients sometimes report that they feel as though they are losing their mind or going crazy (APA, 2013). Panic disorder is defined by recurrent panic attacks combined with persistent worry or concern.

Diagnosis

Because some physical conditions and drug effects can mimic panic disorder, the medical provider may order tests to rule out an organic or pharmacologic basis for symptoms. For example, serum glucose measurements can rule out hypoglycemia, urine catecholamine and vanillylmandelic acid tests can exclude pheochromocytoma, and thyroid function tests can eliminate hyperthyroidism. Urine and serum toxicology tests can rule out the presence of psychoactive substances capable of triggering panic attacks, such as barbiturates, caffeine, and amphetamines (Baldwin, 2013). An official diagnosis of panic disorder is made if the patient meets the criteria set forth by the American Psychiatric Association (APA) in the *Diagnostic and Statistical Manual of Mental Disorders*, 5th Edition (*DSM-5*).

Treatment

Panic disorder is highly treatable with a combination of patient teaching, cognitive or behavioral therapies, and relaxation techniques. Biofeedback can also be of help to these patients. Some patients also require medication.

Patient teaching

Teaching the patient about the disorder and its physiologic effects can help the individual overcome it. Many patients experience some relief simply by understanding exactly what panic disorder is and how many others suffer from it.

Cognitive therapy

Cognitive restructuring can be helpful for patients who worry that their panic attacks mean they're going crazy or are about to have a heart attack. This method teaches them to replace those negative thoughts with more realistic, positive ways of viewing the attacks. It also helps them identify and evaluate the thoughts that precede anxiety and then restructure them to gain a more realistic perception.

Trigger talk

Through cognitive therapy, the patient can identify possible triggers for the panic attacks, such as a particular thought or situation or even a slight change in the heartbeat. Once the patient understands that the panic attack is separate and independent of the trigger, that trigger starts to lose some of its power to induce an attack.

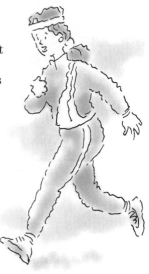

I'm not just jogging. I'm trying to induce tachycardia as part of my interoceptive conditioning.

Panic interrupted

In a technique called *interoceptive conditioning* (or *panic control treatment*), a therapist guides the patient through repeated exposure to the sensations he or she experiences during a panic attack (such as palpitations or dizziness). The feared sensations may be produced using such methods as controlled hyperventilation or physical exertion (such as running up a flight of stairs to cause tachycardia). Through this approach, the patient learns that these sensations needn't progress to a full-blown attack.

"Cognitive-behavioral therapy (CBT) was as effective as pharmacotherapy and demonstrated significantly lower drop-out rates. . . . Combined treatment with CBT and medication improves short-term outcomes better than CBT alone, but medication discontinuation posttreatment can actually lead to poorer outcomes than CBT alone" (Prenoveau & Craske, 2010, pp. 81 and 89).

Baby steps

Behavioral therapy also can help the patient deal with the situational avoidance associated with panic attacks. In one behavioral technique called *systematic desensitization*, a trained therapist helps the patient break down a fearful situation into small, manageable steps. The patient then performs the steps one at a time until he or she can master the most difficult step.

Relaxation techniques

Relaxation techniques help the patient cope with a panic attack by easing physical symptoms and directing the patient's attention elsewhere. These techniques include:
• deep-breathing exercises, which also reduces the risk of hyperventilation (a contributing factor for anxiety)
• progressive relaxation, which involves conscious tightening and relaxation of the skeletal muscles in a sequential fashion
• positive visualization or guided imagery, in which the patient elicits peaceful mental images or some other purposeful thought or action, promoting feelings of relaxation, renewed hope, and a sense of being in control of a stressful situation
• listening to calming music.

Biofeedback

Biofeedback is a technique in which an individual learns how to control physiologic reactions to stress in order to avert a panic attack. This is done with a computer application and equipment, which monitors heart rate variability.

Pharmacologic therapy

For some patients, the medical provider may prescribe antianxiety drugs (e.g., benzodiazepines such as lorazepam [Ativan]) or antidepressants (especially selective serotonin reuptake inhibitors [SSRIs] such as sertraline [Zoloft] or serotonin norepinephrine reuptake inhibitors [SNRIs] such as venlafaxine extended release [Effexor XR]). It may take a few weeks for the SSRI or SNRI to start working (Roy-Byrne, 2013). Combining an antianxiety drug with an antidepressant promotes rapid stabilization of panic symptoms. "This strategy provides rapid symptom relief but avoids the complications associated with long-term benzodiazepine use" (Boyd, 2012, p. 459). Some patients also benefit from beta blockers such as propranalol (Atenolol) and alpha-2 receptor agonists such as clonidine (Catapres), as they suppress the somatic manifestations that can occur with anxiety (Boyd, 2012).

Nursing interventions

These nursing interventions may be appropriate for patients with panic disorder.

During a panic attack
• Stay with the patient until the attack subsides. If left alone, the patient may grow even more anxious.
• If the patient loses control, guide the patient to a smaller, quieter area.

Just breathe

- Instructing the patient to take slow breaths can help to prevent hyperventilation. Breathing in and out slowly and deeply with the patient can help to shift thoughts away from the distressing symptoms (Halter, 2014).

> Keep a panicky patient away from crowds, bright lights, and noise.

Serenity now

- Maintain a calm, serene approach. "Anxiety is contagious and can be transferred from staff to client or vice versa" (Townsend, 2014, p. 544).
- Speak in short, simple sentences, and slowly give the patient one direction at a time. Avoid giving lengthy explanations and asking too many questions.

Out with the extraneous

- Reduce external stimuli, such as groups of people, as this can increase anxiety. Excessive stimuli may be overwhelming. Dim lights if necessary.
- Provide a safe environment, and prevent harm to the patient or others.

Cut the patient some slack

- Encourage the patient to express his or her feelings and to cry, if necessary.
- Administer medication (such as antianxiety medication) as ordered by physician.

Between panic attacks

- Teach relaxation techniques.
- Determine things that increase anxiety such as caffeine and teach the patient how to avoid those substances.
- Encourage the patient to discuss his or her fears. Help the patient identify situations or events that trigger the attacks.
- Ask questions to clarify and dispute illogical thinking:

 What evidence do you have?

 Explain the logic in that.

 Are you basing that conclusion on fact or feeling?

What's the worst thing that can happen? (Halter, 2014, p. 286)

- Discuss alternative coping mechanisms such as the use of positive self-talk. Using positive statements such as "I can control my anxiety" replaces negative self-talk and is an effective form of cognitive restructuring (Halter, 2014).

• Monitor therapeutic and adverse effects of prescribed medications. Teach the patient how to recognize adverse effects and when to use medication for panic attacks and/or anxiety.

• Instruct the patient to notify the medical prescriber before discontinuing medication because abrupt withdrawal could cause severe symptoms.

• Make appropriate referrals to a mental health professional. Dissuade the patient from visiting the hospital emergency room for symptom relief because of the frantic atmosphere.

Agoraphobia

"Agoraphobia is intense, excessive anxiety or fear about being in places or situations from which escape might not be available" (Halter, 2014, p. 284). Patients with agoraphobia worry they won't be able to get somewhere safe and may fear they'll have a panic attack or panic symptoms (such as dizziness, vomiting, loss of control, or difficulty breathing). Eventually, they begin to avoid situations where they feel uncomfortable.

Holed up at home

Without treatment, agoraphobia may get worse. In extreme cases, the person becomes a prisoner in his or her home, too fearful to leave the "safe" zone. In less severe cases, the individual is able to engage in activities or travel if a trusted companion goes along.

Many experts view agoraphobia as an adverse behavioral outcome of repeated panic attacks and the subsequent worry, preoccupation, and avoidance. However, agoraphobia sometimes occurs without a history of panic disorder. (See "Panic disorder," page 196.)

Scary territory

Among agoraphobic patients, common fears include large public spaces (such as parks, malls, theaters, and supermarkets), crowds, and places where the person feels trapped (such as airplanes or driving in rush-hour traffic or on a bridge). Most patients can verbalize what they fear and where they fear it, although some know only that they have a sense of dread.

The facts

"Every year approximately 1.7% of adolescents and adults have a diagnosis of agoraphobia. The disorder is twice as common in women as men" (APA, 2013, p. 219). Age of onset in two-thirds of cases occur before the age of 35 years. In 30% of community samples and 50% of clinic samples that report agoraphobia, panic attacks and panic disorder precede the onset of agoraphobia (APA, 2013, p. 219).

Agoraphobic patients have higher depression and suicide rates than the general population and may be prone to substance use disorders, especially alcohol. Comorbid anxiety disorders are common as is PTSD (APA, 2013, p. 221).

Causes

The exact cause of agoraphobia isn't known. Theories include biochemical imbalances (especially related to neurotransmitters) and environmental factors. The disorder may run in families, suggesting a genetic basis. "Heritability rate for agoraphobia is 61% which is the strongest association of all of the phobias. Negative events in childhood and other stressful events are associated with the onset of agoraphobia" (APA, 2013, p. 220).

McCabe (2013a) states that personality factors such as introversion, anxiety sensitivity, dependent personality traits, lack of perceived control, and low self-efficacy have all been associated with agoraphobia. In addition, cognitive factors include fear of having an illness, bodily preoccupation, and fear that the individual will be trapped or unable to cope due to a physical limitation.

Signs and symptoms

The patient's avoidance of the feared situation significantly impairs daily functioning. "More than one-third of individuals with agoraphobia are completely homebound and unable to work" (APA, 2013, p. 220).

The patient may report or exhibit:
- fear and avoidance of open spaces or public places
- fear or anxiety of enclosed spaces such as theatres or airplanes
- fear of standing in line or being in a crowd
- fear of being outside the home
- concern that help might not be available in public places.

If the patient also has panic disorder, he or she may express concern that a panic attack in public will lead to embarrassment or the inability to escape. (For symptoms of a panic attack, see "Panic disorder," page 196.)

Diagnosis

Agoraphobia is diagnosed when the patient meets the criteria in the *DSM-5*. It is important to note that this is a separate diagnosis from panic disorder. Agoraphobia can exist as an isolate diagnosis or in conjunction with the diagnosis of panic disorder.

Treatment

Treatment usually includes both medication and behavioral therapy. The medical provider may prescribe an SSRI, such as paroxetine (Paxil), or an SNRI, such as duloxetine hydrochloride (Cymbalta). To treat a panic attack in progress, the patient may receive a benzodiazepine, such as alprazolam (Xanax). Treatment is similar to the treatment of panic disorder (see p. 199).

The overexposure cure

One treatment for agoraphobia is desensitization, which gradually exposes the patient to the situation that triggers fear and avoidance. Recently, this has included exposure to internal stimuli (e.g., rapid heart rate, increased respiratory rate), which can precipitate symptoms. Such exposure helps the patient learn to cope with the situation and break the mental connection between the situation and anxiety. The patient may receive antianxiety medications to reduce anxiety during desensitization sessions (Sadock & Sadock, 2007, p. 596).

Implosive therapy has also been used in the treatment of agoraphobia. The patient is presented with anxiety-provoking imagery, which depicts the fear as vividly as possible. This technique is frequently used in conjunction with flooding where a patient is desensitized by being repeatedly exposed to the trigger without breaks until the anxiety subsides. "For example, a patient with ophidiophobia might be presented with a real snake repeatedly until his or her anxiety decreases" (Boyd, 2012, p. 464).

Patients may also benefit from relaxation techniques as well as psychotherapy in which they discuss underlying emotional conflicts with a therapist or support group.

Nursing interventions

For a patient with agoraphobia, these nursing interventions may be appropriate.
• Encourage the patient to discuss the feared object or situation.
• Collaborate with the patient and multidisciplinary team to develop and implement a systematic desensitization program that exposes the patient gradually to the feared situation in a controlled environment.

- Provide training in assertiveness skills to reduce submissive and fearful responses. Such strategies allow the patient to experiment with new coping skills and encourage him or her to discard ineffective ones.
- Administer antianxiety or antidepressant medications, as ordered.
- If the patient is taking a medication for anxiety, stress the importance of complying with prescribed therapy. Teach the patient about adverse drug reactions and what needs to be reported to the prescriber.

Generalized Anxiety Disorder

Occasional anxiety is a normal part of life. However, with GAD, the anxiety and worry is persistent, generalized, and excessive.

Effects of GAD range from mild to severe and incapacitating. To relieve anxiety, many with GAD self-medicate with alcohol and antianxiety drugs.

Constant worrying can feel like the weight of the world on your shoulders. It can cause your heart to be unhappy with a chronic elevated heart rate.

Egad, that's a lot of GAD

GAD affects an estimated 3% of the general population, occurring more often in women than men. The lifetime risk of developing GAD is 9.0%. Age of onset is typically in the early 30s, but all age groups—including children and the elderly—are affected.

Usually, GAD emerges slowly, although occasionally, it's triggered by a stressful event. GAD tends to be chronic, with periods of exacerbation and remission. "Many people with GAD report that they have felt anxious and nervous all of their lives" (APA, 2013, p. 223).

Medley of maladies

Up to 25% of patients with GAD go on to develop panic disorder. Many also have other psychiatric disorders, such as social phobia (34%), specific phobia (35%), depression, or dysthymic disorder (Baldwin, 2013).

Untreated, GAD can cause constant, unremitting tension that ultimately results in immunosuppression, leaving the patient more susceptible to physical illnesses. According to Baldwin (2013), "worrying and GAD have been commonly associated with increased blood pressure, coronary heart disease, and it does not benefit health promoting behaviors."

Causes

The exact cause of GAD is unknown. As with other anxiety disorders, genetic, biochemical, psychosocial, and other factors are suspected.

Genetic factors

"One-third of the risk of experiencing GAD is genetic, and these genetic factors overlap with the risk of neuroticism and are shared with other anxiety and mood disorder, particularly major depressive disorder" (APA, 2013, p. 224).

Biochemical abnormalities

Imbalances in serotonin, norepinephrine, glutamate, and GABA, an amino acid, may play a key role in susceptibility to GAD. Serotonin seems to be vital to feelings of well-being, whereas GABA helps prevent nerve cells from overfiring. Glutamate is an excitatory neurotransmitter. Serotonin is a key neurotransmitter that innervates the amygdala as well as other parts of the brain such as the prefrontal cortex and thalamus, which regulates fear and worry (Stahl, 2013, p. 405). "GABA is the principal inhibitory neurotransmitter in the brain and normally plays an important regulatory role in reducing the activity of many neurons, including those in the amygdala and feedback loops from the prefrontal cortex" (Stahl, 2013, p. 397).

You say there's a glitch in my GABA? Well, that's one more thing for me to worry about.

Psychosocial and environmental factors

Children of anxious parents may learn to see the world as dangerous and uncontrollable, predisposing them to GAD. "Behavioral inhibition, negative affectivity (neuroticism), and harm avoidance have been associated with GAD" (APA, 2013, p. 224).

Death of a loved one, illness, job loss, or divorce can increase a person's stress level and may trigger anxiety or stress responses. However, experts believe stress is merely a trigger for GAD, not the cause.

Risk factors and attention to things that might be scary

Risk factors for GAD include unresolved conflicts, a tendency to misinterpret events, and such behaviors as shyness and avoidance of new situations. In Baldwin (2013), "patients with GAD have been found to allocate extensive attentional resources to threatening stimuli, detect 'threats' rapidly and effectively, and misinterpret ambiguous information as being threatening."

Signs and symptoms

Signs and symptoms of GAD fall into three general categories—excessive physiologic arousal, distorted cognitive processes, and poor coping.

Excessive physiologic arousal

With excessive physiologic arousal, the patient may report or exhibit:
- shortness of breath
- tachycardia or palpitations
- dry mouth
- sweating
- nausea or diarrhea
- inability to relax
- muscle tension, aches, and spasms
- irritability
- fatigue
- restlessness
- trembling
- headache
- cold, clammy hands
- insomnia.

Distorted cognitive processes

Signs and symptoms of distorted cognitive processes include:
- poor concentration
- unrealistic assessment of problems
- excessive anxiety and worry over minor matters
- fears of grave misfortune or death.

Poor coping

A patient with poor coping may exhibit:
- avoidance
- procrastination
- poor problem-solving skills.

Diagnosis

Because anxiety is the central feature of many mental disorders, the patient should undergo a psychiatric evaluation to rule out phobias, OCD, depression, and acute schizophrenia. GAD is characterized by excessive worry lasting more than 6 months that significantly impairs the patient's ability to function in his or her personal and social life. The diagnosis of GAD is confirmed when the patient meets the criteria from the *DSM-5*.

Treatment

For patients with mild anxiety, nonpharmacologic methods should be tried first. Relaxation techniques and biofeedback can decrease arousal. Applied relaxation targets the physiologic effects of anxiety (Wells & Fisher, 2010, p. 33). Psychotherapy helps the patient identify and deal with the cause of anxiety, anticipate the patient's reactions, and plan effective responses to deal with anxiety.

Other treatment options include cognitive therapy and medications.

Cognitive therapy

Cognitive therapy reduces cognitive distortions by teaching the patient how to restructure his or her thoughts and view worries more realistically. Wells and Fisher (2010) assert that "individuals with high levels of anxiety have core beliefs/schemas that overestimate the dangerousness of the world, with a corresponding underestimate of his or her ability to cope" (p. 34).

Worry ledger

In one cognitive therapy approach, the patient is taught to record worries and list evidence that justifies or contradicts each one. The patient also learns that "worrying about worry" maintains anxiety and that avoidance and procrastination are ineffective problem-solving techniques.

Cognitive-behavioral therapy

A review of literature and clinical trials have shown that CBT is a first-line treatment for GAD. This involves both behavior by modifying problematic coping strategies and cognitive approaches (e.g., reality testing negative thoughts) as well as approaches that address the physiologic aspects of GAD (relaxation strategies) (Wells & Fisher, 2010, p. 34–35).

Biofeedback training

Biofeedback training eases physical symptoms of anxiety by teaching the patient how to become aware of—and then consciously control—various body functions (including blood pressure, heart and respiratory rates, skin temperature, and perspiration). Using a biofeedback device, the patient learns when changes in these functions occur. With adequate training, the patient can repeat this response at will, even when not hooked up to the biofeedback device.

Pharmacologic therapy

Drugs may be considered if anxiety significantly impairs the patient's daily functioning. Antianxiety agents, including such benzodiazepines as diazepam, lorazepam, and clonazepam, are commonly prescribed. Benzodiazepines reduce anxiety by decreasing vigilance and easing somatic symptoms (for instance, muscle tension). "Although widely used in patients with GAD, benzodiazepine treatment remains somewhat controversial. If the patient self-medicates, benzodiazepines may complicate because of their addictive qualities" (Boyd, 2012, p. 481). These drugs are most effective when used initially to manage symptoms while waiting for other pharmacologic interventions to "kick in," as many take a few weeks to produce an optimal effect. SSRIs and SNRIs are the preferred medications in the treatment of GAD. First-line medications include the SSRIs paroxetine (Paxil), sertraline (Zoloft), citalopram (Celexa), and escitalopram (Lexapro). Fluoxetine (Prozac) and fluvoxamine (Luvox) have also been found to be effective. SNRIs include venlafaxine extended release (Effexor XR) and duloxetine (Cymbalta) (Bystritsky, 2013). Second-line medications include tricyclic antidepressants (e.g., imipramine), benzodiazepines, buspirone, and certain anticonvulsants (e.g., pregabalin). Other medications that have been found to be helpful include mirtazapine, quetiapine, tiagabine, hydroxyzine (Bystritsky, 2013), and, in practice, gabapentin.

Hangin' in there

Buspirone appears to be as effective as benzodiazepines in treating GAD. It causes less sedation and rarely leads to physical dependence or tolerance. However, onset of action takes several weeks, so patients should be told to expect a delay in symptom relief. The same applies to SSRIs and SNRIs. Benzodiazepines can be used to assist the patient with the symptoms of GAD until the other medication takes effect (Bystritsky, 2013).

Nursing interventions

When caring for a patient with GAD, these nursing interventions may be appropriate.
• Stay with the patient when he or she is anxious. Remain calm and nonjudgmental. Suggest activities that distract the individual from the anxiety symptoms.
• Encourage the patient to discuss his or her feelings.
• Reduce environmental stimuli.

Stress-busting strategies

• Teach the patient progressive muscle relaxation, guided imagery, deep breathing, or other relaxation techniques. Besides easing anxiety, these methods reduce the risk of hyperventilation, help him or her focus on something other than the anxiety, and interrupt the flow of negative or stressful thoughts.

• Provide nutritional counseling to reduce stress and promote health. Advise the patient to avoid caffeine, energy drinks, and alcohol, for instance. A well-balanced diet is also important in decreasing stress.

• Instruct the patient in time-management skills, such as making lists, setting realistic goals, and grouping tasks in batches to help manage anxiety.

• Make appropriate referrals to a mental health professional. Dissuade the patient from visiting the hospital emergency department for symptom relief because of the frantic atmosphere.

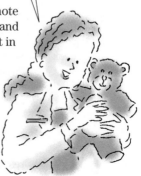

This is kind of embarrassing, but my teddy bear helps me to relax and get my mind off my anxiety.

Drug discussions

• Administer prescribed antianxiety agents, as ordered.

• Inform the patient and family that these drugs may cause adverse reactions, such as drowsiness, fatigue, ataxia, blurred vision, slurred speech, tremors, and hypotension. Instruct the patient to report these to the medical provider.

• Advise the patient not to discontinue medications except with the medical provider's approval because abrupt withdrawal could cause severe symptoms.

Social anxiety disorder (social phobia)

Social anxiety disorder refers to marked, persistent fear or anxiety in social or performance situations. The anxiety causes the one with social anxiety to avoid these situations whenever possible out of fear of embarrassment, scrutiny, humiliation, or ridicule. Common situations that provoke anxiety include speaking or eating in public and using a public restroom. The hallmark physical response is blushing.

Could you be specific?

Social phobia may be limited to performing (e.g., musicians, athletes) or speaking in public (e.g., public officials). It can be generalized where the patient has symptoms almost anytime the individual is with other people (e.g., social situations) and being observed (e.g., drinking and eating).

Spotlight shunners

Many people with social phobia are concerned that others will see their anxiety symptoms (such as sweating or blushing) or will judge them to be weak, stupid, or crazy. Some fear they'll faint, lose bowel or bladder control, or go mentally blank.

Even when around familiar people, they may feel overwhelmed, fearing that others are watching their every move and making negative judgments about them.

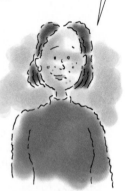

School wouldn't be so bad if the other kids weren't there.

Expecting the worst

Socially phobic people may have anticipatory anxiety for days or weeks before the dreaded event. Such anxiety may further handicap the person's performance and heighten embarrassment.

The disorder can be debilitating, preventing the patient from going to work or school on some days. It can cause loss of a job or job promotion out of fear of speaking in public, or result in continual inconvenience—for instance, from fear of using a public lavatory.

Also of concern

Patients with social anxiety disorder have high rates of substance use disorders and other psychiatric conditions (such as major depression, bipolar disorder, and body dysmorphic disorder) (APA, 2013, p. 208). Avoidant personality disorder is also prevalent. Those with social anxiety disorder have a higher rate of suicide than the general population (Schneier, 2013).

Numeric rundown

An estimated 7% of Americans suffer from social anxiety disorder. More common in women, the disorder typically starts in childhood or adolescence. Median age of onset is 13 years. It rarely develops in adults except for some that develop it after a stressful or humiliating event (APA, 2013, pp. 204–205).

Causes

For many people with social anxiety disorder, it's linked with the traits of shyness and social inhibition, early childhood adversity, and parental/peer influences. "Persons with social anxiety disorder have biased, negative cognitions about their own social performance, others' perceptions of them, and the consequences of those perceptions" (Schneier, 2013).

Female gender and a family history of social anxiety disorder are also linked to this disorder (Schneier, 2013). The interaction of biological and environmental factors can cause a child with a genetic predisposition and expression of high behavioral inhibition to be socially anxious as modeled by parents. First-degree relatives of those with social anxiety disorder have a two to six times greater chance of having this disorder (APA, 2013, p. 205).

Scientists exploring biological aspects of the disorder believe there may be a physiologic basis for increased sensitivity to autonomic arousal (e.g., increased heart rate, trembling). Neurotransmitters implicated in social anxiety disorder include serotonin, possibly dopamine, increased glutamate levels, and peripheral oxytocin. Others are investigating the role of the amygdala, a brain structure that controls fear responses. The amygdala plays a role in the hyperactivity of limbic and paralimbic fear circuits. The medial prefrontal cortex may have decreased activation. The hypothalamic-pituitary-adrenal axis may have increased reactivity to social stressors especially in those with a history of early childhood abuse (Schneier, 2013).

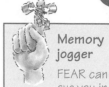

Memory jogger

FEAR can cue you in to signs and symptoms of phobias.

F: Fear of an object or a situation

E: Emotional conflict occurring unconsciously

A: Avoidant behavior demonstrated

R: Reacts with severe anxiety

Signs and symptoms

Signs and symptoms of social anxiety disorder may include:
• fear or avoidance of eating, writing, or speaking in public; being stared at; or meeting strangers
• pronounced sensitivity to criticism
• low self-esteem
• scholastic underachievement because of test anxiety.
    Physical manifestations may include:
• blushing
• profuse sweating
• trembling
• nausea or stomach upset
• difficulty talking.

Worried about looking worried

Visible signs of social anxiety disorder, such as blushing or profuse sweating, heighten the patient's fear of disapproval and may become an additional focus of fear. Thus, a vicious cycle may begin: The more the patient worries about experiencing symptoms of social anxiety disorder, the greater chance of developing symptoms.

Diagnosis

No specific test can diagnose social anxiety disorder. Differential diagnosis to separate this disorder from other related disorders (such as GAD, specific phobias, and panic disorder) is important. An official diagnosis is confirmed if the patient meets the criteria in the *DSM-5*.

Treatment

A mental health professional may use desensitization therapy to gradually reintroduce the feared situation while coaching the patient on relaxation techniques.

Relaxation techniques, such as progressive muscle relaxation, deep-breathing exercises, or listening to calming music, may be helpful, too. By role-playing in guided imagery, the patient rehearses ways to relax while confronting a feared object or situation.

CBT have been demonstrated to produce positive results in the treatment of social anxiety disorder. A combination of exposure and cognitive techniques has been the most useful (Jakatdar & Heimberg, 2010).

A model for behavior

Modeling behavior and assertiveness training also can be valuable. In modeling behavior, the patient observes someone modeling, or demonstrating, appropriate behavior when confronted with the feared situation.

Thought police

A behavioral technique called *negative thought-stopping* can reduce the frequency and duration of disturbing thoughts by interrupting them and substituting competing thoughts. In thought-stopping, the patient is taught to recognize negative thoughts and then use an intense distracting stimulus (such as snapping a rubber band around the wrist) to stop the thought. With practice, the patient can control thoughts without this distracting stimulus.

Stop right there, negative thought! I'm making a citizen's arrest!

Pharmacologic therapy

SSRIs are the most commonly prescribed medication in the treatment of social anxiety disorder. Paroxetine (Paxil) was the first SSRI approved by the U.S. Food and Drug Administration (FDA) for the treatment of social anxiety disorder. Other SSRIs approved by the FDA are fluvoxamine (Luvox), sertraline (Zoloft), and venlafaxine XR (Effexor XR) (Stahl, 2011).

Alpha-2-delta ligands such as gabapentin (Neurontin) and pregabalin (Lyrica) have also been first-line choices for some prescribers (Stahl, 2013, p. 418).

Beta adrenergic blockers (e.g., propranolol) are used for performance-type social anxiety disorder. It is not effective in generalized social anxiety disorder. Benzodiazepines (e.g., clonazepam [Klonopin], lorazepam [Ativan]) have very limited usefulness for generalized social anxiety disorder but some use in performance-type social anxiety disorder, as sedation and potential for abuse and dependence are very real risks in the use of these types of medications (Stein, 2011).

Nursing interventions

These nursing interventions may be appropriate for patients with social anxiety disorder.
• No matter how illogical the patient's phobia seems, avoid the urge to trivialize the fears. Remember that the behavior represents an essential coping mechanism. A simplistic pep talk or ridicule may cause more alienation or worsen preexisting low self-esteem.
• Keep in mind that the patient fears criticism. Encourage the individual to interact with others and provide continuous support and positive reinforcement.
• Teach the patient progressive muscle relaxation, guided imagery, or thought-stopping techniques as appropriate.
• Gradual desensitization to the anxiety-provoking situation can be useful.
• Ask the patient how he or she normally copes with the fear. When the patient is able to face the fear, encourage the individual to verbalize and explore personal strengths and resources with you.
• Suggest ways to channel energy and relieve stress, such as running and creative activities.
• Don't let the patient withdraw completely. If the patient is being treated as an outpatient, suggest small steps to help overcome fears. *Ask the patient what will help him or her overcome the anxiety.*
• If the patient is taking a medication for the anxiety, stress the importance of complying with prescribed therapy. Teach the patient about adverse drug reactions and what needs to be reported to the prescriber.

Specific phobia

In specific phobia (also called *simple phobia*), a person experiences intense, irrational anxiety when exposed to a specific feared object (such as a snake) or situation (such as being in an enclosed space). The exposure can take place either in real life or through images from movies, television, photographs, or the imagination.

For many, the anxiety leads to avoidance or disabling behavior that interferes with activities or even confines them to the home. Anxiety may reach panic levels, especially if there's no apparent escape from the feared thing or situation.

Just can't help feeling that way

Although adults with specific phobias realize their fears are irrational and out of proportion to any actual danger, they still experience severe anxiety or panic attacks when facing (or perhaps even thinking about) the feared object or situation. Most try to avoid the stimulus or endure exposure to the stimulus with great difficulty. Some even make important career or personal decisions to avoid the object of their fears.

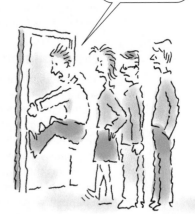

I'm terrified of enclosed spaces! Let me out of here!

Types of specific phobias

(APA, 2013, p. 198)

The *DSM-5* classifies specific phobias into five main groups:
- natural environment type (e.g., heights, storms, water)
- animal type (e.g., spiders, insects, dogs)
- blood-injection-injury type (e.g., needles, invasive medical procedures)
- situational type (e.g., airplanes, elevators, enclosed spaces)
- other type (e.g., situations that may lead to choking or vomiting; in children, e.g., loud sounds or costumed characters).

Many people have multiple specific phobias. (See *The phobia file.*)

Phobia figures

Specific phobias affect about 9.4% to 12.5% of the U.S. population. They're more common in women than men. Onset occurs in childhood or early adolescence with the majority developing the phobia before 10 years old (Koerner, Rogojanski, & Antony, 2010, pp. 60–61). Age of onset varies with the type of phobia.

Most specific phobias persist for years or even decades. Mean duration of the disorder is 20 years. Only about 20% remit spontaneously without treatment (McCabe, 2013b).

Comorbidities associated with specific phobia include other anxiety disorders, mood disorders, and alcohol dependence. Individuals with specific phobia are often phobic of multiple things or situations (McCabe, 2013b). "Individuals with blood-injection-injury phobia show a unique propensity to vasovagal syncope (faint) in the presence of the phobic stimulus" (APA, 2013, p.200).

The phobia file (http://phobialist.com/index.html)

You name it, and somebody somewhere is afraid of it. In the list here (which is by no means all-inclusive), you can read up on phobias for almost every letter of the alphabet.

A

Ablutophobia: Fear of washing

Acarophobia: Fear of itching or insects that cause itching

Acerophobia: Fear of sourness

Achluophobia: Fear of darkness

Aerophobia: Fear of drafts

Ailurophobia: Fear of cats

Antlophobia: Fear of floods

Apiphobia: Fear of bees

Arachnophobia: Fear of spiders

Astrapophobia: Fear of lightning

B

Bacteriophobia: Fear of bacteria

Bathmophobia: Fear of stairs or steep slopes

Bathophobia: Fear of depth

Blennophobia: Fear of slime

Bogyphobia: Fear of the bogeyman

Botanophobia: Fear of plants

Bromidrosiphobia or bromidrophobia: Fear of body smells

C

Cacophobia: Fear of ugliness

Cancerophobia: Fear of cancer

Carnophobia: Fear of meat

Catagelophobia: Fear of being ridiculed

Catapedaphobia: Fear of jumping from high or low places

Cathisophobia: Fear of sitting

Chaetophobia: Fear of hair

Coprastasophobia: Fear of constipation

D

Demophobia: Fear of crowds

Didaskaleinophobia: Fear of going to school

Dikephobia: Fear of justice

Dishabiliophobia: Fear of undressing in front of someone

Domatophobia or oikophobia: Fear of houses

Dysmorphophobia: Fear of deformity

Dystychiphobia: Fear of accidents

E

Ecclesiophobia: Fear of church

Ecophobia: Fear of home

Eisoptrophobia: Fear of mirrors or seeing oneself in a mirror

Emetophobia: Fear of vomiting

Enochlophobia: Fear of crowds

F

Febriphobia: Fear of fever

Frigophobia: Fear of cold or cold things

G

Gamophobia: Fear of marriage

Gerascophobia: Fear of growing old

Geumaphobia or geumophobia: Fear of taste

Glossophobia: Fear of speaking in public

Gynephobia or gynophobia: Fear of women

H

Heliophobia: Fear of the sun

Herpetophobia: Fear of reptiles or creepy, crawly things

Heterophobia: Fear of the opposite sex

Hierophobia: Fear of religious or sacred things

Hippophobia: Fear of horses

Hippopotomonstrosesquippedaliophobia: Fear of long words

Hypsiphobia: Fear of height

I

Iatrophobia: Fear of doctors

Ichthyophobia: Fear of fish

Ideophobia: Fear of ideas

Illyngophobia: Fear of vertigo or feeling dizzy when looking down

Insectophobia: Fear of insects

Iophobia: Fear of poison

Isolophobia: Fear of solitude

K

Kainolophobia: Fear of novelty

Kainophobia: Fear of anything new, novelty

Kakorrhaphiophobia: Fear of failure or defeat

Katagelophobia: Fear of ridicule

Kathisophobia: Fear of sitting down

Kopophobia: Fear of fatigue

L

Levophobia: Fear of objects to the left

Ligyrophobia: Fear of loud noises

Lilapsophobia: Fear of tornadoes and hurricanes

Logophobia: Fear of words

M

Macrophobia: Fear of long waits

Mageirocophobia: Fear of cooking

Maieusiophobia: Fear of childbirth

Medomalacuphobia: Fear of losing an erection

Menophobia: Fear of menstruation

Metallophobia: Fear of metal

Microbiophobia: Fear of microbes

Myctophobia: Fear of darkness

Myrmecophobia: Fear of ants

N

Neopharmaphobia: Fear of new drugs

Neophobia: Fear of anything new

Nephophobia: Fear of clouds

Noctiphobia: Fear of the night

(continued)

The phobia file (continued)

Nostophobia: Fear of returning home

Novercaphobia: Fear of one's stepmother

O

Ochlophobia: Fear of crowds or mobs

Ochophobia: Fear of vehicles

Oenophobia: Fear of wines

Olfactophobia: Fear of smells

Ombrophobia: Fear of rain

Optophobia: Fear of opening one's eyes

Ornithophobia: Fear of birds

P

Pagophobia: Fear of ice or frost

Panphobia: Fear of everything

Panthophobia: Fear of suffering and disease

Pediculophobia: Fear of lice

Pedophobia: Fear of children

Phalacrophobia: Fear of becoming bald

Photophobia: Fear of light

Pogonophobia: Fear of beards

Potamophobia: Fear of rivers

Prosophobia: Fear of progress

Psellismophobia: Fear of stuttering

Pyrophobia: Fear of fire

R

Ranidaphobia: Fear of frogs

Rhypophobia: Fear of defecation

Rhytiphobia: Fear of getting wrinkles

Rupophobia: Fear of dirt

S

Sciophobia: Fear of shadows

Scoleciphobia: Fear of worms

Scolionophobia: Fear of school

Scotophobia: Fear of darkness

Scriptophobia: Fear of writing in public

Selachophobia: Fear of sharks

Selaphobia: Fear of light flashes

Sesquipedalophobia: Fear of long words

Siderodromophobia: Fear of trains

Syngenesophobia: Fear of relatives

T

Thaasophobia: Fear of sitting

Thalassophobia: Fear of the sea

Thanatophobia: Fear of death

Thermophobia: Fear of heat

Tocophobia: Fear of pregnancy or childbirth

Triskaidekaphobia: Fear of the number 13

Trypanophobia: Fear of injections

U

Uranophobia: Fear of heaven

Urophobia: Fear of urine or urinating

V

Vaccinophobia: Fear of inoculations

Verbophobia: Fear of words

Verminophobia: Fear of germs

Vestiphobia: Fear of clothing

W

Wiccaphobia: Fear of witches and witchcraft

X

Xanthophobia: Fear of the color yellow or the word yellow

Xenophobia: Fear of strangers or foreigners

Xerophobia: Fear of dryness

Xylophobia: Fear of wooden objects; fear of forests

Xyrophobia: Fear of razors

Z

Zelophobia: Fear of jealousy

Zoophobia: Fear of animals

Causes

No one knows what causes specific phobias. Because they seem to run in families (especially those involving blood or injury), researchers suspect that genetic predisposition plays a role. Neurobiological factors that could play a role in specific phobias include hyperactivation in the amygdala and insula (McCabe, 2013b).

Other factors that may predispose a person to a specific phobia include:

- experiencing or observing a trauma
- repeated warnings of danger about the feared object or situation

- panic attacks when exposed to the feared object or situation
- disgust sensitivity (the tendency to experience disgust in response to certain stimuli)
- anxiety sensitivity (believing that the physical sensations of anxiety are harmful)
- increased attentional biases to perceived threats.

> Phobias involving blood tend to run in families.

Role models in fear

Family members may have phobias and the patient may have learned to adopt them. Spontaneous, unexpected panic attacks also appear to play a role in development of specific phobia. Cognitive and perceptual distortions consistent with the phobia support continuation of the phobia. Direct conditioning, vicarious acquisition, and informational transmission are other factors in the development of a specific phobia. Direct conditioning is "experiencing a traumatic event in the phobic situation such as being hurt of frightened. . . . Vicarious acquisition involves observing someone behave fearfully in the phobic situation or witnessing a traumatic event (e.g., seeing someone being bit by a dog). . . . Informational transmission involves learning to be fearful through information obtained verbally from others or through the media" (McCabe, 2013b). "Visual and somatic mental imagery may also play a role in the maintenance of specific phobia" (Koerner et al., 2010, p. 64).

Suicide risk

"Individuals with specific phobia are up to 60% more likely to make a suicide attempt than individuals without the diagnosis. This may be due to comorbidity with personality disorders and other anxiety disorders," (APA, 2013, p. 201).

Signs and symptoms

The patient experiences severe anxiety when confronted with the feared thing or situation. If the individual routinely avoids the object of the phobia, the person may have low self-esteem; depression; and feelings of weakness, cowardice, or ineffectiveness.

Diagnosis

Specific phobia diagnosis is considered when the patient has a history of anxiety when exposed to a specific object or situation. This anxiety can also occur with anticipation of the object or situation. Official diagnosis hinges on the patient meeting the criteria in the *DSM-5*. As mentioned previously, diagnosis of specific phobia is further specified into one of five types (animal, natural environment, blood-infection-injury, situational, other) (APA, 2013, p. 198).

Treatment (Koerner et al., 2010, pp. 64–65, 67)

First-line treatment is CBT in combination with exposure treatment (Swinson & McCabe, 2012). Successful treatment usually involves desensitization or exposure therapy in which a mental health professional and a trusted companion gradually exposes the patient to the feared object of situation (p. 67). "The majority of patients benefit significantly from such treatment" (p. 64). It can be especially helpful for phobias involving driving, flying, heights, bridges, or elevators. Applied tension has been shown to be the most effective for phobias involving blood injection. The muscular tension applied temporarily increases blood pressure and prevents fainting.

Other techniques

Relaxation, breathing exercises, and thought-stopping can reduce anxiety symptoms. Role-playing in guided imagery teaches the patient to relax while confronting a feared object or situation.

Pharmacologic therapy

"The consensus has been that psychotropic medication, either in isolation or in combination with psychological treatment, does not lead to appreciable improvement in specific phobia" (Koerner et al., 2010, p. 64).

No proven drug treatments for specific phobias exist, but the medical provider may prescribe medications to reduce anxiety symptoms in advance of a phobic situation, such as flying in an airplane. Benzodiazepines (e.g., lorazepam [Ativan]) are most often used in this situation (Swinson & McCabe, 2012). SSRIs (e.g., sertraline [Zoloft]) have also been used as a second-line treatment for specific phobia. Current research is showing that D-cycloserine shows promise as an effective augmentation for exposure therapy in the treatment of specific phobia and other anxiety disorders. Hydrocortisone is also being studied as an augmentation medication (Swinson & McCabe, 2012).

Nursing interventions

These nursing interventions may be appropriate for patients with specific phobia.

• Encourage the patient to discuss the feared object or situation.

• Collaborate with the patient and the multidisciplinary team to develop and implement a systematic desensitization program in which the patient is systematically exposed to the feared object or situation in a controlled environment.

• Teach the patient assertiveness skills to help reduce submissive, fearful responses. Such strategies enable the patient to experiment with new coping skills and discard coping skills that haven't worked in the past.

• Instruct the patient in relaxation and thought-stopping techniques as appropriate.

• To increase self-esteem and reduce anxiety, explain to the patient that the phobia is a way of coping with anxiety.

• Administer medications as ordered.

Posttraumatic Stress Disorder

PTSD is considered a trauma- and stressor-related disorder. There is a close relationship between anxiety disorders and PTSD. However, there are marked differences that place PTSD in a different diagnostic category (APA, 2013). PTSD can occur after someone experiences or witnesses a serious traumatic event, such as wartime combat, a natural disaster, rape, murder, childhood sexual abuse, or torture. The disorder is characterized by persistent nightmares, recurrent flashbacks, intrusive thoughts, hypervigilance, and sleep disturbance—along with the avoidance of reminders related to the traumatic event(s).

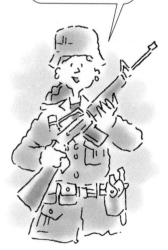

A patient with PTSD may become hypervigilant and easily startled.

Impairments caused by PTSD can be mild to severe, affecting nearly every aspect of the person's life. Those with PTSD are irritable, anxious, fatigued, forgetful, and socially withdrawn. Those who survived a catastrophe that took many lives may also have survivor guilt.

Inordinately alert

To avoid stimuli that trigger memories of the traumatic event, the patient with PTSD may become hypervigilant, easily aroused, and easily startled.

PTSD by the numbers (Ciechanowski & Katon, 2013)

An estimated 6.8% to 12.3% of adult Americans experience PTSD at some time in their lives. Women are four

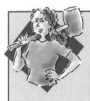

Myth busters

Posttraumatic stress disorder: Not just for war veterans

When some people hear the term PTSD, the image of a male war veteran pops into mind. However, the typical victim is more likely to be female.

Myth: Most PTSD victims are war veterans.

Reality: "PTSD is more prevalent in females than among males across the lifespan" (APA, 2013, p. 278).

In women, the traumatic events most often linked with PTSD are rape, sexual molestation, physical attacks, being threatened with a weapon, and childhood physical abuse. In men, the most common traumatizing events are rape, combat exposure, childhood neglect, and childhood physical abuse.

times more likely to be affected than men. (See *Posttraumatic stress disorder: Not just for war veterans.*) Higher rates of PTSD have been found in Native Americans living on reservations (14.2% to 16.1%) and refugees from countries where traumatic events were commonplace (62% in Cambodian refugees).

Patients with PTSD are at increased (80%) risk for developing other anxiety, mood, and substance-related disorders—especially alcohol abuse. Mild traumatic brain injury (mTBI) has been comorbid with PTSD at a rate of 48% in Iraq and Afghanistan war veterans (APA, 2013, p. 280).

Causes

A traumatic event (or events, such as in chronic childhood sexual abuse) is the trigger for PTSD. Some people, however, may be biochemically predisposed to the disorder. Serotonin may have a role in PTSD and glutamate (excitatory neurotransmitter) has been proposed to also have a role in the development and continued symptoms of PTSD (Ravindran & Stein, 2009). According to Ciechanowski and Katon (2013), the central alpha-2 adrenergic receptor response that inhibits stress-induced release of central norepinephrine is impaired in PTSD patients. This "hyperactivation can lead to anxiety, panic attacks, tremors, sweating, tachycardia, hyperarousal, and nightmares" (Stahl & Grady, 2010, p. 47). MRI scans have shown a decrease in hippocampal and left amygdala volume among volume decreases in other brain structures (Ciechanowski & Katon, 2013; Stahl & Grady, 2010, p. 35).

Risk factors

Risk factors for PTSD include (Ciechanowski & Katon, 2013):

- limited social supports
- parental neglect
- high anxiety levels
- low self-esteem
- initial severity of reaction to the traumatic event
- history of psychiatric disorders (personal or in the family)
- lower socioeconomic status.

Although preexisting psychopathology may predispose a person to this disorder, PTSD can develop in anyone—especially if the stressor is extreme. Genetic factors may also play a role.

Signs and symptoms

Common signs and symptoms of PTSD may include:

- anger
- poor impulse control
- chronic anxiety and tension
- avoidance of people, places, and things associated with the traumatic experience
- emotional detachment or numbness
- depersonalization (loss of personal identity)
- difficulty concentrating
- difficulty falling or staying asleep
- hypervigilance, hyperarousal, and exaggerated startle reflex
- inability to recall details of the traumatic event
- labile affect (rapid, easily changing affective expression)
- social withdrawal
- decreased self-esteem
- loss of sustained beliefs about people or society
- hopelessness
- sense of being permanently damaged
- relationship problems
- survivor's guilt.

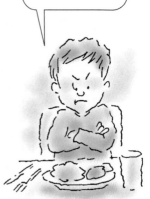

If they keep serving me this awful food, they'll traumatize me for life!

No thanks for the memories

Although the patient may be unable to recall specific aspects of the traumatizing event, the person may experience the trauma in flashbacks, dreams, or thoughts when cues to the event occur.

The psychosocial history may reveal early life experiences, interpersonal factors, military experiences, or other incidents that suggest the precipitating event.

Diagnosis

Diagnosing a patient with PTSD is based on a comprehensive clinical interview where numerous screening tools are used. The diagnosis is confirmed if the patient meets the criteria for the disorder listed in the *DSM-5*.

Treatment

Nonpharmacologic treatment options include interoceptive exposure, desensitization (systematic desensitization, eye movement desensitization and reprocessing), relaxation techniques, CBT, and psychotherapy.

Individual psychotherapy gives the patient a chance to talk through the traumatic experience with a nonthreatening person and thus gain some perspective. Promoting feelings of loss, grief, and anxiety may aid in resolving the emotional numbness associated with PTSD.

Group therapy helps the patient realize that they are not alone. A skilled group therapist can assist group members in confronting stressful feelings in a supportive environment.

CBT is "considered the gold standard of care for PTSD." However, as with all therapies, there is room for improvement (Fuse, Salters-Pedneault, & Litz, 2010, p. 110).

Pharmacologic treatment (Stahl & Grady, 2010)

First-line medications for the treatment of PTSD are the SSRIs and SNRIs. The SSRIs paroxetine (Paxil) and sertraline (Zoloft) are FDA approved for the treatment of PTSD. Other SSRIs and SNRIs are commonly used off-label in the treatment of PTSD. Studies have shown these other medications such as fluoxetine (Prozac), citalopram (Celexa), fluvoxamine (Luvox), and escitalopram (Lexapro) to be effective (Ravindran & Stein, 2009). SNRIs used off-label include venlafaxine XR (Effexor XR), desvenlafaxine (Pristiq), duloxetine (Cymbalta), and milnacipran (Savella).

Second-line medications used off-label in the treatment of PTSD include tricyclic antidepressants, monoamine oxidase inhibitors (MAOIs), gabapentin (Neurontin) and pregabalin (Lyrica), and anxiolytic benzodiazepines. Caution must be used when benzodiazepines are prescribed, as these are very addictive medications and there is already a high comorbidity between PTSD and substance use disorders. An alpha-adrenergic receptor blocker, prazosin (Minipress), has been used successfully to reduce nightmares and improve sleep in those with PTSD (Stein, 2013).

Suicide risk

"Traumatic events such as childhood sexual abuse increase a person's suicide risk. PTSD is associated with suicidal ideation and suicide attempts, and presence of PTSD may indicate which individuals with ideation eventually make a suicide plan or actually attempt suicide," (APA, 2013, p. 278).

Nursing interventions

These nursing interventions may be appropriate for patients with PTSD.

• A patient with a history of trauma may be suspicious of others in his or her care environment. Work to establish a trusting relationship and build rapport with the patient. Assign the same care providers whenever possible. Promote an attitude of openness and acceptance (Townsend, 2014, p. 566).

• Stay with the patient during flashbacks and nightmares. The patient needs reassurance from a trusted person that he or she is not "going crazy" (Townsend, 2014, p. 566).

• Encourage the patient to express his or her grief, complete the mourning process, and gain coping skills to relieve anxiety and desensitize the person to memories of the traumatic event.

• Teach relaxation techniques.

• Reassure the patient of his or her ability to return to a previous level of functioning.

• Use crisis intervention techniques as needed.

Anger adjustment

• Deal constructively with the patient's displays of anger. Encourage the patient to assess angry outbursts by identifying how the anger escalates.

• Help the patient regain control over angry impulses by identifying situations in which the patient lost control and by talking about past and precipitating events.

• Provide a safe, staff-monitored room where the patient can safely deal with urges to commit physical violence or self-abuse by displacement (such as pounding and throwing clay or destroying selected items).

• Encourage the individual to move from physical to verbal expressions of anger.

• Use a direct, nonjudgmental approach in discussing suicide (Halter, 2014, p. 312).

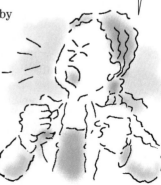

Aagghh! My therapist wants me to verbalize my anger!

Perspective correctives

- Help the patient relieve shame and guilt precipitated by real actions (such as killing or mutilation) that violated a consciously held moral code.
- Help the individual put his or her behavior into perspective, recognizing isolation and self-destructive behavior as forms of atonement, and accept forgiveness from self and others.
- Carefully review the healing process with the patient. Remind the individual not to equate setbacks with treatment failure.

Prescription erudition

- Administer prescribed medications, as ordered.
- Teach the patient about prescribed medications and adverse effects. Advise the individual not to discontinue medication without first consulting the doctor.
- Evaluate the patient's response to the prescribed drug regimen.
- Be aware that although benzodiazepines are fast acting, they may lose their effectiveness with prolonged use.

Reference rendering

- Refer the patient to clergy and community resources as appropriate.
- Refer the individual to group therapy with other victims for peer support and forgiveness.

Acute stress disorder

Acute stress disorder is a syndrome of anxiety and behavioral disturbances that occurs within 4 weeks of an extreme trauma, such as combat, rape, or a near-death experience in an accident. Generally, symptoms start during or shortly after the trauma and impair functioning in at least one key area (e.g., social, occupational). This may include dissociative, reexperiencing, avoidance, and arousal symptoms.

Unlike PTSD, acute stress disorder resolves within 4 weeks. (If symptoms last longer than 4 weeks, the diagnosis changes to PTSD.) Acute stress disorder may begin as early as 2 days after the trauma. Duration of symptoms is 3 days to 1 month.

"Prevalence of acute stress disorder following trauma has been estimated between 5% and 20% depending on the type of severity of the trauma." Risk factors for acute

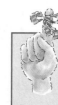

Memory jogger

The word acute is the key to remembering the difference between acute stress disorder and PTSD. Both cause similar symptoms but differ in their timing: Acute stress disorder happens shortly after the trauma (acute). PTSD takes a bit longer to emerge (delayed).

stress disorder are similar to those of PTSD (e.g., history of a psychiatric disorder, female gender, avoidant coping) (Bryant, 2012a).

Progression

Prognosis depends on such factors as severity and duration of the trauma and the patient's level of functioning. With immediate psychological care and much social support, recovery may be more rapid. If untreated, acute stress disorder may progress to PTSD, which can lead to substance abuse or major depression. About half of those who are diagnosed with acute stress disorder develop PTSD (APA, 2013, p. 284).

Causes

Exposure to trauma is the major precipitant of acute stress disorder. The trauma may involve serious physical or emotional injury or threats to one's life. It is not clear what specific factors cause acute stress disorder. However, reactivity to trauma and "catastrophic appraisals of the traumatic experience, often characterized by exaggerated appraisals of future harm, guilt, or hopelessness, are strongly predictive of acute stress disorder" (APA, 2013, p. 284). "Panic plays a role in the cause of acute stress disorder . . . Fear conditioning models state that the fear elicited during a traumatic event results in conditioning in which subsequent reminders of the trauma elicit anxiety in response to trauma reminders" (Bryant, 2012a). Panic attack reactions and the proposed cause of this symptom have been discussed in an earlier section of this chapter.

Signs and symptoms

Signs, symptoms, and clinical features of acute stress disorder, which are similar to PTSD, include:
• generalized anxiety
• hyperarousal
• avoidance of reminders of the traumatic event
• persistent, intrusive recollections of the traumatic event in flashbacks, dreams, or recurrent thoughts or visual images
• irritability
• physical restlessness
• sleep disturbances
• exaggerated startle reflex
• poor concentration.

Outside oneself

A hallmark of acute stress disorder is dissociation—a defense mechanism in which the patient separates anxiety-provoking thoughts and emotions from the rest of the psyche. The world may seem dreamlike or unreal to the patient, or the patient may feel like he or she is observing himself or herself from a distance or that a body part has somehow changed.

Dissociation may be accompanied by poor memory of the traumatic event or even complete amnesia of it.

> When I'm feeling outside myself like this, it usually means I'm experiencing acute stress.

Diagnosis

The patient has a recent history of trauma. Physical examination helps rule out organic causes of signs and symptoms.

The patient is diagnosed with acute stress disorder if he or she meets the criteria in the *DSM-5*.

Treatment

Treatment of acute stress disorder may include social supports, psychotherapy, CBT, and pharmacotherapy. A patient experiencing hyperarousal may benefit from relaxation techniques and deep-breathing exercises. "First-line treatment for acute stress disorder is trauma-focused CBT. . . . The aim is to curtail symptoms and prevent development into PTSD" (Bryant, 2012b).

Supportive counseling or short-term psychotherapy helps the patient examine the trauma in a supportive environment, strengthen previously helpful coping mechanisms, and learn new coping strategies.

CBT may involve trauma education, cognitive restructuring of the traumatic event to help the patient see it from a different perspective, and gradual reexposure with less avoidance (Bryant, 2012b).

When all else fails . . .

Drugs may be used if nonpharmacologic methods aren't effective. The medical provider may prescribe short-term use of benzodiazepines (e.g., clonazepam), although use of longer than 2 weeks may increase the risk of developing PTSD. Other medications that have been studied in the treatment of acute stress disorder are antidepressants, propranolol, and morphine (Bryant, 2012b).

Nursing interventions

These nursing interventions may be appropriate for patients with acute stress disorder.

- Encourage the patient to discuss the stressful event and identify it as traumatic. This validates that the situation was indeed beyond the individual's personal control.
- Urge the patient to talk about the feelings of anxiety and feelings about the trauma. This helps the individual cope with the reality of the event.
- Encourage the patient to identify any feelings of survivor guilt, inadequacy, or blame. Expressing these feelings helps the person understand that survival may have been due to chance and not related to any personal action or inaction.
- Teach relaxation techniques, such as progressive muscle relaxation.
- Administer antianxiety medications, as ordered.
- If the patient is taking a medication for the anxiety, stress the importance of complying with prescribed therapy. Teach the patient about adverse drug reactions and what needs to be reported to the prescriber.

With survivor's guilt, your patient may feel better if they understand that their survival was due to chance alone.

Obsessive-compulsive disorder

OCD is characterized by unwanted, recurrent, and intrusive thoughts or images (obsessions), which the person tries to alleviate through repetitive behaviors or mental acts (compulsions). The compulsions are meant to reduce the anxiety or prevent some dreaded event from happening. The person has rules in the compulsion that must be applied in a rigid fashion.

Obsessions and compulsions may be simple or complex and ritualized. Compulsions include both overt behaviors, such as hand washing or checking, and mental acts, such as praying or counting. Although anxiety disorder is closely related to OCD, there are marked differences that have spurned the classification of obsessive-compulsive and related disorders in the *DSM-5*. OCD is not considered an anxiety disorder.

Run-on rituals

Obsessive-compulsive behaviors and activities take up more than 1 hour per day. For some patients, compulsive rituals take hours to complete and become the major life activity.

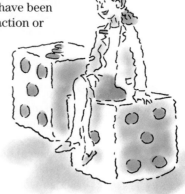

Not surprisingly, OCD causes significant distress and may severely impair occupational and social functioning. Compulsive behaviors also can endanger health and safety. For example, severe dermatitis or a skin infection may result from compulsive hand washing.

But then, who's counting? (APA, 2013, p. 239)

OCD affects about 2% of the general population, striking men and women equally. In males, it typically begins in adolescence to young adulthood; in females, in young adulthood. "In the United States, the mean age of onset is 19.5 years and 25% of the cases start by the age of 14 years" (APA, 2013, p. 239). The onset usually is gradual—over months or years.

For most patients, the disorder takes a fluctuating course, with exacerbations linked to stressful events. In some cases, psychosocial functioning steadily deteriorates.

To make matters worse . . . (Sadock & Sadock, 2007, p. 605)

Many of those with OCD also have major depressive disorder (67%), panic disorder, social phobia (25%), specific phobia, eating disorders, substance abuse, or personality disorders.

In clinical samples, approximately 20% to 30% of patients with OCD report a past history of tics; about 5% to 7% meet the full criteria for Tourette syndrome (a neurobehavioral disorder characterized by sudden, involuntary motor and vocal tics). "About 90% of those with Tourette syndrome meet the diagnostic criteria for OCD" (Sadock & Sadock, 2007, p. 610).

Causes

Genetic, biological, and psychological factors may be involved in OCD development. (See *The strep connection.*)

The strep connection (Simpson, 2013)

Researchers have found an association between OCD and beta-hemolytic streptococci infection. Studies of children have linked the sudden appearance of obsessions, compulsions, and motor or vocal tics with streptococcal throat infection.

Possibly, an autoimmune response to the infection occurs, in which antibodies attack both healthy and infected cells. This could cause inflammation of the basal ganglia, a brain region involved in movement and motor control.

Sad syndrome, cute name

The syndrome, called *pediatric autoimmune neuropsychiatric disorders associated with streptococcal infections* (PANDAS), typically affects children aged 5 to 11 and has a dramatic, sudden onset. In some of these children, OCD symptoms respond to prompt antibiotic treatment.

"The concept of PANDAS is debated in the literature; in other words, the researchers are looking at other infectious agents also as a precipitant to a similar neuropsychiatric syndrome."

Genetic factors

OCD tends to run in families. The risk of OCD is two times higher among first-degree relatives. Even worse, the risk of OCD in first-degree relatives is 10-fold when the onset of OCD for the patient occurred in childhood or adolescence (APA, 2013, p. 240).

Biological aspects

Biological evidence is strong, too. MRI and computed tomography scans show enlarged basal ganglia in some OCD patients. Positron emission tomography scans found increased glucose metabolism in a particular part of the basal ganglia. The cortico-striato-thalamo-cortical circuit has been implicated in OCD. Abnormalities in the serotonin and dopamine signaling have also been hypothesized to play a role in OCD. "Several studies found OCD subjects aberrantly recruited the hippocampus in a learning task, whereas healthy participants recruited the striatum" (Simpson, 2013).

Psychological factors

Whittal and Robichaud (2010, pp. 93–94) state in cognitive theory, "appraisal of the thought that fuels OCD, wherein sufferers view intrusions as meaningful and catastrophic; it is this interpretation that leads to anxiety and distress. . . . In response to these feelings, individuals with OCD engage in a variety of neutralizing acts (i.e., compulsions) that are designed to reduce the distress."

Risk factors

In the *DSM-5* (pp. 239–240), temperamental traits in childhood such as greater internalizing symptoms, higher negative emotionality, and behavioral inhibition may lead to an increased risk of developing OCD. Physical and sexual abuse in childhood and other stressful/traumatic events also increase the risk of developing OCD.

Suicide risk

"Suicidal thoughts occur at some point in as many as about half of individuals with OCD. Suicide attempts are also reported in up to one-quarter of individuals with OCD." Risk is increased in those with comorbid major depression (APA, 2013, p. 240).

Signs and symptoms

"Symptom dimensions" or themes of OCD are present in the patient. A patient often has multiple dimensions to his or her disorder. Symptom dimensions include (Simpson, 2013):
• Cleaning: fears of contamination and cleaning rituals (e.g., hand washing)
• Symmetry: symmetry obsessions and repeating, ordering and counting compulsions

- Forbidden or taboo thoughts: examples include aggressive, sexual, and religious obsessions and related compulsions
- Harm (e.g., thoughts or images about harm befalling oneself or other and checking compulsions)
- Hoarding (hoarding obsessions and compulsions)
    A patient with OCD may exhibit or report:
- repetitive thoughts that cause stress (obsessions)
- repetitive behaviors (compulsions), such as hand washing, counting, or checking and rechecking whether a door is locked
- social impairment caused by preoccupation with obsessions and compulsions
- perceived need to achieve perfection
- avoidance of people, places, or things that trigger the obsession and compulsion.

They know it's weird

Most patients are aware that their obsessions are excessive or irrational and interfere with normal daily activities. In fact, many hide their symptoms out of embarrassment. However, a minority don't perceive their obsessions and compulsions as irrational. (See *Cultural practices and OCD*.)

Diagnosis

The diagnosis of OCD is confirmed if the patient meets the criteria listed in the *DSM-5*. (See *Diagnostic criteria: Obsessive-compulsive disorder*.)

Treatment

Treatment options for OCD include:
- behavioral techniques
- relaxation techniques, such as deep breathing, progressive muscle relaxation, meditation, imagery, or music
- support groups, which decrease the patient's isolation
- partial hospitalization and day treatment programs
- medication.

Behavior therapy

The behavioral technique of exposure and response prevention (ERP) may be used to treat patients with OCD. This is the treatment of choice for mild to moderate OCD. For moderate

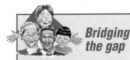

Bridging the gap

Cultural practices and OCD

Don't mistake certain cultural or religious practices for OCD. In some cultures, for instance, people pray repetitively or mourn a loved one's death with intensely ritualized behavior that seems obsessive or compulsive to an observer. For this reason, always assess the patient within the context of cultural and religious background.

Crucial criteria
Remember—culturally prescribed ritual behavior in itself doesn't signal OCD unless it:
- exceeds cultural norms
- occurs at times and places that others in the culture would judge inappropriate
- interferes with the patient's social role functioning.

Diagnostic criteria: Obsessive-compulsive disorder

A. Presence of obsessions, compulsions, or both:

Obsessions are defined by (1) and (2):

1. Recurrent and persistent thoughts, urges, or images that are experienced, at some time during the disturbance, as intrusive and unwanted and that in most individuals cause marked anxiety or distress

2. The individual attempts to ignore or suppress such thoughts, urges, or images or to neutralize them with some other thought or action (i.e., by performing a compulsion).

Compulsions are defined by (1) and (2):

1. Repetitive behaviors (e.g., hand washing, ordering, checking) or mental acts (e.g., praying, counting, repeating words silently) that the individual feels driven to perform in response to an obsession or according to rules that must be applied rigidly

2. The behaviors or mental acts are aimed at preventing or reducing anxiety or distress or preventing some dreaded event or situation; however, these behaviors or mental acts are not connected in a realistic way with what they are designed to neutralize or prevent or are clearly excessive. (Note: Young children may not be able to articulate the aims of these behaviors or mental acts).

B. The obsessions or compulsions are time-consuming (e.g., take more than 1 hour per day) or cause clinically significant distress or impairment in social, occupational, or other important areas of functioning.

C. The obsessive-compulsive symptoms are not attributable to the physiologic effects of a substance (e.g., a drug of abuse, a medication) or another medical condition.

D. The disturbance is not better explained by the symptoms of another mental disorder (e.g., excessive worries, as in generalized anxiety disorder; preoccupation with appearance, as in body dysmorphic disorder; difficulty discarding or parting with possessions, as in hoarding disorder; hair pulling, as in trichotillomania (hair-pulling disorder); skin picking, as in excoriation disorder; stereotypies, as in stereotypic movement disorder; ritualized eating behavior, as in eating disorders; preoccupation with substances or gambling, as in substance-related and addictive disorders; preoccupation with having an illness, as in illness anxiety disorder; sexual urges or fantasies, as in paraphilic disorders; impulses, as in disruptive, impulse-control, and conduct disorders; guilty ruminations, as in major depressive disorder; thought insertion or delusional preoccupations, as in schizophrenia spectrum and other psychotic disorders; or repetitive patterns of behavior, as in autism spectrum disorder.

Specify if:

With good or fair insight: The individual recognizes that OCD beliefs are definitely or probably not true or that they may or may not be true.

With poor insight: The individual thinks OCD beliefs are probably true.

With absent/delusional beliefs: The individual is completely convinced that OCD beliefs are true.

Specify if:

Tic-related: The individual has a current or past history of a tic disorder.

to severe OCD, medication and ERP is the treatment of choice. This method exposes the patient to the object or situation that triggers the obsessions—but then asks the individual to refrain from engaging in the usual compulsive response. The patient writes down what happens as a result of the behavioral restraint and comes to realize that not performing the ritual doesn't bring distressing outcomes. Eventually, the individual learns to manage his or her intense anxiety until it subsides (Whittal & Robichaud, 2010).

ERP therapy proves effective in about 56% of patients (Whittal & Robichaud, 2010, p. 95). Its success rate has led to its use in telephone-access therapy, in which OCD patients call in and get computer-generated response-prevention therapy.

Pharmacologic therapy

Pharmacologic interventions used in the treatment of OCD include SSRIs, clomipramine, and venlafaxine (Simpson, 2011). The FDA has approved the use of clomipramine (Anafranil), fluoxetine (Prozac), fluvoxamine (Luvox), paroxetine (Paxil), and sertraline (Zoloft) in the treatment of OCD. Fluvoxamine controlled release (Luvox) has shown to be superior in recent trials with good remission rates for both OCD and social anxiety disorder (Stahl, 2013, p. 299).

Nursing interventions

These nursing interventions may be appropriate for patients with OCD (Cawley, 1998, p. 385).
* Approach the patient unhurriedly. Ask specific questions about the thoughts and behaviors, especially if you note physical cues, such as chafed or reddened hands or hair loss due to compulsive pulling (trichotillomania).
* Identify disturbing topics of conversation that reflect underlying anxiety or terror.
* Keep the patient's physical health in mind. For example, compulsive hand washing may cause skin breakdown; rituals or preoccupations may cause inadequate food and fluid intake and exhaustion. Provide for basic needs, such as rest, nutrition, and grooming, if the patient becomes involved in ritualistic thoughts and behaviors to the point of self-neglect. If skin breakdown is an issue related to compulsions, consider replacing harsh antibacterial soap with a moisturizing alternative.

Isn't it tiring?

* Let the patient know you're aware of his or her behavior. For example, you might say, "I noticed you've made your bed three times today. That must be very tiring for you."
* Help the patient explore feelings associated with the behavior. For example, ask, "What do you think about while you perform your chores?" Listen attentively, offering feedback.
* Explore patterns leading to the behavior or recurring problems.

Don't be shocked

- Maintain an accepting attitude.
- Don't show shock, amusement, or criticism of the ritualistic behavior.
- Understand that OCD is irrational and will not be changed by logical explanations.

Don't try to block

- Give the patient time to carry out the ritualistic behavior (unless it's dangerous) until he or she can be distracted by some other activity. Be aware that blocking such behavior could increase the anxiety to an intolerable level.
- Allow the patient to have some control over anxiety-provoking situations. Never force the individual to do something.
- Make reasonable demands and set reasonable limits—and make their purpose clear. Avoid creating situations that increase frustration and provoke anger, which may interfere with treatment.

Diversionary tactics

- Encourage active diversions, such as exercise or playing a game with another individual, to divert attention from the unwanted thoughts and promote a pleasurable experience.
- Explain how to channel emotional energy to relieve stress (e.g., through creative endeavors).
- Engage the patient in activities that create positive accomplishments and raise self-esteem and confidence.

Time's up!

- Assist the patient in exploring new ways to solve problems and developing more effective coping skills by setting limits on unacceptable behavior (e.g., by limiting the number of times per day the individual may participate in the compulsive behavior). Gradually shorten the time allowed. For the remainder of the time, help the individual focus on other feelings or problems.
- Identify insight and improved behavior (reduced compulsive behavior and fewer obsessive thoughts). Evaluate behavioral changes by your own and the patient's reports.
- Observe when interventions don't work; reevaluate and recommend alternative strategies.
- Help the patient identify progress and set realistic expectations.

Memory jogger

To help the patient cope with OCD, remember the word COPING.

C: Concerns and feelings are discussed.

O: Offer a structured routine that allows time for rituals.

P: Practice thought-stopping skills.

I: Initiate a behavioral contract to decrease rituals and reward nonritualistic behaviors.

N: Nurture effective ways to problem-solve stressful situations.

G: Get the patient to perform relaxation techniques.

In one OCD intervention, you shorten the time that the patient may engage in compulsive behavior.

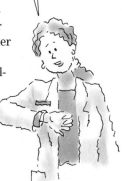

- Encourage the use of appropriate coping mechanisms to relieve loneliness and isolation.
- Monitor the patient for suicidal behaviors and thoughts. Hopelessness and helplessness may overwhelm the individual as he or she realizes the absurdness of the behavior but feels powerless to control it.
- Monitor for desired and adverse effects of prescribed drugs.

Meds matters

Pharmacologic therapy for anxiety disorders (Stahl, 2011)

This chart highlights FDA-approved drugs used to treat anxiety disorders.

Drug	Adverse effects	Contraindications	Nursing considerations
Antihistamine			
Hydroxyzine (Atarax, Vistaril)	• Dry mouth • Sedation • Tremor Rare: • Convulsions • Cardiac arrest (intramuscular [IM] only) • Bronchodilation • Respiratory depression	• Early stages of pregnancy; proven allergy to hydroxyzine	• Dose reduction and close monitoring of elderly patients due to increased risk of confusion and oversedation • Evaluate alertness; sedation may occur (tell patient not to drive or engage in other potentially dangerous activities). • If on a high dose, monitor oral hydration and increase fluids as necessary. • No concomitant use of alcohol • If the patient has also been given central nervous system (CNS) depressants, dose reduction will be needed in the depressant and the patient needs to be monitored closely.
Antipsychotic			
Trifluoperazine (Stelazine)	• Neuroleptic-induced deficit syndrome • Akathisia • Rash • Priapism • Extrapyramidal symptoms • Galactorrhea	• CNS depression • Presence of blood dyscrasias • Bone marrow depression • Liver disease	• Observe closely for signs of neuroleptic malignant syndrome. • Administer cautiously in patients in alcohol withdrawal or seizure history. • Respiratory disorders • Glaucoma • Urinary retention • Avoid extreme sunlight and heat exposure.

Pharmacologic therapy for anxiety disorders *(continued)*

Drug	Adverse effects	Contraindications	Nursing considerations
Benzodiazepines			
Alprazolam (Xanax) Chlordiazepoxide (Librium) Clonazepam (Klonopin) Clorazepate (Tranxene) Diazepam (Valium) Lorazepam (Ativan) Oxazepam (Serax)	• Ataxia • Confusion • Constipation • Double or blurred vision • Dry mouth • Sedation • Skin reactions (rash, urticaria, photosensitivity) • Vertigo • Weight change	• Acute alcohol intoxication • Acute angle-closure glaucoma or untreated open-angle glaucoma • Coma • Depression or psychosis without anxiety • Pregnancy or breast-feeding • Shock • Within 14 days of taking an MAOI	• Monitor closely after giving each dose because of a possible disinhibitory effect (excitement) rather than calming effect. • Administer cautiously in the elderly and in patients with epilepsy, myasthenia gravis, impaired hepatic or renal function, history of substance abuse, or other CNS depressant use. • Assess for unexplained bleeding. • Monitor liver function and blood counts. • Instruct patient to avoid alcohol, antidepressants, and anticonvulsants. • Caution patient not to drive or operate hazardous machinery until drowsiness subsides. • Stress the importance of avoiding abrupt drug withdrawal.
Beta-adrenergic blocking agent			
Propranolol (Inderal)	• Bradycardia • Dizziness • Emotional lability • Fatigue • Fever • GI disturbances • Heart block • Hypotension • Impaired concentration • Impotence and decreased libido • Mental depression • Skin rash • Shortness of breath • Sore throat • Worsening of angina	• Concomitant use of reserpine, MAOIs, digoxin, calcium channel blockers, theophylline, norepinephrine, or dopamine • Compromised cardiac function • Diabetes • Respiratory disease	• Take patient's apical pulse for 1 full minute after giving dose. • Monitor blood pressure. Take blood pressure prior to administration and after administration of medication. • Monitor cardiac function (fluid intake and output, daily weight, serum electrolytes). • Assess patient for signs and symptoms of depression. • Advise patient not to change dose or stop drug without doctor's approval. • Instruct patient to report weight gain of more than 2 lb per week. • Inform diabetic patients that drug may mask hypoglycemia symptoms. • Instruct patient to take drug with food to minimize GI disturbance. • Teach patient which adverse effects to report.

(continued)

Pharmacologic therapy for anxiety disorders *(continued)*

Drug	Adverse effects	Contraindications	Nursing considerations
SNRIs			
Duloxetine (Cymbalta) Venlafaxine (Effexor)	• GI (nausea, diarrhea, decreased appetite, dry mouth, constipation) • Insomnia, sedation, dizziness • Sexual dysfunction • Increase in blood pressure (2 mm Hg) • Urinary retention • Rare seizures • Rare induction of hypomania • Rare activation of suicidal ideations and behavior	• Uncontrolled narrow angle-closure glaucoma • Substantial alcohol use • If patient is taking thioridazine or an MAOI • Proven allergy to duloxetine	• Give in the morning with or without food. • Monitor for weight loss if nausea occurs. • Instruct patient to avoid alcoholic beverages. • Monitor blood pressure. • Tell patient to report adverse effects, especially rash or itching. • Advise patient that stopping medication abruptly may cause serotonin withdrawal syndrome.
SSRIs			
Escitalopram (Lexapro) Fluoxetine (Prozac) Fluvoxamine (Luvox) Paroxetine (Paxil) Sertraline (Zoloft)	• Insomnia • Nausea • Nervousness • Vertigo	• Within 14 days of taking an MAOI	• Give in the morning with or without food. • Monitor for weight loss if nausea occurs. • Instruct patient to avoid alcoholic beverages. • Tell patient to report adverse effects, especially rash or itching. • Advise patient that stopping medication abruptly may cause serotonin withdrawal syndrome.

Pharmacologic therapy for anxiety disorders (continued)

Drug	Adverse effects	Contraindications	Nursing considerations
Tricyclic antidepressants			
Clomipramine (Anafranil) Doxepin (Sinequan)	• Agranulocytosis • Arrhythmias • Blurred vision • Bone marrow depression • Constipation • Dry mouth • Esophageal reflux • Galactorrhea • Hallucinations • Heart failure • Increased or decreased libido • Jaundice and fatigue • Mania • MI • Orthostatic hypotension or hypertension • Palpitations • Shock • Slowing of intracardiac conduction • Urinary hesitancy • Weight gain	• Concomitant use of MAOIs • Recent myocardial infarction (MI) • Renal or hepatic disease	• Monitor blood pressure and pulse for signs of orthostatic hypotension. • Monitor patient for suicidal thoughts and behaviors. • Supervise drug ingestion. • Know that special monitoring is required if patient has a history of angle-closure glaucoma or seizure disorder. • Monitor for adverse effects. • Monitor liver function and complete blood counts. • Tell patient to change positions slowly. • Instruct patient to avoid driving or hazardous machinery if drowsiness occurs. • Teach patient to avoid alcohol and over-the-counter (OTC) agents unless the doctor approves. • Inform patient that desired drug effects may take up to 4 weeks to appear.
Other antianxiety agent			
Buspirone (BuSpar)	• Dizziness • Excitement • Headache • Light-headedness • Nausea • Nervousness	• Concomitant MAOI therapy • Renal or hepatic impairment	• Assist with ambulation if needed. • Instruct patient to inform all health care providers of all prescription, OTC, and recreational drug use. • Caution patient against driving or operating machinery until drowsiness subsides. • Instruct patient to report adverse effects. • Inform the patient that improvement may take 3 to 4 weeks. • Advise patient to have liver and kidney tests periodically.

References

American Psychiatric Association. (2013). *Diagnostic and statistical manual of mental disorders* (5th ed.). Arlington, VA: Author.

Baldwin, D. (2013). *Generalized anxiety disorder: Epidemiology, pathogenesis, clinical manifestations, course, assessment, and diagnosis.* Retrieved from http://www .uptodate.com/contents/generalized-anxiety-disorder-epidemiology-pathogenesis-clinical-manifestations-course-assessment-and-diagnosis

Boyd, M. (2012). *Psychiatric nursing: Contemporary practice* (5th ed.). Philadelphia, PA: Lippincott Williams & Wilkins.

Bryant, R. (2012a). *Acute stress disorder: Epidemiology, clinical manifestations, and diagnosis.* Retrieved from http://www.uptodate.com/contents/acute-stress-disorder-epidemiology-clinical-manifestations-and-diagnosis

Bryant, R. (2012b). *Treatment of acute stress disorder.* Retrieved from http://www.uptodate .com/contents/treatment-of-acute-stress-disorder

Bystritsky, A. (2013). *Pharmacotherapy for generalized anxiety disorder.* Retrieved from http://www.uptodate.com/contents/pharmacotherapy-for-generalized-anxiety-disorder

Cawley, D. (1998). Chapter 20: Anxiety disorders. In C. A. Glod (Ed.). *Contemporary psychiatric-mental health nursing: The brain-behavior connection.* Philadelphia, PA: F.A. Davis.

Ciechanowski, P., & Katon, W. (2013). *Posttraumatic stress disorder: Epidemiology, pathophysiology, clinical manifestations, course, and diagnosis.* Retrieved from http://www .uptodate.com/contents/posttraumatic-stress-disorder-epidemiology-pathophysiology-clinical-manifestations-course-and-diagnosis

Fuse, T., Salters-Pedneault, K., & Litz, B. T. (2010). Post-traumatic stress disorder. In S. G. Hofmann & M. A. Reinecke (Eds.), *Cognitive-behavioral therapy with adults: A guide to empirically-informed assessment and intervention.* Cambridge, United Kingdom: Cambridge University Press.

Halter, M. (2014). *Varicolis' foundation of psychiatric mental health nursing: A clinical approach* (7th ed.). St. Louis, MO: Elsevier.

Jakatdar, T. A., & Heimberg, R. G. (2010). Social anxiety disorder. In S. G. Hofmann & M. A. Reinecke (Eds.), *Cognitive-behavioral therapy with adults: A guide to empirically-informed assessment and intervention.* Cambridge, United Kingdom: Cambridge University Press.

Katon, W., & Ciechanowski, P. (2013). *Panic disorder: Epidemiology, pathogenesis, clinical manifestations, course, assessment, and diagnosis.* Retrieved from http://www .uptodate.com/contents/panic-disorder-epidemiology-pathogenesis-clinical-manifestations-course-assessment-and-diagnosis

Koerner, N., Rogojanski, J., & Antony, M. M. (2010). Specific phobia. In S. G. Hofmann & M. A. Reinecke (Eds.), *Cognitive-behavioral therapy with adults: A guide to empirically-informed assessment and intervention.* Cambridge, United Kingdom: Cambridge University Press.

McCabe, R. E. (2013a). *Agoraphobia in adults: Epidemiology, pathogenesis, clinical manifestations, course, assessment, and diagnosis.* Retrieved from http://www.uptodate. com/contents/agoraphobia-in-adults-epidemiology-pathogenesis-clinical-manifestations-course-and-diagnosis

McCabe, R. E.(2013b). *Specific phobia in adults: Epidemiology, clinical manifestations, course and diagnosis*. Retrieved from http://www.uptodate.com/contents/specific-phobia-in-adults-epidemiology-clinical-manifestations-course-and-diagnosis

National Institute of Mental Health. (2014). Anxiety disorders. Retrieved from http://www.nimh.nih.gov/health/topics/anxiety-disorders/index.shtml

Prenoveau, J. M., & Craske, M. G. (2010). Panic disorder and agoraphobia. In S. G. Hofmann & M. A. Reinecke (Eds.), *Cognitive-behavioral therapy with adults: A guide to empirically-informed assessment and intervention*. Cambridge, United Kingdom: Cambridge University Press.

Ravindran, L. N., & Stein, M. B. (2009). Pharmacotherapy of PTSD: Premises, principles, and priorities. *Brain Research, 1293*, 24–39. http://dx.doi.org/10.1016/j.brainres.2009.03.037

Roy-Byrne, P. P. (2013). *Pharmacotherapy for panic disorder*. Retrieved from http://www.uptodate.com/contents/pharmacotherapy-for-panic-disorder

Sadock, B. J., & Sadock, V. A. (2007). *Kaplan and Sadock's synopsis of psychiatry: Behavioral sciences/clinical psychiatry* (10th ed.). Philadelphia, PA: Lippincott Williams & Wilkins.

Schneier, F. R. (2013). *Social anxiety disorder: Epidemiology, clinical manifestations, and diagnosis*. Retrieved from http://www.uptodate.com/contents/social-anxiety-disorder-epidemiology-clinical-manifestations-and-diagnosis

Simpson, H. B. (2011). *Pharmacotherapy for obsessive-compulsive disorder*. Retrieved from http://www.uptodate.com/contents/pharmacotherapy-for-obsessive-compulsive-disorder

Simpson, H. B. (2013). *Obsessive-compulsive disorder in adults: Epidemiology, pathogenesis, clinical manifestations, course, and diagnosis*. Retrieved from http://www.uptodate.com/contents/obsessive-compulsive-disorder-in-adults-epidemiology-pathogenesis-clinical-manifestations-course-and-diagnosis

Stahl, S. M. (2011). *Stahl's essential psychopharmacology: The prescriber's guide* (4th ed.). Cambridge, United Kingdom: Cambridge University Press.

Stahl, S. M. (2013). *Stahl's essential psychopharmacology: Neuroscientific basis and practical application* (4th ed.). Cambridge, United Kingdom: Cambridge University Press.

Stahl, S. M., & Grady, M. M. (2010). *Stahl's illustrated: Anxiety, stress, and PTSD*. Cambridge, United Kingdom: Cambridge University Press.

Stein, M. B. (2011). *Pharmacotherapy for social anxiety disorder*. Retrieved from http://www.uptodate.com/contents/pharmacotherapy-for-social-anxiety-disorder

Stein, M. B. (2013). *Pharmacotherapy for posttraumatic stress disorder*. Retrieved from http://www.uptodate.com/contents/pharmacotherapy-for-posttraumatic-stress-disorder

Swinson, R., & McCabe, R. E. (2012). *Pharmacotherapy for specific phobia in adults*. Retrieved from http://www.uptodate.com/contents/pharmacotherapy-for-specific-phobia-in-adults

Townsend, M. (2014). *Psychiatric mental health nursing: Concepts of care in evidenced-based practice* (8th ed.). Philadelphia, PA: F.A. Davis.

Wells, A., & Fisher, P. (2010). Generalized anxiety disorder. In S. G. Hofmann & M. A. Reinecke (Eds.), *Cognitive-behavioral therapy with adults: A guide to empirically-informed assessment and intervention*. Cambridge, United Kingdom: Cambridge University Press.

Whittal, M. L., & Robichaud, M. (2010). Obsessive-compulsive disorder. In S. G. Hofmann & M. A. Reinecke (Eds.), *Cognitive-behavioral therapy with adults: A guide to empirically-informed assessment and intervention*. Cambridge, United Kingdom: Cambridge University Press.

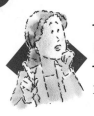

Quick quiz

1. Signs and symptoms of acute stress disorder may occur:
A. for at least 3 days and last no more than 1 month.
B. several months after the traumatic event.
C. on and off again for years.
D. whenever the trigger is experienced.

Answer: A. Acute stress disorder lasts no more than one month. If symptoms persist after one month, the diagnosis is PSTD.

2. Fear of situations or places that may be difficult or embarrassing to leave describes:
A. social phobia.
B. panic disorder.
C. agoraphobia.
D. GAD.

Answer: C. Agoraphobia is the fear and avoidance of situations or places that may be difficult or embarrassing to leave.

3. Characteristics of GAD include:
A. dissociation, avoidance, and repeated hand washing.
B. onset is shortly after an event, fear of leaving home, and fear of spiders.
C. difficulty concentrating, easily fatigued, and occurs for at least 6 months.
D. fear of performing a task in public, fear of a specific object, and fear of losing control.

Answer: C. Some of the GAD criteria are listed. The other answers all are inconsistent with GAD.

4. The fear of losing one's mind or having a heart attack is most likely to occur in:
A. social phobia.
B. panic disorder.
C. GAD.
D. myctophobia.

Answer: B. Anxiety severe enough to cause the patient to fear he or she's losing his or her mind or having a heart attack occurs with panic disorder. Social phobia, GAD, and myctophobia may have a panic component to the patient, but the anxiety is less severe.

5. Flashbacks of an unpleasant, terrifying, or painful experience may occur in:
   A.   PTSD.
   B.   panic disorder.
   C.   agoraphobia.
   D.   OCD.

Answer: A. Flashbacks are characteristic of PTSD. They aren't major components of panic disorder, agoraphobia, or OCD.

6. Fear of embarrassing oneself in public characterizes:
   A.   GAD.
   B.   panic disorder.
   C.   specific phobia.
   D.   social phobia.

Answer: D. Social phobia is characterized by a dread of being scrutinized and subsequently being embarrassed in public.

7. A patient with a history of panic attacks says he or she feels trapped after an attack. The patient most likely fears:
   A.   loss of maturity.
   B.   loss of control.
   C.   loss of memory.
   D.   loss of identity.

Answer: B. People who fear loss of control during a panic attack commonly make statements about feeling trapped, getting hurt, or having little or no personal control over their situations.

Scoring

☆☆☆   If you answered all seven items correctly, terrific! We're sending you on a worry-free vacation to the Sea of Tranquility.

☆☆   If you answered five or six items correctly, relax. You have nothing to be anxious about when it comes to understanding anxiety disorders.

☆   If you answered fewer than five items correctly, no need to panic. Just breathe deeply, relax, stop those negative thoughts—and then reexpose yourself to the chapter for further study.

7

Somatic symptom and related disorders

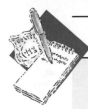

Just the facts

In this chapter, you'll learn:

◆ how stress can be converted to physical symptoms

◆ differences between conversion disorder and factitious disorders

◆ proposed causes of somatic symptoms

◆ signs and symptoms of somatic and related disorders

◆ assessment and interventions for individuals with somatic symptoms and related disorders.

A look at somatic symptoms and related disorders

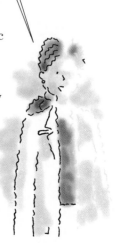

I seem to be disappearing, but I'm trying not to let it preoccupy me.

Somatic symptoms and related disorders are a group of psychiatric disorders in which the individual has persistent somatic (physical) complaints associated with significant distress and impairment. This category is characterized by distressing somatic symptoms combined with abnormal thoughts, feelings, and behaviors in response to the somatic symptoms. There may be a diagnosed medical disorder or medically unexplained symptoms as in conversion disorder or pseudocyesis (false pregnancy). The American Psychiatric Association previously called this diagnostic category *psychosomatic disorders* or *somatoform disorders*. Because of the high degree of overlap between past diagnoses, the terms *somatic symptom and related disorders* have been adopted for use (American Psychiatric Association [APA], 2013). Somatic disorders are seen more frequently in medical primary care offices or consultation-liaison practices than in mental health settings. It is important to note that in this diagnostic category, these somatic symptoms cannot be attributed to substance misuse or another mental disorder. Instead, the symptoms are linked to psychological factors. Distress and preoccupation with the symptoms can lead to occupational, academic, social, and other impairments (APA, 2013).

This chapter discusses the somatic symptom disorder as well as illness anxiety disorder, conversion disorder, factitious disorder, and psychological factors affecting other medical conditions

They're not faking it

Individuals with somatic disorders don't feign their symptoms (as in malingering or conscious "faking"). Because they don't produce the symptoms intentionally or feel a sense of control over them, they have trouble accepting that the symptoms have a psychological origin.

Researchers have identified several factors that affect vulnerability to these disorders. Early life events such as being separated from mother, a history of childhood maltreatment, recent stressors, and long-standing subtle stressors have all been reported to increase vulnerability to somatic disorders. The individual experiences too much stress and/or does not have adequate coping skills to deal with the predisposing factors. Which individuals cope adequately or develop somatic disorders is determined by personality factors, genetic determinants, and environmental factors such as social support. Individuals who have these predisposing factors and do not develop symptoms or develop symptoms but quickly recover and return to previous level of functioning are referred to as being resilient.

Converting stress into symptoms

Somatization refers to the unconscious conversion of emotional or mental states into bodily symptoms (Phoenix & Johnson, 2013). Individuals with somatic symptom disorders internalize their anxiety, stress, and frustration. Instead of confronting these feelings directly, they express them unconsciously through physical symptoms. (See *The scoop on somatic symptom disorders*, page 246)

All in the head—not!

Health care professionals who can't find a physical basis for an individual's symptoms may tell the patient that the illness is

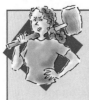

Myth busters

The scoop on somatic symptom disorders

Many people misunderstand the nature of somatic symptom disorders. To separate yourself from the masses, read on.

Myth: In patients with illness anxiety disorder (hypochondriasis), the primary emotional feature is fear.

Reality: Although patients with illness anxiety disorder may fear they have a life-threatening disease, many also struggle with depression, severe anxiety, and obsessive-compulsive symptoms.

Myth: In somatic disorders with prominent pain, no medical evidence of a pathologic process exists.

Reality: In some patients with somatic symptom disorder, diagnostic tests identify evidence of a pathologic process, such as a musculo-skeletal condition or cancer. Nonetheless, psychological factors play a predominant role in the severity, exacerbation, and maintenance of the pain.

"all in your head." Failure to recognize somatization and manage it appropriately, however, can lead to frustrating, costly, and potentially dangerous tests and treatments as well as more distress for the individual.

Many individuals go to multiple health care providers in search of a diagnosis and treatment with minimal relief.

Coexisting disorders

Other disorders such as depression or anxiety may initially present with somatic symptoms and this other diagnosis may account for the somatic symptoms or may occur simultaneously with the somatic disorder. This comorbidity often results in more severe disability and treatment resistance.

Some of the common combinations include the following:
• Individuals with somatic symptom disorder often develop panic attacks or agoraphobia.
• Illness-related anxiety disorder and somatic disorders with prominent pain often exists concomitantly with depression and an increased risk for suicide.

Cultural and ethnic factors

"In many cultures, the expression of physical discomfort is more acceptable than acknowledging psychological distress. The disruption of routine body cycles, such as digestion, menstruation, or sleep is more socially acceptable than having emotional responses related to interpersonal relationships, economic crises, adjustment to marriage, infertility, or the death of a spouse." (Boyd, 2012, p. 537). Interestingly, the relationships that exist between somatic symptoms and depression is very similar around the world and even between varied cultures within the same country (APA, 2013).

> ### Bridging the gap
>
> ## How culture influences treatment choices
>
> An individual's cultural or ethnic background may influence his or her treatment preferences and choices. Some cultures may be suspicious of alternative medicine, whereas those from other cultures may often use alternative techniques—but hesitate to disclose this. Their hesitancy may arise from previous experiences with skeptical health care professionals.

Causes

The precise causes of somatic disorders remain mostly a mystery. When there is a medical disorder, it is difficult to determine which came first, the excessive worry or the medical symptoms. There are several possible factors contributing to somatic symptom disorders. An increased sensitivity to pain from genetic and biological factors, early childhood trauma, and the societal stigma associated with psychological suffering but not physical suffering may all influence the development of somatic disorders.

Family stress

Among children and adolescents, family stress is thought to be a common cause of somatic disorders. For instance, a child may unconsciously reflect or imitate a parent's behavior—especially if the parent reaped considerable secondary gain (such as attention) from the symptoms. (See *Primary and secondary gain,* page 248.). Furthermore, multiple somatic symptoms have been reported to indicate child physical or sexual abuse and children with somatic symptoms often experience depression and anxiety as adults.

Learned responses

Behavioral theorists view psychosomatic symptoms as responses that the patient has consciously learned and subsequently maintains because they bring some type of reward. The symptoms, for instance, may allow the patient to:
- gain concern or sympathy
- avoid unpleasant tasks
- explain or justify failures.

Psychobiological mechanisms

Some experts describe four independent psychobiological mechanisms at work in somatization:

- heightened body sensations
- increased autonomic arousal
- identification of the "patient" within a family
- perceived need to be sick.

An individual patient may show evidence of a single mechanism or any combination of the four.

Heightened body sensations

Somatic symptom disorders may be linked to a heightened awareness of normal body sensations. Paired with a cognitive bias, this heightened awareness may predispose the patient to interpret any physical symptom as a sign of physical illness.

An individual who is worried about physical disease may focus attention on common variations in bodily sensations (hunger, pressure, stiffness, etc.)—to the point that these sensations become disturbing and unpleasant. The patient thinks the sensations confirm the suspected presence of physical disease. The perception of such altered sensations exacerbates his or her concerns, further increasing his or her anxiety and amplifying the sensations.

Increased autonomic arousal

Some patients with somatoform disorders may have heightened autonomic arousal. Such arousal may be associated with the effects of body chemicals that cause norepinephrine release, resulting in such symptoms as tachycardia or gastric hypermotility. Heightened autonomic arousal also may cause pain and muscle tension associated with muscular hyperactivity, as in muscle tension headache.

Identification of the "patient" within a family

In a family under stress, identifying one member as the "patient" may provide a focus that relieves anxiety for the family system. With a single member taking on the "sick" role, family behavior patterns may become dysfunctional. Health care providers may reinforce this dynamic by focusing medical attention on the "sick" family member's disability and illness.

Primary and secondary gain

Primary gain refers to relief of the unconscious psychological conflict, wish, or need that's causing the physical symptom. As the individual's anxiety increases and threatens to emerge into consciousness, they unconsciously "convert" it to physical symptoms. This relieves the pressure to deal with it directly and decreases the level of anxiety.

Secondary gain, in contrast, refers to the benefit, resources, or advantages that come from having the symptom—such as avoiding difficult situations, work, or getting emotional support or sympathy that the individual might not otherwise receive.

Perceived need to be sick

Individuals with somatic disorders may seek the "sick" role because it provides relief from stressful interpersonal expectations and, in most societies, offers attention and caring.

Somatic symptom disorder

Somatic symptom disorder is characterized by multiple and often vague physical complaints that are distressing and interfere with daily functioning. There are excessive thoughts, feelings, and behaviors related to the somatic symptoms. Typically, the symptoms are recurrent.

Complaints may involve any body system and often persist for years. They may begin or get worse after a job loss, death of a close relative or friend, or some other loss. Stress tends to intensify the symptoms.

Sickly life story

Patients with somatic symptom disorder may have impairments in occupational, social, and other functioning and may become extremely dependent in their relationships. Patients may seek medical care from multiple physicians, which can lead to confusion in treatment and conflicting treatment plans (Townsend, 2014). Even when presented with medical evidence to the contrary, patients with somatic symptom disorder will still think the worst about their health assuming a high degree of medical seriousness associated with their presenting symptoms (APA, 2013).

Commonly, the patient undergoes repeated medical evaluations, which (unlike the symptoms themselves) can be potentially damaging and debilitating. When the patient grows dissatisfied with the medical care he or she is receiving, the patient finds another provider and may continue to press for more tests and treatments. These patients may even undergo unnecessary surgery. However, unlike the individual with illness anxiety disorder, this patient isn't preoccupied with the belief that he or she has a specific disease.

Prevalence and onset

Somatic symptom disorder affects an estimated 0.2% to 2% of the general population (APA, 2013). It's 10 times more common in females—possibly reflecting cultural pressures on women or greater social "permission" for women to be physically weak or sickly. Symptoms begin before age 30, often in adolescence or early adulthood. Somatic symptom disorder is a chronic condition of fluctuating course and a poor prognosis. Complete, spontaneous remission is rare.

Ever-present illness

Symptoms may be most obvious during early adulthood, but few patients are entirely asymptomatic or go more than 1 or 2 years without seeking medical attention.

Somatic symptom disorder often co-exists with other psychiatric conditions, including major depression and anxiety. These patients are at an increased risk for substance abuse disorders involving prescription medications, as well as drug interactions from prescriptions written by multiple providers (Townsend, 2014).

> This is your third admission to the hospital this year, isn't it?

Causes

Somatic symptom disorder has no specific cause but genetic, biological, environmental, and psychological factors may contribute to its development. These causes are discussed more on page 247 in the overview of somatic disorders.

Signs and symptoms

Signs and symptoms may involve any body system but most commonly involve the gastrointestinal (GI), neurologic, cardiopulmonary, or reproductive systems. Many patients complain of multiple symptoms at the same time. (See *Common assessment findings in somatic symptom disorder.*)

An important clue to this disorder is a history of multiple medical evaluations by different providers at different health care facilities (sometimes simultaneously)—without significant findings. Unfortunately, it is common for the patient to have dissatisfaction with the health care provider. This dissatisfaction leads to "doctor shopping" and contributes to the cycle of misdiagnosis and treatment (Sharma & Manjula, 2013).

Advice from the experts

Common assessment findings in somatic symptom disorder

Signs and symptoms of somatic symptom disorder may mimic actual disorders and are just as real to the individual as the physical disorders that can cause them. They most often involve a few key body systems.

Cardiopulmonary symptoms
- Chest pain
- Dizziness
- Palpitations
- Shortness of breath (without exertion)

Female reproductive signs and symptoms
- Excessive menstrual bleeding
- Irregular menses
- Vomiting throughout pregnancy

GI signs and symptoms
- Abdominal pain (excluding menstruation)

- Diarrhea
- Flatulence
- Intolerance to foods
- Nausea and vomiting (excluding motion sickness)

Pain
- In extremities
- In the back
- During urination

Pseudoneurologic signs and symptoms
- Amnesia
- Blindness

- Difficulty walking, paralysis, or weakness
- Double or blurred vision
- Dysphagia
- Dysuria or urinary retention
- Fainting or loss of consciousness
- Loss of voice or hearing
- Seizures

Sexual signs and symptoms
- Burning sensation in sexual organs or rectum (except during intercourse)
- Dyspareunia or lack of pleasure during sex
- Impotence
- Sexual indifference

It is important to remember that in somatic symptom disorder, "somatic symptoms are not under the individual's voluntary control" (Halter, 2014, p. 331). The individual tends to report complaints and previous medical evaluations in a dramatic or exaggerated fashion. The patient may have a complicated medical history in which many physical diagnoses have been considered. They may also seem quite knowledgeable about tests, procedures, and medical jargon.

> What a complicated medical history! It's typical for a patient with somatic symptom disorder.

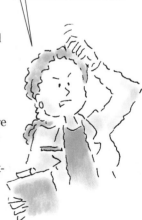

Diagnosis

Diagnosis of somatic symptom disorder is challenging. There is no specific test that reveals the disorder, and because the nature of the illness is related to physical complaints, these must be ruled out. The patient should undergo a physical examination and some diagnostic testing to rule out physical conditions that may produce vague, confusing symptoms (such as multiple sclerosis, hypothyroidism, hyperparathyroidism, systemic lupus erythematosus, or chronic fatigue syndrome).

A psychological evaluation can rule out related psychiatric disorders, including:
- depression
- schizophrenia with somatic delusions
- illness anxiety disorder
- malingering.

Ultimately, the diagnosis is confirmed if the patient meets the criteria in the *Diagnostic and Statistical Manual of Mental Disorders*, 5th Edition (*DSM-5*), which revolve around persistent physical symptoms that "result in significant disruption of daily life" (APA, 2013, p. 311).

Treatment

Somatic symptom disorder is one of the "most difficult disorders to manage because the symptoms tend to change, are diffuse and complex, moving from one body system to another" (Boyd, 2012, p. 537). The individual isn't likely to acknowledge any psychological aspect of the symptoms or consider psychiatric treatment.

The goal is control

The goal of treatment is to help the patient learn to control and cope with symptoms rather than eliminate them completely (Phoenix & Johnson, 2013). Telling the patient that his or her symptoms are imaginary won't help. It is very important to develop a relationship and trusting rapport with the patient. Part of developing trust is validating feelings while also presenting factual information and supportive care. For example, the nurse may say, "You do not have a serious illness but I will continue to provide care to help you and ease your symptoms."

A single gatekeeper

Management also focuses on preventing unnecessary medical and surgical interventions and turning the patient's attention away from the symptoms. Successful management of this disorder often takes a multidisciplinary team. The key to success is communication between the team, as this helps to create consistency and decreases the opportunity for unnecessary medical intervention (Halter, 2014). The multidisciplinary team should work together to support healthy and adaptive behaviors and encourage the patient to move beyond the somatization and work toward effective management of life.

Pharmacologic treatment

There is unclear evidence regarding the use of medications in the treatment of somatic symptom disorder. If the patient has a coexisting depressive or anxiety disorder, he or she may benefit from antidepressant drugs, such as selective serotonin reuptake inhibitors (SSRIs), to ease his or her preoccupation with symptoms. Short-term antianxiety medication may also be used. However, the decision to treat pharmacologic requires balancing the benefit with the chance that these patients may abuse the medication or take it erratically (Saddock & Saddock, 2008 as cited in Halter, 2014).

Nursing interventions

These nursing interventions may be appropriate for a patient with somatic symptom disorder.

• Acknowledge the individual's symptoms and support his or her efforts to function and cope despite distress. Don't tell the patient that the symptoms are imaginary—but do inform him or her of diagnostic test results and their implications.

• Encourage the patient to keep a symptom journal. This validates what the patient is feeling. Have the patient bring the journal with him or her to his or her next appointment and look for symptomatic patterns. This is helpful in educating the patient and also increases feelings of control over the symptoms (Boyd, 2012).

• Negotiate a plan of care with input from the patient and, if possible, the family.

Strength in positive statements

• Emphasize the patient's strengths. For example, say "It's good that you can still work even though you're in pain. You can be pleased with that accomplishment."

• Gently point out the link between stressful events and the onset of physical symptoms.

• Keep in mind that your goal is to help the individual manage symptoms, not eliminate them.

• Because these patients seek medical care so frequently, they often associate health care providers as their support network versus looking to develop healthy relationships with family and friends. Work to establish a trusting rapport while fostering their independence by helping the patient strengthen social relationships (Boyd, 2012).

> Emphasize the individual's strengths and point out accomplishments.

Attitude assessment

• Check your own feelings and attitudes periodically. If you think you've developed an attitude that says, "This person doesn't really want to get better, so why should I waste my time?" acknowledge your feelings honestly. Be sure that your body language does not display frustration or anger toward the patient. It is important to remember that the patient really does believe what he or she is feeling is real even though there is no physical basis for the symptoms. Caring for these patients can be very trying and at times unsatisfying for the nurse. Care conferences (team or unit-based meetings) are a great way to discuss care and the nurse's feelings associated with care as well as provide a more consistent level of overall care to the patient (Halter, 2014).

> **Memory jogger**
>
> SIGNS of somatic disorders
>
> **S:** Sexual or reproductive symptoms
>
> **I:** Intense pain
>
> **G:** GI problems
>
> **N:** Neurologic symptoms
>
> **S:** Symptoms of high anxiety about physical symptoms or health

Evaluation and treatment

Accurate diagnosis of somatic symptom disorder can prevent unnecessary laboratory tests, surgery, and other procedures. The individual should undergo a thorough physical workup to identify and treat medical and neurologic conditions and, in patients with pain, to assess and treat pain severity. Other psychiatric disorders that resemble somatic disorders as well as substance misuse must be identified also. Currently, this diagnosis is used when there are distressing somatic symptoms with abnormal thoughts, feelings, and behaviors in response to the somatic symptoms.

One-stop shopping

Ideally, an individual with a somatic disorder should develop a long-term relationship with a single, trusted primary health care provider. This helps guard against unnecessary tests and treatments. It is best when the primary care provider works in conjunction with a supportive mental health team to provide multidisciplinary care. However, many with this diagnosis are reluctant to seek help from a mental health provider. Referrals to mental health professionals should be handled with great sensitivity in order to avoid feelings of "abandonment" from the primary provider.

The manner in which the diagnosis is explained is very important to avoid more distress and embarrassment. For example, an explanation about the physiologic effects of extreme or chronic stressors or the analogy of a circuit breaker shutting down when overloaded may be helpful. The explanation that "it's all in your head" should always be avoided.

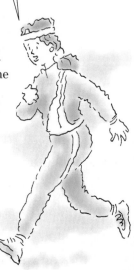

> I tell my patients that regular exercise gives them a sense of control—and I like to practice what I preach.

Patient's role

The individual should take an active role in treatment and be willing to take responsibility for moving forward with the treatment plan (such as by keeping a diary of symptoms and activities). Also, he or she should be encouraged to attend physical therapy or get regular exercise because self-initiated physical activity fosters responsibility and a sense of control. Periodic conferences should be scheduled with the patient and his or her family to provide a forum for communication and education. Patients with this disorder often find comfort in having a regularly scheduled appointment with their health provider. If a regular appointment is scheduled, it may decrease the number of "urgent" visits related to somatic symptomology.

Therapeutic approaches

"Cognitive-behavioral therapy is one the most frequently examined treatment methods used in somatic symptom disorders and endorses the strongest and consistent evidence for its efficacy" (Kroenke & Swindle, 2007 as cited in Sharma & Manjula, 2013, p. 120). The goal with behavioral therapy is to reduce symptoms and restore social relationships as well as stabilize the personality. Psychoanalysis and other forms of insight-oriented psychotherapy are less effective, although some patients may benefit from group therapy or support groups.

Family therapy

Family therapy may be recommended for children or adolescents with somatic disorders, particularly if the parents seem to be using the child to divert attention from other difficulties.

Alternative therapies

Alternative therapies may relieve stress, pain, and other symptoms, not just on a physical level but also on a mental, emotional, and spiritual level (Ornbol, Wald, Rehfeld, Schroder & Fink, 2013). These therapies include:
- acupuncture
- hydrotherapy
- therapeutic massage
- meditation
- botanical medicine
- homeopathic treatment.

Illness anxiety disorder

Illness anxiety disorder is marked by the persistent conviction that one has or is likely to get a serious disease—despite medical evidence and reassurance to the contrary. You may recognize the previous terminology used for this disorder as hypochondriasis. There is a very high level of anxiety about health status even though significant symptoms are not present. This individual focuses on the fear of having or developing a serious physical illness as opposed to the individual with somatic symptom disorder who focuses on the symptoms. "Individuals with illness anxiety disorder are extremely conscious of bodily sensations and changes and may become convinced that a rapid heart rate indicates they have heart disease or that a small sore is skin cancer" (Townsend, 2014, p. 584).

> Have I ever overlooked organic disease in a patient with chronic unfounded physical complaints?? I hope not, but I can't be sure.

Illness anxiety disorder may lead to physical illness

A long history of previously unfounded complaints may contribute to the health care provider overlooking a serious organic disease. The individual is also at risk for complications from multiple evaluations, tests, and invasive procedures.

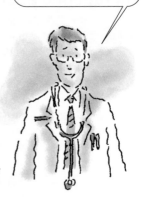

Prevalence and onset

In general medical clinic populations, the prevalence of illness anxiety disorder is between 3% and 8%. Illness anxiety disorder affects as many men as women. Onset of illness

---

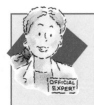

Advice from the experts

Assessing elderly patients for illness anxiety or somatic symptom disorders

Elderly individuals may perceive themselves to be in poor health even if they have no significant physical impairments. Their tendency to present with somatic complaints poses a challenge to assessment and management.

As a first step, the individual should undergo a comprehensive medical evaluation (and laboratory tests, as needed) to check for a physical basis for complaints. Cognitive and psychiatric examinations may be warranted, too.

Essential assessment data

When assessing an elderly patient for a somatic disorder, always gather a complete history. Be sure to obtain:
- past level of functioning
- extent of current ability
- cognitive deficits
- manifestations of emotional distress.

Also assess the patient's psychosocial status, including:
- living situation
- social supports
- role within the family
- key support persons outside the family.

To verify the individual's information, obtain a collaborative history from family members, if possible.

Family stress and abuse

Be aware that the family may respond to the patient's somatic symptoms by giving the patient more time and attention. In some cases, however, family members become angry and frustrated as conflicts arise and escalate. The individual may even suffer neglect and abuse. If you suspect this is happening, make sure it's reported to the proper authorities.

anxiety disorder is early to mid adulthood, and prevalence seems to increase with age (APA, 2013).

Illness anxiety disorder is considered a chronic and relapsing condition (APA, 2013). Flare-ups often follow stressful events and the specific feared illness may vary. It is relevant to note that some cases of illness anxiety disorder are transient and are associated with more medical comorbidity versus psychological morbidity (APA, 2013). In other words, for some people, the disorder is less severe and does not carry a long-term psychological component.

Causes

The exact cause of illness anxiety disorder isn't known. There are numerous potential causative factors discussed on page 247.

Just like Mommy or Daddy

Most likely, psychological factors play a role. For instance, children may complain of physical symptoms that resemble those of other family members.

Sick excuse

In adults, illness anxiety disorder may reflect self-centeredness or a wish to be taken cared of. The condition enables the patient to take on a dependent sick role and thereby escape responsibilities or postpone unwelcome challenges.

Angry, then ill

Emotionally, the individual's symptoms may be linked to— or may be an expression of—anger or guilt.

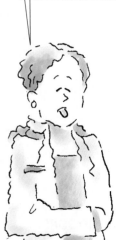

They want me to work a double shift tomorrow— but I think I feel the flu coming on.

Contributing factors

Factors that may contribute to illness anxiety disorder include:
- death of a loved one
- family member or friend with a serious illness
- a history of serious illness.

In elderly people, illness anxiety disorder may be associated with depression, grief, or loneliness. (Refer to the advice from the experts on page 256).

Signs and symptoms

Signs and symptoms of illness anxiety disorder range from specific to general complaints. Usually, the patient has multiple complaints that involve a single body system that reflect a preoccupation with normal body functions for a minimum of 6 months. The individual may have excessive contact with health care providers or totally avoid contact.

Mountains from molehills

Physical sensations and symptoms commonly misinterpreted as signs of organic disease include:
• borborygmi (rumbling sounds caused by gas and fluids moving through the intestines)
• abdominal bloating
• crampy discomfort
• cardiac awareness
• sweating.

Doting on details

Typically, the individual describes the symptom's location, quality, and duration in minute detail. Yet, these symptoms rarely follow a recognizable pattern of organic dysfunction and usually aren't associated with abnormal physical findings. As medical evaluation proceeds, the individual's complaints may change.

Don't confuse me with the facts

Examination and reassurance by a health care provider doesn't relieve the patient's concerns. Instead, the patient tends to believe the provider has failed to find the real cause of the disorder.

Other findings

Other assessment findings in patients with illness anxiety disorder may include:
• abnormal focus on bodily functions and sensations
• anger, frustration, and depression
• frequent visits despite assurance from health care providers that the individual is healthy
• intensified symptoms when around sympathetic people
• rejection of the notion that symptoms are stress or psychologically related
• use of symptoms to avoid difficult situations.

Diagnosis

Just like somatic symptom disorder, diagnosis of illness anxiety disorder is challenging. Patient symptoms change frequently and are often associated with normal bodily functioning (such as abdominal pain from flatulence). A complete history, with an emphasis on current psychological stressors, is helpful. Tests to rule out underlying organic disease may be used, although invasive procedures should be minimized. Typically, test results are inconsistent with the complaints and physical findings.

Let's make it official

Although history and physical findings may suggest illness anxiety disorder, the diagnosis is official only if the patient meets the criteria in the *DSM-5*. These criteria are basically a milder form of somatic symptom disorder. There is a persistent preoccupation of having or acquiring a serious disease without symptoms present. The disturbance lasts at least 6 months and is not explained by another mental disorder.

Treatment

The goal of treatment is to help the individual lead a productive life despite distressing symptoms and fears. Appropriate teaching and a supportive relationship with a single competent, trusted health care professional are crucial.

Breaking the not-so-awful news

After the medical evaluation is complete, the individual should be told that he or she doesn't have a serious disease but continued follow-up will help control symptoms. Although providing a diagnosis may not make illness anxiety disappear, it may ease some of the anxiety.

Linking the diagnosis to psychological stressors also can prove therapeutic. On the other hand, telling the patient that his or her symptoms are imaginary is counterproductive.

Follow-up care

Besides aiding detection of organic illness, regular outpatient follow-up care can help the patient deal with symptoms. That's important because up to 30% of individuals with illness anxiety later develop organic disease.

Psychotherapy

Most patients with illness anxiety disorder don't acknowledge any psychological influence on their symptoms and resist psychiatric treatment. However, a patient who's willing to try psychotherapy may be treated individually, in a group, or as part of a family.

• *Individual* psychotherapy uses psychodynamic principles to help the patient understand unconscious conflicts.

• *Group* therapy provides support to help the patient learn to cope with symptoms and to improve social skills.

• *Family* therapy focuses on improving family members' awareness of their interaction patterns and on enhancing their communication with each other.

Cognitive and behavioral therapy

Other therapeutic approaches to illness anxiety disorder include cognitive and behavioral techniques. Behavior modification provides incentives, motivation, and rewards to control symptoms.

Pharmacologic therapy

Drugs prescribed for patients with illness anxiety disorder may include:
- benzodiazepines, such as lorazepam (Ativan) or alprazolam (Xanax) for short-term use
- antidepressants in the SSRI group
- tricyclic antidepressants, such as amitriptyline (Elavil) or imipramine (Tofranil).

Medication can be especially helpful for patients with overlapping psychiatric conditions, such as depression or other anxiety disorders.

Nursing interventions

Because there is a close relationship between somatic symptom disorder and illness anxiety disorder, the nursing care often overlaps. In addition to the nursing interventions discussed on page 253 for somatic symptom disorder, these nursing interventions may also be appropriate for a patient with illness anxiety disorder.
- Help the individual expand coping skills and attend to altered health maintenance.
- Assess the patient's level of knowledge about the effects of emotions and stress on physiologic functioning. Provide appropriate teaching.
- Encourage the patient to express his or her feelings to deter emotional repression, which can have physical consequences.

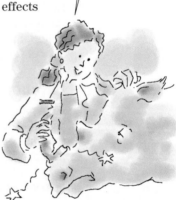

Enough about your symptoms. Let's talk about mine!

Change the subject

- Respond to the individual's symptoms in a matter-of-fact way to reduce the secondary gain that the patient gets from talking about them.
- Engage the individual in conversations that focus on something other than physical maladies.
- Create a supportive relationship that helps the patient feel cared for and understood.
- Keep in mind that the patient with illness anxiety disorder experiences real distress. Don't deny his or her symptoms or challenge behavior. Instead, help the patient find new ways to deal with stress other than developing physical symptoms.

Relaxation techniques

If your patient has symptoms related to stress or anxiety, relaxation techniques may help. Simple relaxation techniques include:
• deep breathing, in which the patient takes a series of slow, deep breaths and releases each breath slowly
• meditation, in which the patient either clears his or her mind or focuses on a single soothing thought, image, or sound.

Deep breathing

To teach your patient how to perform deep breathing, first instruct his or her to sit in a comfortable position with his or her eyes closed. Next, tell the patient to focus on a peaceful sound or image, and then breathe in through his or her nose to a count of 4.

Have the patient hold his or her breath for a count of 2. Then instruct him or her to breathe out through his or her mouth for a count of 6. The patient should repeat this cycle for 30 seconds to 5 minutes.

Meditation (Ornbol et al., 2013)

Meditation may offset some of the negative physiologic effects of stress through a mechanism called the *relaxation response*. Meditating takes about 20 minutes and can be done anywhere at any time—or it may be done as a scheduled activity. Tell the patient that learning to meditate takes some practice—ideally, he or she should practice it daily.

Techniques include concentrative and mindful meditation. For *concentrative* meditation, instruct the patient to focus on a peaceful image, thought, sound, or his or her own breathing.

For *mindful* meditation, instruct the patient to remain aware of all sensations, feelings, images, thoughts, sounds, and smells that pass through his or her mind—without actually thinking about them.

Whichever technique the patient uses, encourage him or her to make a conscious effort to relax his or her muscles and maintain a comfortable posture as he or she meditates. Closing the patient's eyes can help him or her focus on inner peace.

Don't get mad

• Recognize that the patient will probably never be symptom-free, and don't get angry when the patient doesn't give up his or her symptoms. Such anger can drive the patient away to yet another unnecessary medical evaluation.
• Help the patient learn nonpharmacologic strategies to reduce distress, such as imagery, relaxation, hypnosis, biofeedback, and massage. (See *Relaxation techniques.*) Also, teach assertiveness techniques, if appropriate.

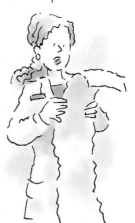

Yikes! This patient's history is as long as Billy the Kid's rap sheet!

Conversion disorder

Conversion disorder, also referred to as *functional neurologic symptom disorder*, is marked by the loss of or change in voluntary motor or sensory functioning (for instance, blindness, paralysis, or anesthesia) that suggests a physical illness but has no demonstrable physiologic basis. The symptom likely has a psychological basis, although it may not be readily identifiable. Previous diagnostic criteria inferred that there must be a psychological stressor to cue the conversion symptoms. This criterion has been removed from the *DSM-5*. "The potential etiologic relevance of stress or trauma may be suggested by a close temporal relationship. However, although assessment for stress and trauma is important, the diagnosis should not be withheld if none is found" (APA, 2013, p. 319–320).

The conversion symptom itself isn't life-threatening and usually has a short duration. However, it's clinically significant and distressing enough to disrupt social, occupational, or other important areas of functioning.

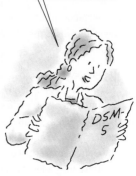

The more I read about conversion disorder, the more fascinated I am.

No fakery involved

The symptom isn't under the individual's voluntary control. Unlike in factitious disorders or malingering, the patient with a conversion disorder doesn't feign or intentionally produce the symptoms, although they may have the unconscious motives of primary or secondary gain. (See *Facts about factitious disorders*, page 268.)

Complications and consequences

Conversion symptoms can severely impede the individual's normal activities. "The severity of the disability can be similar to that experienced by individuals with comparable medical disease" (APA, 2013, p. 321).

Prevalence and onset

"Transient conversion symptoms are common, but the precise prevalence of the disorder is unknown" (APA, 2013, p. 320). This disorder is not usually diagnosed in primary care but rather in the secondary care environment. The disorder is found in up to 5% of the referrals made to neurology clinics. Conversion disorder affects two to three times more females than males.

It can happen at any age

Onset of conversion disorder can occur at any age. Conversion disorder is rarely chronic. In hospitalized patients, symptoms generally improve within 2 weeks. About 90% of patients recover within 1 month. However, about 20% to 25% of patients have recurrent symptoms within 1 year. In a few, symptoms become chronic.

Conversion disorders in children

Among children and adolescents, conversion disorder often reflects stress in the family or in school rather than a long-term psychiatric problem.

According to some experts, children and adolescents with conversion disorders have an overprotective or overinvolved parent with a subconscious need to see their child as sick. The child's symptoms then become the center of attention in the family.

Causes

Conversion disorder may have biological, environmental, and psychological components.

Psychological factors

Psychodynamic theory explains conversion disorder as a defense mechanism that absorbs and neutralizes the anxiety evoked by an unacceptable impulse or wish. The patient represses unconscious intrapsychic conflicts and converts anxiety into a physical symptom. For example, the patient may lose his or her voice in a circumstance where he or she is afraid to speak. Thus, the symptom gets the patient out of an unpleasant situation.

Biological factors

There may be a connection between neurobiologic changes in the brains of those with conversion disorder. These subtle changes may cause the lack of sensation or movement control (Boyd, 2012).

Seeing no evil

Often, conversion symptoms arise suddenly—soon after the patient experiences a traumatic conflict, he or she may feel as though he or she cannot cope. Two theories may explain why this occurs:

The patient achieves a primary gain as the symptoms keep the psychological distress out of conscious awareness.

The patient achieves a secondary gain by avoiding a traumatic activity. For example, a soldier may develop a "paralyzed" hand that prevents entry into combat.

Risk factors

Risk factors for conversion disorder include a history of maladaptive personality traits (such as excessive emotionality and attention seeking). Also, children are more likely to have conversion disorder if their family members have a history of the disorder or are seriously ill or in chronic pain. In some children and adolescents, conversion disorder is linked to physical or sexual abuse within the family.

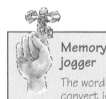

Memory jogger

The word convert is your clue to what happens in conversion disorder. Convert means to change from one form or function to another. Patients with conversion disorder convert stress into physical symptoms.

Signs and symptoms

The patient's history may reveal the sudden onset of a single, debilitating sign or symptom that prevents normal function of the affected body part, such as weakness, paralysis, or sensation loss in a specific body part.

Aphonia means loss of the voice. If only my dog would come down with it right now!

Other common conversion symptoms include:
• pseudoseizures (seizure-like attacks that are thought to be psychogenically produced)
• loss of a special sense, such as vision (blindness or double vision), hearing (deafness), or touch
• aphonia (inability to use the voice) or slurring of speech
• dysphagia (difficulty swallowing)
• impaired balance or coordination
• weakness or paralysis
• urinary retention.

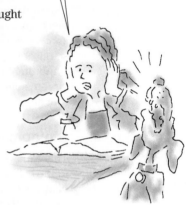

The patient may report that the symptom began after a traumatic event.

La belle indifférence

Oddly, many individuals with conversion disorder don't show concern over the symptoms or their functional limitations. Called la belle indifférence (French for "the beautiful indifference"), this apathy is associated with conversion disorder but should not be used as an isolate indicator of the disorder (APA, 2013).

Things just don't add up

Conversion symptoms rarely conform fully to the known anatomic and physiologic mechanisms underlying a true physical disorder. Here are three examples:

 Tendon reflexes may be normal in a "paralyzed" body part.

Reported loss of function fails to follow anatomic patterns of innervation.

Normal pupillary responses and evoked potentials are present in an individual who complains of blindness.

Diagnosis

With many individuals, the diagnosis of conversion disorder is considered only after extensive physical examination and laboratory tests fail to reveal a physical disorder that fully accounts for their symptoms. Nonetheless, early consideration of the disorder may avoid tests that increase patient costs and risks. What's more, unnecessary, painful, or invasive testing may reinforce and cause fixation of the individual's symptoms.

Process of elimination

Depending on the individual's symptoms, he or she may undergo a neurologic evaluation to rule out physical illnesses that affect sensory function (for instance, blindness or anesthesia) or voluntary motor function (such as paralysis or the inability to walk or stand). Diseases with a vague onset (such as multiple sclerosis or systemic lupus erythematosus) must also be ruled out.

Laboratory tests can identify such conditions as:
- hypoglycemia or hyperglycemia
- electrolyte disturbances
- renal failure
- systemic infection
- toxins
- effects of prescribed, over-the-counter, or illicit drugs.

Scans, X-rays, and punctures

Some individuals may undergo diagnostic procedures, including:
- computed tomography or magnetic resonance imaging scans to exclude a space-occupying lesion in the brain or spinal cord
- chest X-ray to rule out neoplasms
- lumbar puncture for spinal fluid analysis, which can rule out infection and other causes of neurologic symptoms
- electroencephalogram to help distinguish pseudo-seizures from true seizures.

Inconsistency's the key

In conversion disorder, physical and diagnostic findings are inconsistent with the complaints. The diagnosis is confirmed if the individual fulfills the diagnostic criteria listed in the *DSM-5* (APA, 2013). (See *Diagnostic criteria: Conversion disorder*.) The diagnosis can be further specified as acute or persistent and with or without a psychological stressor.

A chest X-ray may be ordered to rule out neoplasms in an individual with suspected conversion disorder.

Diagnostic criteria: Conversion disorder

The diagnosis of conversion disorder is confirmed when the patient meets these criteria from the *DSM-5*.

The criteria include one or more symptoms of altered motor or sensory function incompatible with recognized conditions and not explained by another medical or mental disorder.

Using biofeedback

Biofeedback training promotes relaxation and may relieve conversion symptoms by teaching the individual how to consciously control body functions—such as blood pressure, heart and respiratory rates, temperature, and perspiration. It involves the use of an electronic device that informs the patient when changes in these functions occur.

    Biofeedback has more than 150 applications for prevention of disease and restoration of health. It's often used for stress-related disorders and has many applications in therapy.

Treatment

A trusting clinician–patient relationship is essential. In many cases, simply reassuring the individual that the symptom doesn't indicate a serious underlying disorder makes him or her feel better and leads to symptom disappearance.

    Psychotherapy, family therapy, relaxation training, behavior modification, biofeedback training, or hypnosis may be used alone or in combination to treat conversion disorder. (See *Using biofeedback.*) However, none of these methods are uniformly effective. For a child or adolescent, family therapy is the treatment of choice.

Exploratory spell

In hypnosis, the clinician identifies and explores psychological issues with the hypnotized individual. Hypnosis in and of itself is not a treatment. It is a procedure that can help to facilitate other treatment methods (American Psychological Association, 2014). The discussion continues after hypnosis when the patient is fully alert.

Pharmacologic therapy

Benzodiazepines, such as lorazepam and alprazolam, have proven useful in treating some individuals with conversion disorder.

Nursing interventions

- Establish a supportive relationship that communicates acceptance of the individual but keeps the focus away from the symptoms. Doing this helps the patient learn to recognize and express anxiety.
- Don't force the individual to talk, but convey a caring attitude that encourages him or her to share feelings.
- Encourage the patient to seek psychiatric care if he or she is not already receiving it.

Hint at emotional links

- Help the individual identify any emotional conflicts that preceded symptom onset to help clarify the link between the conflict and the symptom. But don't imply that the symptoms are all in the patient's head.
- Help the individual increase his or her coping ability, reduce anxiety, and enhance self-esteem.
- Use measures to maintain the integrity of the affected body system or part. For instance, regularly exercise a "paralyzed" limb to prevent muscle wasting and contractures. Frequently change a bedridden individual's position to prevent pressure ulcers.

Ditch the insistence

- Don't insist that the individual use the affected body part or body system. This would only anger the patient and impede a therapeutic relationship.
- Ensure adequate nutrition even if the individual complains of GI distress.
- Promote social interaction to decrease the individual's self-involvement.

Call for a casting change

- Identify constructive coping mechanisms to encourage the individual to use practical coping skills and relinquish the "sick" role.
- Include the family in the patient's care. Not only may they be contributing to the perceived stress; they're also essential in providing support and helping the patient regain normal function.

Psychological factors affecting other medical conditions

This diagnosis is appropriate when psychological or behavioral factors adversely affect a medical disease. This may include poor adherence to treatment, denial of symptoms, psychological distress, or negative coping styles. The result is exacerbation or delayed recovery from medical condition, interference with treatment, or influence the underlying pathology such as anxiety inducing an asthma attack.

Facts about factitious disorders

Factitious disorders (FDs) are conditions in which a patient deliberately produces or exaggerates symptoms of a physical or mental illness to assume the role of a sick person. These disorders aren't a form of malingering (pretending illness for a clear benefit, such as financial gain). Instead, the patient has a deep-seated need to be seen as ill or injured.

Patients create their symptoms using various methods—injecting themselves with bacteria to produce infections, contaminating urine samples with blood, taking hallucinogens, or other behaviors.

There are two types of FD. The first type is referred to as *factitious disorder imposed on self*. (This diagnosis was previously referred to as *Munchausen syndrome*.) This means that the individual falsifies physical or psychological symptoms or induces illness on themselves. The second type is referred to as *factitious disorder imposed on another*. (This diagnosis was previously referred to as *Munchausen syndrome by proxy* or *factitious disorder by proxy*) This is the same process but is imposed on another person (in this case, a victim). The key element of both is deception.

Factitious disorder imposed on self
In FD imposed on self, the individual convincingly presents with intentionally feigned physical symptoms. These symptoms may be:
• fabricated (e.g., acute abdominal pain without underlying disease)
• self-inflicted (e.g., deliberately infecting an open wound)
• an exacerbation or exaggeration of a preexisting disorder (e.g., taking penicillin despite a known allergy to it)
• a combination of the previously discussed.

Some patients with this type of FD go so far as to have major surgery repeatedly.

History lessons
The patient with an FD may have a history of the following:
• multiple admissions to various hospitals, typically across a wide geographic area
• extensive knowledge of medical terminology
• pathologic lying
• shifting complaints, signs, and symptoms
• poor interpersonal relationships
• refusal of psychiatric examination
• psychoactive substance or analgesic use
• eagerness to undergo hazardous, painful procedures
• evidence of previous treatments, such as surgery
• discharge against medical advice to avoid detection.

Factitious disorder imposed on another
In this type, the same patterns of behavior or symptomatology may be present but in the caregiver versus the patient. The illness is being imposed on another (the victim) by the person with the disorder. "The perpetrator, not the victim, is given the diagnosis. The victim may be given an abuse diagnosis" (APA, 2013, p. 325). It is important to remember with this disorder that there is no external reward associated with this behavior. For example, if a caregiver lies to cover up child abuse to prevent punishment, then they are not diagnosed with an FD. With this disorder, the " deceptive behavior is evident even in the absence of external rewards" (APA, 2013, p. 325).

The individual (typically, a parent) intentionally produces or causes a physical illness in another person (most often a child) through such actions as:
• falsifying the child's medical history
• tampering with laboratory tests to make the child appear sick
• injecting toxic substances into the child
• tampering with treatments (for instance, intravenous or ventilator settings)
• biting or mutilating the child.

References

American Psychiatric Association. (2013). *Diagnostic and statistical manual of mental disorders* (5th ed.). Arlington, VA: Author.

American Psychological Association. (2014). *Hypnosis today: Looking beyond the media portrayal.* Retrieved from http://www.apa.org/topics/hypnosis/media.aspx#

Boyd, M. (2012). *Psychiatric nursing: Contemporary practice* (5th ed.). Philadelphia, PA: Lippincott Williams & Wilkins.

Halter, M. (2014). *Varicolis' foundation of psychiatric mental health nursing: A clinical approach* (7th ed.). St. Louis, MO: Elsevier.

Ornbol, E., Wald, H., Rehfeld, E., Schroder, A., & Fink, P. (2013). Mindfulness therapy for somatization disorder and functional somatic syndromes: Randomized trial with one year follow up. *Journal of Psychosomatic Research, 74*(1), 31–40.

Phoenix, B., & Johnson, K. (2013). Integrative management of anxiety. In K. Tusaie & J. Fitzpatrick (Eds.), *Advanced practice psychiatric nursing: Integrating psychotherapy, pharmacotherapy and complementary/alternative approaches* (pp. 158–181). New York, NY: Springer.

Sharma, M., & Manjula, M. (2013). Behavioural and psychological management of somatic symptom disorders: An overview. *International Review of Psychiatry, 25*(1), 116–124. doi:10.3109/09540261.2012.746649

Townsend, M. (2014). *Psychiatric mental health nursing: Concepts of care in evidence-based practice* (8th ed.). Philadelphia, PA: F.A. Davis.

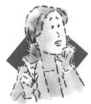

Quick quiz

1. Manifestation of physical symptoms caused by psychological distress is termed:

    A.   pain disorder.

    B.   somatization.

    C.   conversion disorder.

    D.   psychosomatic.

Answer: B. Somatization occurs when a psychological state causes or contributes to the development of physical symptoms.

2. An individual overly concerned with physical symptoms that lead to behaviors and thoughts that interfere with functioning may have which disorder?

    A.   Somatic symptom disorder

    B.   Conversion disorder

    C.   Illness anxiety disorder

    D.   Factitious disorder imposed on self

Answer: A. Somatic symptom disorder.

3. A therapeutic technique which is used in cognitive-behavioral therapy is:
  A.   thought stopping.
  B.   aversion therapy.
  C.   implosion therapy.
  D.   response prevention.

Answer: A. Cognitive-behavioral therapy uses techniques such as thought stopping and thought reframing to assist with changes in thoughts and behaviors.

4. A patient who reports paralysis with no specific cause but has a history of a recent stressful event has a probable diagnosis of:
  A.   hypochondriasis.
  B.   somatic illness.
  C.   conversion disorder.
  D.   pain disorder.

Answer: C. In conversion disorder, symptoms suggest a physical disorder, but physical examination and diagnostic tests find no physiologic cause.

5. Misinterpretation of bodily sensations or symptoms is a chief feature of:
  A.   conversion disorder.
  B.   somatization.
  C.   malingering.
  D.   illness anxiety disorders.

Answer: D. A patient with illness anxiety disorder misinterprets the severity and significance of bodily sensations or symptoms as indications of illness.

Scoring

☆☆☆   If you answered all five items correctly, kudos! You've obviously converted all the information in this chapter to your brain!

☆☆   If you answered three or four items correctly, nice job! There's nothing factitious about your understanding of somatoform disorders.

☆   If you answered fewer than three items correctly, don't convert your disappointment into symptoms. Just flood yourself with the concepts in this chapter, and then give it another try.

8

Dissociative disorders

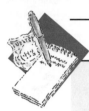

Just the facts

In this chapter, you'll learn:

♦ general characteristics of dissociation

♦ diagnostic tools used to evaluate dissociative disorders

♦ proposed causes of dissociative disorders

♦ signs and symptoms of dissociative disorders

♦ assessment and interventions for patients with dissociative disorders.

A look at dissociative disorders

Dissociative disorders are marked by disruption of the fundamental aspects of waking consciousness—memory, identity, consciousness, and the general experience and perception of oneself and the surroundings. Dissociation is used as an unconscious defense mechanism to separate anxiety-provoking feelings and thoughts from the conscious mind (American Psychiatric Association [APA], 2013).

Actually, dissociation is a common occurrence that ranges from normal to pathologic. Normal types of dissociation include daydreams, highway hypnosis (a trancelike feeling that can occur when driving), and getting "lost" in a book, movie, or television program to the point that someone fails to notice the time or surroundings. Pathologic dissociation occurs in dissociative disorders (APA, 2013).

This chapter discusses depersonalization/derealization disorder, dissociative amnesia, and dissociative identity disorder (DID). Depersonalization/derealization disorder alters the experience and perception of oneself.

> One type of dissociation is highway hypnosis, a trancelike feeling that occurs when driving.

Dissociative amnesia affects mainly memory, whereas dissociative amnesia with dissociative fugue and DID affect both identity and memory (APA, 2013).

Too awful to remember

Usually, dissociative disorders result from overwhelming stress caused by a traumatic event that has been experienced or witnessed or by intolerable psychological conflict. The disorder occurs as the mind isolates the unacceptable information and feelings.

Dissociation is a poorly understood phenomenon, and many question it's existence (Brand, Classen, McNary, & Zaveri, 2009). Dissociative disorders (especially dissociative amnesia) gained significant interest in the past related to "forgotten" childhood traumas and repressed memories. Some experts believe dissociation is a common defense mechanism used by a child who's traumatized, especially by abuse. Controversy and lawsuits have arisen over the accuracy of "recovered" childhood memories (Rhodes, 2011; Spiegel et al., 2013). Dissociative disorders are rare and affect more females than males. Symptoms may arise suddenly or gradually. Many dissociative episodes are transient. But if they persist, such episodes may cause functional impairments (APA, 2013).

> My brain helps me escape unpleasant situations by dissociation.

Causes

There are several theories that propose to explain dissociative disorders and they include psychological, biological, and learning theories.

Psychological theories

According to psychological theories, dissociative disorders are a response to severe trauma or abuse. To cope with the trauma or abuse, the patient tries to repress the unpleasant experience from awareness. If repression fails, dissociation occurs as a defense mechanism: The patient separates the experience from the conscious mind because it's too traumatic to integrate it (Foote, 2013; Sadock & Sadock, 2007; Wheeler, 2008). (See *Delving into dissociation.*)

Biological theories

Biological theories are most closely linked with depersonalization/derealization disorder. Researchers point out that this disorder

Myth busters

Delving into dissociation

Dissociation is a mysterious and often misunderstood phenomenon.
Myth: A person who experiences dissociation or derealization after a traumatic event can consciously control the dissociation.
Reality: Dissociation and derealization occur because the traumatic event has overwhelmed the person's ability to cope using any other method. They are beyond conscious control.
Myth: People in dissociative fugue states behave in a confused manner.
Reality: Most people in dissociative fugue states behave in a normal manner.

shares a key symptom—a sense of loss of one's own reality—with certain neurologic disorders (such as epilepsy and tumors), several psychiatric disorders, and the effects of certain drugs (most notably, barbiturates, benzodiazepines, hallucinogens, and marijuana) (Sadock & Sadock, 2007).

Learning theory

According to learning theory, dissociative disorders represent a learned response of avoiding stress and anxiety. With opportunity and practice, a person can become highly skilled at dissociating. This learned behavior of forcing the memory from awareness is common in people with a history of abuse (Allen & Smith, 1993).

Evaluation

Because a dissociative disorder can mimic a physical illness or another psychiatric disorder, the patient should undergo a complete physical examination.

Trials of trauma

In addition, a mental health professional should obtain a careful personal history from the patient and family members. The interview should include questions about childhood and adult trauma and abuse as well as any of these experiences:
• blackouts or "lost" time
• fugues—travel away from home with no memory of what happened on these trips

> A patient with a dissociative disorder may find himself or herself far from home with no memory of how he or she got there.

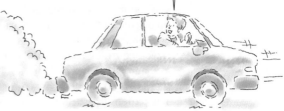

- unexplained possessions
- relationship changes
- fluctuations in skills and knowledge
- unclear or spotty recollection of the life history
- spontaneous trances
- spontaneous age regression
- out-of-body experiences
- awareness of other personalities within oneself.

Diagnostic toolbox

Patients with dissociative disorders may be evaluated with any of these diagnostic tools.

• Dissociative Experiences Scale (DES). This brief self-report scale measures the frequency of dissociative experiences. The patient quantifies his or her experiences for each item (Bernstein & Putnam, 1986). If the patient scores high, he or she may undergo further evaluation using the Dissociative Disorders Interview Schedule, the Multidimensional Inventory of Dissociation, or the Structured Clinical Interview for Dissociative Disorders (MacPhee, 2013).

• Dissociative Disorders Interview Schedule. This highly structured interview is used to diagnose trauma-related disorders. The patient answers questions that the examiner must ask in a precisely designated order. The interview takes 30 to 45 minutes (Tupper, 1996).

• Structured Clinical Interview for Dissociative Disorders (SCID-D). This semi-structured interview assesses the nature and severity of five dissociative symptoms—amnesia, depersonalization, derealization, identity confusion, and identity alteration. It also enables the clinician to diagnose a dissociative disorder based on *Diagnostic and Statistical Manual of Mental Disorders* criteria (Rhodes, 2011).

• Cambridge Depersonalization Scale. This self-report scale requires that the patient rate the frequency and duration of 29 types of depersonalization and derealization experiences. A high score of 70 or above indicates that his or her experiences are not better explained by various mood, anxiety, or neurologic disorders (Simeon, 2013a).

• Multidimensional Inventory of Dissociation. This self-report scale consists of 218 items that are ranked on a scale of "never" to "always." It can take up to 90 minutes to complete and the results can be categorized according to potential diagnoses (Chu, 2011).

• Diagnostic Drawing Series. This test is used by art therapists to aid diagnosis of dissociative disorders. The patient is instructed to draw a tree and a picture of how he or she's feeling (Cohen, 1983).

> An art therapist may use the Diagnostic Drawing Series to help diagnose a dissociative disorder.

Depersonalization/derealization disorder

Depersonalization/derealization disorder is marked by a persistent or recurrent feeling that one is detached from one's own mental processes or body or by feelings of detachment from other persons, objects, or their surroundings. The patient seldom loses touch with reality completely. However, depersonalization episodes may cause severe distress and sometimes impair functioning (APA, 2013).

Honey, I've shrunk!

During episodes of depersonalization, self-awareness (or a portion of it) is altered or lost temporarily. The sense of depersonalization may be restricted to a single body part, such as a limb—or it may encompass the whole self. The patient may feel as if a body part or the entire body has shrunk or grown.

Honey, you've shrunk!

During episodes of derealization, the patient's awareness of others is temporarily altered. Another person, object, or his or her surroundings may seem veiled or flat and seemingly artificial or lifeless, or other persons or objects may seem larger, smaller, closer, or farther away than they really are, much as Alice experienced after falling down the rabbit hole (APA, 2013).

Watching the world go by

The patient may perceive the change in consciousness as a barrier between himself or herself and the outside world. The patient may feel as if he or she's passively watching his or her mental or physical activity or as if the external world is unreal or distorted (APA, 2013).

We're all space cadets

Although depersonalization/derealization disorder is rare, the experience of depersonalization or derealization isn't. It occurs in many "normal" people for brief periods and shouldn't be confused with a psychiatric disorder.

For example, many people occasionally feel "spaced out" or as if they're in a dream or looking at themselves from the outside. When intoxicated, some people feel they're out of control of their actions. Depersonalization or derealization symptoms also can arise from meditation or certain religious practices (APA, 2013). (See *Dissociation/derealization and cultural considerations*, page 276.)

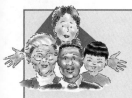

Bridging the gap

Dissociation/derealization and cultural considerations

If your patient has symptoms of a dissociative disorder, make sure to find out about his or her cultural and religious practices before drawing conclusions about his or her mental state.

Possession trances
Meditative and trancelike practices are a part of some religions and cultures. Some of these practices may resemble a dissociative disorder (particularly depersonalization disorder).

For instance, certain cultural groups in Indonesia, Malaysia, the Arctic, Latin America, and India may experience "possession trances." During the trance, a person's customary identity is replaced with a new identity, which is attributed to the influence of a deity, spirit, or power. In many cases, people in these trances make stereotyped "involuntary" movements, which they experience as being beyond their control (Ross, Schroeder, & Ness, 2013; Spiegel et al., 2013).

More of it than you'd think

Actually, the experience of depersonalization or derealization is common and often follows life-threatening danger, such as accidents, assaults, and serious illnesses and injuries. It can occur as a symptom in many other psychiatric disorders as well as in physical alterations of health such as seizure disorders (APA, 2013; Sadock & Sadock, 2007).

Although the *symptoms* of depersonalization or derealization are brief and have no lasting effect, depersonalization/derealization *disorder* is a chronic illness (Simeon, 2013a).

Prevalence and onset

The prevalence of depersonalization/derealization disorder is believed to be about 2%. Males and females are equally affected. Onset can be sudden or gradual, usually in childhood or adolescence. It rarely occurs after age 40 (APA, 2013).

The disorder often progresses and becomes chronic, with exacerbations and remissions. Exacerbations can be caused by stress and overstimulation (APA, 2013).

Causes

As a separate disorder, depersonalization/derealization disorder hasn't been studied widely and its exact cause is unknown. It typically occurs in people who have experienced early life complex trauma or severe stress or trauma such as combat, violent crime, accidents, or natural disasters (APA, 2013; Sadock & Sadock, 2007).

Other factors linked to its development include:

- immature defense mechanisms
- sensory deprivation
- neurophysiologic factors, such as epilepsy or a concussion
- history of physical or mental abuse or neglect
- history of substance abuse
- history of emotional abuse or neglect.

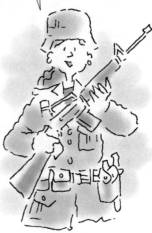

Combat experiences may lead to depersonalization/derealization disorder in some people.

Signs and symptoms

A patient with depersonalization/derealization disorder may report that he or she feels emotionally numb and detached from his or her entire being and body, as if he or she were a robot or was watching himself or herself from a distance or living in a dream. The patient may report that he or she feels as if he or she were in a fog or dream and that either his or her vision and/or hearing are distorted (APA, 2013).

Rumination and disconsolation

Other signs and symptoms may include:

- obsessive rumination
- depression
- anxiety
- fear of going insane
- disturbed sense of time
- slow recall
- physical complaints, such as dizziness
- impaired social and occupational functioning.

Diagnosis

The medical provider must rule out physical disorders, substance abuse, and other dissociative disorders (Simeon, 2013a). Psychological tests and special interviews may aid diagnosis. Standard tests include the Dissociative Experiences Scale and the Dissociative Disorders Interview Schedule, both of which can demonstrate the presence of dissociation. The Cambridge Depersonalization Scale is the most specific scale to the diagnosis of depersonalization/derealization (Simeon, 2013a).

The diagnosis is confirmed if the patient meets the criteria established in the *DSM-5*. (See *Diagnostic criteria: Depersonalization/derealization disorder*, page 278.)

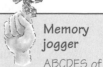

Memory jogger

ABCDES of depersonalization

A: Altered perceptions of self

B: Belief that one is observing oneself from outside the body

C: Characteristics of the body are perceived as altered

D: Detachment from the environment

E: Errors in the perceived sense of time

S: Sense of unreality

Diagnostic criteria: Depersonalization/derealization disorder

The diagnosis of depersonalization disorder is confirmed when the patient meets these criteria from the *Diagnostic and Statistical Manual of Mental Disorders*, 5th Edition (*DSM-5*).

• The patient has persistent or recurrent experiences of depersonalization, as indicated by a feeling of being detached from his or her mind or body (as if observing himself or herself from the outside) or feeling as if he or she's in a dream, or of derealization, as indicated by a feeling that other persons or objects are visually distorted or not real.

• During the depersonalization or derealization episode, the patient isn't psychotic and is able to perceive or discern the qualities of the surroundings.

• The disturbances cause clinically significant distress or impairment in social, occupational, or other important areas of functioning.

• The disturbances do not stem from direct physiologic effects of a substance or a neurologic or general medical condition.

• The depersonalization or derealization experience doesn't occur only during the course of another mental disorder (such as schizophrenia, panic disorder, acute stress disorder, or another dissociative disorder) and doesn't result from the direct physiologic effects of a substance or a general medical condition.

Treatment

Even without treatment, many patients recover completely. Treatment is warranted, however, if the disorder is persistent, recurrent, or distressing.

    Treatment measures include supportive psychotherapy and psychoeducation that give the patient information about the disorder, reduce associated guilt and stigma, and provide hope for the future. Cognitive-behavioral therapy and hypnosis may also be useful if the patient also experiences anxiety and/ or depression (Simeon, 2013a; 2013b).

Untangling the trauma

If depersonalization/derealization disorder is linked to a traumatic event, psychotherapy focuses on helping the patient recognize the event and anxiety it has evoked. Then, the therapist teaches the patient to use reality-based coping strategies instead of detaching from the situation (Simeon, 2013b).

Pharmacologic therapy

In addition to psychotherapy, a selective serotonin reuptake inhibitors (SSRIs) may be used when depressive symptoms are severe, or a benzodiazepine may be used for excessive anxiety. Patients who experience emotional

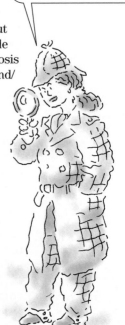

For treatment to succeed, all stressors linked to onset of the disorder must be identified.

numbing that does not respond to psychotherapy may benefit from an opioid antagonist (naltrexone or naloxone) (Sadock & Sadock, 2007; Simeon, 2013b).

Nursing interventions

Nursing interventions that may be appropriate for a patient with depersonalization disorder include:
• Establish a therapeutic, nonjudgmental relationship with the patient.
• Encourage the patient to recognize that depersonalization is a defense mechanism being used to deal with anxiety caused by a traumatic event.
• Help the patient recognize and deal with anxiety-producing experiences by implementing behavioral techniques to cope with stressful situations, if appropriate.
• Assist the patient in establishing supportive relationships (Stuart, 2013).

Dissociative amnesia

The key feature of dissociative amnesia is an inability to recall important personal information (usually of a stressful nature) that can't be explained by ordinary forgetfulness. Commonly, the patient forgets basic autobiographical information, such as his or her name, people he or she spoke to recently, and what he or she said, thought, experienced, or felt recently.

In most cases, an acute memory loss is triggered by a severe psychological stress. Recovery is usually complete and recurrence is rare, although the patient may be unable to recall certain life events. (See *Myths about memory lapses*, page 280.)

When dissociative amnesia is accompanied by sudden, unexpected travel away from one's home or workplace as well as the inability to recall one's past and confusion about one's personal identity (or assumption of a new identity) it is called *dissociative amnesia with dissociative fugue.* The travel during a fugue may range from brief trips lasting hours or days to complex wandering for weeks or months. In some cases, the person travels thousands of miles (APA, 2013). (See memory jogger for dissociative fugue in the following text.)

During the fugue state, the patient may appear normal and attract no attention. However, confusion about identity—or the return to original identity—may make the patient aware of the memory loss or may cause distress.

Memory jogger

The word TRAIL is your clue to ineffective coping in patients with dissociative amnesia with dissociative fugue.

T: Temporarily assumes a new identity or personality

R: Runs away or travels to escape severe distress

A: Amnesia occurring as memory gaps or memory loss

I: Intense, overwhelming anxiety

L: Low self-esteem

A rough landing

Although the patient may be asymptomatic during a fugue, he or she may experience various symptoms when it ends—depression, discomfort, grief, shame, intense conflict, or even suicidal or aggressive impulses. Failure to remember the events that took place during the fugue may cause confusion, distress, or even terror.

Types of dissociative amnesia

Dissociative amnesia occurs in five main types.

In *localized amnesia*, the patient can't remember events that took place during a specific period of time— usually, the first few hours after an extremely stressful or traumatic event.

In *selective amnesia*, the patient can recall some, but not all, of the events during a circumscribed time period. For instance, a soldier may be able to recall only some parts of a violent combat experience.

In *generalized amnesia*, the patient suffers prolonged loss of memory—possibly encompassing an entire lifetime.

In *continuous amnesia*, the patient forgets all events from a given time forward to the present.

In *systematized amnesia*, the patient's memory loss is limited to a specific type of information. For instance, he or she may have no memories related to a specific person (APA, 2013).

Time warp

Most patients with dissociative amnesia are aware that they have "lost" some time. But a few have "amnesia for amnesia"—they realize they have lost time only after seeing evidence that they have done things they don't recall. Some patients are distressed over their amnesia; others aren't (APA, 2013).

Unlike other types of amnesia, dissociative amnesia doesn't result from an organic disorder (such as a stroke or dementia) (APA, 2013).

Prevalence and onset

The prevalence of dissociative amnesia is believed to be about 1.8%, about twice as high for women than men. Most common in adolescents and young women, the disorder is also seen in young men after combat. It usually comes on suddenly but may be delayed for hours, days, or longer following a traumatic event. It may resolve quickly but sometimes becomes chronic (APA, 2013).

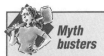

Myth busters

Myths about memory lapses

Myth: Memory lapses are a sign of insanity.
Reality: Occasional, brief memory lapses are common—and normal—experiences. If these lapses recur often and cause impairment, they may reflect an injury or an underlying psychiatric or physical disorder.

Unfilled memory voids

The prognosis depends mainly on life circumstances, particular stresses and conflicts associated with the amnesia, and the patient's overall psychological adjustment. (See *Patient safety and family strain*.) Although most patients recover, some never break through the barriers to reconstruct their missing past, and those persons usually remain impaired in both their relationships and vocations. Persons who experience amnesia with dissociative fugue are particularly at risk for poorer outcomes (APA, 2013).

Causes

Dissociative amnesia probably results from severe stress associated with a traumatic experience, major life event, or severe internal conflict (APA, 2013).

Factors that may contribute to development of this disorder include:
- history of a traumatic event or repeated trauma
- history of physical, emotional, or sexual abuse, particularly in childhood
- mild traumatic brain injury.

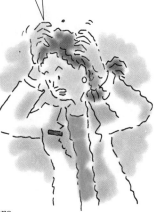

During an amnesiac episode, the person may wander aimlessly, seeming disoriented and perplexed.

Signs and symptoms

During an amnesiac episode, the patient may seem perplexed and disoriented, wandering aimlessly, especially if experiencing a fugue. The patient is unable to remember the event that precipitated the episode and usually doesn't even recognize the inability to recall information. The patient may have mild to severe social impairment.

Patient safety and family strain

During an episode of dissociative amnesia or fugue, the patient may pose a safety risk to himself or herself because of his or her impaired memory and reduced awareness of surroundings. Not only is the patient at high risk for falls and other injuries—if he or she appears obviously confused, he or she's also easy prey for con artists and criminals. His or her self-care may suffer, too.

Family strain
If the patient experiences frequent amnesia or fugue episodes, his or her family may feel helpless to cope with his or her behavior. Concerned for his or her well-being, they may change their daily routines—a burden that could lead to strained relationships and, possibly, abuse.

Once the amnesia episode ends, the patient usually isn't aware that there has been a memory disturbance. However, the patient may gradually recall some memories and may experience distress or symptoms of posttraumatic stress disorder (PTSD) and may develop self-destructive or suicidal behaviors (APA, 2013).

Diagnosis

The patient should undergo a thorough physical examination to rule out an organic cause for the symptoms. Blood and urine tests may be done to rule out drug use and other conditions. Electroencephalography (EEG) can exclude a seizure disorder. A history of past head trauma should be explored (DynaMed, 2012).

Say it in pictures

The patient also should undergo a psychiatric examination. Psychological tests help characterize the nature of his or her dissociative experiences. These tests include the Diagnostic Drawing Series, Dissociative Experiences Scale, and Dissociative Disorders Interview Schedule (Bernstein & Putnam, 1986; Cohen, 1983; Tupper, 1996).

The diagnosis of dissociative amnesia is confirmed if the patient meets the criteria in the *DSM-5*. (See *Diagnostic criteria: Dissociative amnesia.*) However, when dissociative amnesia occurs as a symptom of another psychiatric disorder, it isn't diagnosed separately.

Treatment

Sometimes, the amnesia resolves by itself. If not, psychotherapy is used to help the patient recognize the traumatic event that triggered the amnesia and the anxiety it has produced. A supportive, trusting therapeutic relationship is essential to achieving this goal. An accepting environment may in itself enable the patient to gradually recover his or her missing memories. The psychotherapist subsequently attempts to teach his or her reality-based coping strategies (MacPhee, 2013.)

Recovery and clarification

Filling in the memory gaps can be useful in restoring the continuity of the patient's identity and sense of self. Once these gaps have been filled, treatment helps the patient clarify the trauma or conflicts and resolve the problems associated with the amnesic episode (MacPhee, 2013).

Diagnostic criteria: Dissociative amnesia

The diagnosis of dissociative amnesia is confirmed when the patient meets these criteria from the *DSM-5*.

• The main disturbance is an episode marked by the sudden inability to recall important personal information (usually of a stressful or traumatic nature) that's too extensive to attribute to normal forgetfulness.

• Symptoms cause clinically significant distress or impairment of social, occupational, or other areas of functioning.

• The disturbance doesn't stem from direct physiologic effects of a substance or a neurologic or general medical condition.

• The disturbance cannot be explained as DID, acute stress disorder, PTSD, somatic symptom disorder, or a neurologic disorder

Mission: Memory retrieval

When the need to recover memories is urgent, the patient may be questioned under hypnosis or in a drug-induced semihypnotic state, which may help the patient to relax enough to recall forgotten information. However, such memory retrieval techniques must be used cautiously because the circumstances that triggered the memory loss are likely to be highly distressing to the patient (Sadock & Sadock, 2007).

Also, the validity of "recovered" memories is controversial, and external corroboration is required to validate their accuracy. (See *First do no harm.*)

Pharmacologic therapy

Drugs used during treatment for dissociative amnesia may include short-acting barbiturates such as thiopental (Pentothal) and sodium amobarbital (Amytal) or benzodiazepines, such as alprazolam (Xanax) and lorazepam (Ativan) (DynaMed, 2012).

Advice from the experts

First do no harm

Dissociative amnesia usually arises as a reaction to a trauma too overwhelming for the patient to integrate into waking consciousness. In other words, the patient has experienced something he or she wants to forget.

Although you may encourage the patient to express feelings, don't try to elicit forgotten memories. Only a mental health professional with special competence in addressing unconscious memories should attempt to do this. The techniques used to elicit memories, such as hypnosis, guided imagery, and free association, carry certain risks and could prove harmful to the patient.

Nursing interventions

These nursing interventions may be appropriate for a patient with dissociative amnesia.

• Establish a therapeutic, nonjudgmental relationship.
• Encourage the patient to verbalize feelings of distress.
• Help the patient to recognize that memory loss is a defense mechanism used to deal with anxiety and trauma.
• Help the patient deal with anxiety-producing experiences.
• Teach and assist the patient in using reality-based coping strategies under stress rather than strategies that distort reality.
• If the patient is resolving a dissociative fugue state, monitor for signs of overt aggression toward self or others.

Dissociative identity disorder

Formerly called *multiple personality disorder*, DID is marked by two or more distinct identities or subpersonalities (or alters) that recurrently take control of the patient's consciousness and behavior. Each identity may exhibit unique behavior patterns, memories, and social relationships (APA, 2013).

Made famous by movies and books such as *Sybil* and *The Three Faces of Eve*, DID is the most severe type of dissociative disorder (Spiegel et al., 2013).

Sugar or spice, naughty or nice

In many cases, the primary personality is religious with a strong moral sense, whereas the subpersonalities are radically different. They may behave aggressively and lack sexual inhibitions. They may have a different gender, sexual orientation, religion, or race than the primary personality—and may even differ in hand dominance, vocal qualities, intelligence level, and EEG readings (Foote, 2013).

The primary personality may be unaware of the subpersonalities and may wonder about lost time and unexplained events. Subpersonalities are more likely to be aware of the existence of the other personalities and may even interact with one another (Gentile, Dillon, & Gillig, 2013).

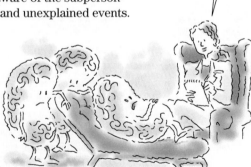

OK, which one of you subpersonalities swiped my stethoscope?

About face!

The transition from one personality to another often is triggered by stress or a meaningful social or environmental cue. Although usually sudden (seconds to minutes), the transition can take hours or days. The switch from one personality to another is often accompanied by trancelike behavior, a change in posture, and/or rolling or blinking of the eyes (APA, 2013; Gentile et al., 2013).

Prevalence and onset

It is estimated that 1.5% of adults suffer from DID. Men are affected at a slightly higher rate (1.6%) than women (1.4%) (APA, 2013).

It can get very complicated

DID may lead to severe social and occupational impairment, depending on the nature of the subpersonalities and their interrelationships. Often, one or more of the subpersonalities has an overlapping mental disorder, such as generalized anxiety disorder, borderline personality disorder, or mood disorder. Suicide attempts, self-mutilation, externally directed violence, and psychoactive drug dependence may occur (Gentile et al., 2013).

Causes

No known single cause for DID exists, but many experts believe the disorder results primarily from trauma, extreme stress, or severe physical and sexual abuse—especially in childhood. Symptoms may become apparent at any age. Some people—such as those who are easily hypnotized—may be predisposed to DID (APA, 2013; Foote, 2013).

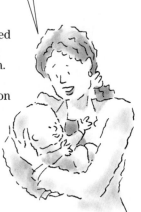

Be kind to your kids. A child who suffers trauma may develop multiple personalities.

Survival through splitting

Some psychiatrists believe victims of severe trauma and abuse develop DID as a survival mechanism. A child exposed to overwhelming trauma may evolve multiple personalities to dissociate himself or herself from the traumatic situation. The dissociated contents then become linked with one of many possible influences that shape personality organization (APA, 2013).

Besides emotional, physical, or sexual abuse, factors that may contribute to DID include:
- genetic predisposition
- lack of nurturing experiences to assist in recovering from abuse
- removal of the original stressor
- combat or a traumatic event
- prison conditions (APA, 2013).

Signs and symptoms

Signs and symptoms of DID may include:
- lack of recall about personal past history beyond ordinary forgetfulness
- inability to recall how to perform past skills, such as how to read or use a computer
- confrontation with evidence of activity they do not recall or "awakening" during an activity they do not remember initiating
- hallucinations, particularly auditory and visual
- posttraumatic symptoms, such as flashbacks, nightmares, and an exaggerated startle response
- recurrent depression
- sexual dysfunction and difficulty forming intimate relationships
- sleep disorders
- eating disorders
- somatic pain disorders
- substance abuse
- guilt and shame
- self-mutilation
- suicidal tendencies or other self-harming behaviors, such as excessive risk taking; unprotected sex with multiple partners; self-neglect; or excessive drinking, smoking, or eating (APA, 2013).

Baffling vacillations

The patient's history may include unsuccessful psychiatric treatment, periods of amnesia, and disturbances in time perception. Family members and friends may describe incidents that the patient can't recall as well as pronounced changes in his or her facial presentation, voice, and behavior (Sadock & Sadock, 2007).

Diagnosis

Many patients with DID spend months or even years in the mental health system before they're diagnosed correctly. Common misdiagnoses are psychotic disorders, PTSD, substance abuse disorder, and bipolar disorder (Spiegel et al., 2013).

The medical provider must rule out physical disorders and substance abuse. Standard tests for DID include the Diagnostic Drawing Series, DID, Dissociative Disorders Interview Schedule, and the SCID-D (Bernstein & Putnam, 1986; Cohen, 1983; Rhodes, 2011; Tupper, 1996). These tests all demonstrate the presence of dissociation.

The diagnosis is confirmed if the patient fulfills the criteria in the *DSM-5*. (*See Diagnostic criteria: Dissociative identity disorder.*)

Diagnostic criteria: Dissociative identity disorder

The diagnosis of DID is confirmed when the patient meets these criteria from *DSM-5*.

• Two or more distinct identities or personality states (each with its own relatively lasting pattern of perceiving, relating to, and thinking about the self and the environment) that results in a disruption in identity that the patient reports or others may observe. In some cultures, this may be described as "possession."

• The patient's experience of recurrent gaps in personal information and/or personal and traumatic events that go beyond normal forgetting.

• The symptoms are distressing or disrupt important areas of functioning, such as social life or occupations.

• The symptoms are not normally accepted as a cultural or religious practice, and for children, they are not explained as imaginary play-mates or other play fantasies.

• The disturbance doesn't stem from direct physiologic effects of a substance or a general medical condition.

Treatment

Treatment of DID is a long-term complex process, taking 5 or more years. The goal of therapy is to integrate all of the patient's personalities and to help with understanding that the different presenting affects can be expressed within a single personality (APA, 2013; Gentile et al., 2013; MacPhee, 2013).

Can't they all just get along?

Experts recommend a staged treatment approach. After first stabilizing the patient and decreasing the degree of dissociation, the therapist tries to identify the personality that remembers the trauma and enhance cooperation and co-consciousness among the subpersonalities, and ultimately merge them into one personality (Gentile et al., 2013).

Unifying the parts

Although the therapist may address the different personalities separately, an increased connectedness is the measure of success. Treatment success is linked to the strength of the therapist's relationship with each subpersonality (DynaMed, 2009; Gentile et al., 2013).

Whether disagreeable or congenial, all of the patient's personalities must be treated with equal respect and empathetic concern

Advice from the experts

Promoting recovery from dissociative identity disorder

Integrating the subpersonalities is the goal of therapy for a patient with DID. Certain actions by the therapist and caregivers can promote connectedness among the subpersonalities, but the following actions are counterproductive:

• *Don't* encourage the patient to create additional subpersonalities.

• *Don't* suggest that the patient adopt names for unnamed subpersonalities.

• *Don't* encourage subpersonalities to function more autonomously.

• *Don't* encourage the patient to ignore certain subpersonalities.

• *Don't* exclude unlikable subpersonalities from therapy.

(Gentile et al., 2013). (See *Promoting recovery from dissociative identity disorder.*)

Respecting boundaries

Clearly delineating boundaries is also important in treating patients with DID. Many grew up in environments without clear boundaries or where personal boundaries weren't always respected.

Family focus

Family and couples therapy also may be indicated (Sadock & Sadock, 2007). Many patients have difficulty parenting and admit to being abusive toward their children.

Hypnosis

Some therapists may use hypnosis for the purpose of:
• obtaining additional history
• identifying previously unrecognized identity
• inducing abreactions (Burnand, 2013). (See memory jogger for ABREACTIONS.)

Tiffs over trances

However, the role of hypnosis in ongoing DID treatment is controversial. For one thing, patients and therapists may become overconfident in the accuracy of information arrived at during a hypnotic trance (Powell & Gee, 1999). To reduce the risk that the patient will alter details of what is recalled during hypnosis, the therapist must minimize the use of leading questions.

Informed consent should be obtained before the use of hypnosis, and its benefits, risks, and limitations should be discussed. Also, the therapist should tell the patient that anything recalled while in a trance isn't likely to be admissible evidence used in legal actions (Cannell, Hudson, & Pope, 2001).

Pharmacologic interventions

Drugs used to treat DID include antidepressants and anxiolytics and sometimes anticonvulsants such as carbamazepine (Tegretol). Experts disagree on using antipsychotics; if they are used, they should be atypical or second-generation drugs that block both dopamine and serotonin receptors (Gentile et al., 2013; Sadock & Sadock, 2007).

Nursing interventions

These nursing interventions may be appropriate for a patient with DID.
• Establish a trusting relationship with each subpersonality. If the patient has a history of abuse, be aware that it may cause difficulty trusting others.
• Promote interventions that help the patient identify each subpersonality, with the goal of integration.
• Encourage the patient to identify emotions that occur under stress.
• Recognize even small gains that the patient makes.
• Teach the patient effective defense mechanisms and coping skills, including use of available social support systems.

Preach patience

• Stress the importance of continuing with psychotherapy. Prepare the patient to expect the need for prolonged therapy, with alternating successes and failures, and the possibility that one or more of the subpersonalities may resist treatment.
• Monitor the patient for violence directed at others.
• Monitor the patient for suicidal ideation and behavior. Implement precautions as needed (MacPhee, 2013).

Memory jogger

ABREACTION refers to the purging of distressing memories or feelings. This term will help you remember key interventions for patients with DID.

A: Abuse is identified

B: Blend or integrate all the personalities into one personality

R: Recall the trauma in detail and process it

E: Encourage the patient to maintain a safe environment

A: Anxiety is decreased

C: Conflict resolution is taught

T: Talk about the patient's feelings, especially guilt and shame

I: Inform the patient about the use of hypnosis to help mobilize memories

O: Orient the patient to surroundings as necessary

N: New coping strategies are developed

References

Allen, J. G., & Smith, W. H. (1993). Diagnosing dissociative disorders. *Bulletin of the Menninger Clinic, 57*(3), 328–343.

American Psychiatric Association. (2013). *Diagnostic and statistical manual of mental disorders* (5th ed.). Washington, DC: Author.

Bernstein, C., & Putnam, F. W. (1986). Development, reliability and validity of a dissociative scale. *Journal of Nervous and Mental Disease, 174*, 727–735.

Brand, B. L., Classen, C. C., McNary, S. W., & Zaveri, P. (2009). A review of dissociative disorders treatment studies. *Journal of Nervous and Mental Disease, 197*(9), 646–654.

Burnand, G. (2013). A right hemisphere safety backup at work: Hypotheses for deep hypnosis, post-traumatic stress disorder, and dissociation identity disorder. *Medical Hypotheses, 81*(3), 383–388.

Cannell, J., Hudson, J. L., & Pope, H. G., Jr. (2001). Standards for informed consent in recovered memory therapy. *Journal of the American Academy of Psychiatry and the Law, 29*(2), 138–147.

Chu, J. A. (2011). Appendix 3: The multidimensional inventory of dissociation (MID). In J. A. Chu (Ed.), *Rebuilding shattered lives: Treating complex PTSD and dissociative disorders* (2nd ed., pp. 287–298). Retrieved from http://onlinelibrary.wiley.com/doi/10.1002/9781118093146.app3/pdf

Cohen, B. M. (1983). Diagnostic drawing series. In S. L. Brooke (Ed.), *Tools of the trade: A therapist's guide to art therapy assessments* (2nd ed., pp. 56–65). Springfield, IL: Charles C. Thomas.

DynaMed. (2009). *Dissociative identity disorder.* Retrieved from http://web.b.ebscohost.com.proxy.lib.uiowa.edu/dynamed/detail?vid=3&sid=c9cb0278-67b9-4857-aac2-a677053c8d55%40sessionmgr198&hid=114&bdata=JkF1dGhUeXBlPWlwLGNvb2tpZSx1aWQsdXJsJnNpdGU9ZHluYW1lZC1saXZlJnNjb3BlPXNpdGU%3d#db=dme&AN=114524

DynaMed. (2012). *Dissociative amnesia.* Retrieved from http://web.b.ebscohost.com.proxy.lib.uiowa.edu/dynamed/detail?vid=3&sid=014606ef-480e-42cb-97a2-eccb6e3c3c5f%40sessionmgr113&hid=120&bdata=JkF1dGhUeXBlPWlwLGNvb2tpZSx1aWQsdXJsJnNpdGU9ZHluYW1lZC1saXZlJnNjb3BlPXNpdGU%3d#db=dme&AN=114936&anchor=anc-2051443402

Foote, B. (2013). Dissociative identity disorder: Epidemiology, pathogenesis, clinical manifestations, course, assessment, and diagnosis. Retrieved from http://www.uptodate.com/contents/dissociative-identity-disorder-epidemiology-pathogenesis-clinical-manifestations-course-assessment-and-diagnosis

Gentile, J .P., Dillon, K. S., & Gillig, P. M. (2013). Psychotherapy and pharmacotherapy for patients with dissociative identity disorder. *Clinical Neuroscience, 10*(2), 22–29.

MacPhee, E. (2013). Dissociative disorders I medical settings. *Current Psychiatric Reports, 15*(398), 1–9.

Powell, R. A., & Gee, T. L. (1999). The effects of hypnosis on dissociative identity disorder: A reexamination of the evidence. *Canadian Journal of Psychiatry, 44*(9), 914–916.

Rhodes, J. (2011). *Clinical consult to psychiatric mental health care.* New York, NY: Springer.

Ross, C. A., Schroeder, E., & Ness, L. (2013). Dissociation and symptoms of culture-bound syndromes in North America: A preliminary study. *Journal of Trauma and Dissociation, 14*(2), 224–235.

Sadock, B. J., & Sadock, V. A. (2007). *Kaplan & Sadock's synopsis of psychiatry* (10th ed.). Philadelphia, PA: Lippincott Williams & Wilkins.

Simeon, D. (2013a). *Depersonalization disorder: Epidemiology, pathogenesis, clinical manifestations, course and diagnosis.* Retrieved from http://www.uptodate.com/contents/depersonalization-disorder-epidemiology-pathogenesis-clinical-manifestations-course-and-diagnosis

Simeon, D. (2013b). *Treatment of depersonalization derealization disorder.* Retrieved from http://www.uptodate.com/contents/treatment-of-depersonalization-derealization-disorder

Spiegel, D., Lewis-Fernandez, R., Lanius, R., Vermetten, E., Simeon, D., & Friedman, M. (2013). Dissociative disorders in DSM-5. *Annual Review of Clinical Psychology, 9*, 299–326.

Stuart, G. W. (2013). Self concept responses and dissociative disorders. In G. W. Stuart (Ed.), *Principles and practice of psychiatric nursing* (10th ed., pp. 262–288). St. Louis, MO: Elsevier.

Tupper, J. E. (1996). *The self report dissociative disorders interview schedule: Reliability and validity.* West Chester, PA: West Chester University.

Wheeler, K. (2008). *Psychotherapy for the advanced practice psychiatric nurse.* St. Louis, MO: Mosby.

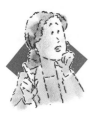

Quick quiz

1. In patients with dissociative disorders, the nurse understands that defense mechanisms are often used to block traumatic experiences. These are called:

    A.   passive aggression.

    B.   reaction formation.

    C.   denial.

    D.   repression.

Answer: D. Repression is the defense mechanism used most often to block traumatic experiences. Neither reaction formation nor denial are relevant in these disorders.

2. Feelings of a dreamlike state or of being a detached observer typically can occur in a patient experiencing which of the following?

    A.   Dissociative fugue

    B.   Dissociative amnesia

    C.   Depersonalization disorder

    D.   DID

Answer: C. Depersonalization disorder is characterized by a sense of being in a dreamlike state or being a detached observer.

3. The nurse is caring for a patient who describes having "multiple personality disorder." The nurse knows this is now referred to as what name?

    A.   Dissociative fugue

    B.   Depersonalization disorder

    C.   Dissociative amnesia

    D.   DID

Answer: D. DID was formerly known as multiple personality disorder.

4. Factors that may contribute to DID include all of these except:
  A. history of seizures.
  B. emotional, physical, or sexual abuse.
  C. genetic predisposition.
  D. extreme stress and trauma.

Answer: A. A history of seizures hasn't been linked to the development of DID.

5. Signs and symptoms of dissociative amnesia with dissociated fugue are most pronounced:
  A. weeks before the fugue episode.
  B. during the fugue episode.
  C. after the fugue episode.
  D. hours before the fugue episode.

Answer: C. After a fugue, the patient may experience depression, grief, shame, intense conflict, confusion, terror, or suicidal or aggressive impulses. In contrast, a fugue in progress is rarely recognized. There are no warning signs of an impending fugue episode.

Scoring

✩✩✩ If you answered all five items correctly, unreal! You've integrated all aspects of dissociative disorders into your conscious mind.

✩✩ If you answered three or four items correctly, fantastic! It's all coming together for you nicely.

✩ If you answered fewer than three items correctly, don't go to pieces! Just thumb through the chapter again and try to fill in those memory gaps.

9

Personality disorders

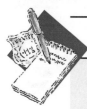

Just the facts

In this chapter, you'll learn:

♦ major features of personality disorders

♦ proposed causes of personality disorders

♦ assessment findings and nursing interventions for patients with personality disorders

♦ recommended treatments for patients with personality disorders.

A look at personality disorders

Merriam-Webster (Personality, n.d.) defines personality as "the set of emotional qualities, ways of behaving, etc., that makes a person different from other people." In other words, your personality defines who you are and how you relate to others. A personality disorder occurs when behavior patterns and relationship patterns become maladaptive. Personality disorders affect the way a person perceives the environment and has an impact on the person's cognition, behavior, and interactions with others. Many who have a personality disorder have inadequate coping mechanisms and may have trouble dealing with everyday stresses. "By definition, a personality disorder is an enduring pattern of thinking, feeling, and behaving" that is not consistent with the cultural norms (American Psychiatric Association [APA], 2013, p. 647). The pattern is generally inflexible and creates some degree of impairment in every area of life.

Currently, the American Psychiatric Association (2013) recognizes 10 different personality disorders. These disorders are then clustered into three groups based on similarities. In this chapter, an overview of personality disorders will be discussed as well as specifics related to each cluster of disorders.

Cluster A	Behavior is odd or eccentric (paranoid, schizoid, schizotypal personality disorders).
Cluster B	Behavior is emotional and dramatic (antisocial, borderline, histrionic, narcissistic personality disorders).
Cluster C	Behavior is fearful or anxious (avoidant, dependent, obsessive-compulsive personality disorders).

Stress, symptoms, and sequelae

Personality disorders are often overlapping with other psychiatric disorders. In addition, it is common for individuals to experience a co-occurring personality disorder from another cluster.

Mild symptoms of personality disorder may have little effect on a person's social, family, or work life. However, when symptoms get worse—as they commonly do during times of increased stress—the disorder can seriously interfere with emotional, psychological, social, and occupational functioning. Severe symptoms may result in hospitalization, poor work performance, and lost productivity. Their emotional toll—unhappiness, domestic violence, child abuse, imprisonment, and even suicide—is equally staggering.

> Severe personality disorders impose a hefty financial and emotional burden.

Relationship woes

People with personality disorders have trouble in their relationships with others. Others are forced to adjust to them.

Myth busters

The fix is in

Relationship problems may arise if the patient's family and friends don't understand the nature of personality disorders.

Myth: If someone with a personality disorder seems normal, that means he or she is capable of changing his or her behavior.

Reality: With a personality disorder, personality traits are fixed and not conducive to change. Yet with a mild personality disorder, the patient's behavior seems normal, so friends and family may assume he or she can easily change behavior. When the patient doesn't change, they may think that he or she is not willing to—when the problem is that he or she *can't.*

When others don't or can't adjust, the person with the disorder may become angry, frustrated, depressed, or withdrawn. This sets up a vicious cycle of interaction in which the person with the disorder persists with their maladaptive behavior until their needs are met, which can further anger those around them. (See *The fix is in.*)

Common features

To one degree or another, most people with personality disorders share the following features:
- disturbances in self-image
- inappropriate range of emotions
- poor impulse control
- maladaptive ways of perceiving themselves, others, and the world
- long-standing problems in personal relationships, ranging from dependency to withdrawal
- reduced occupational functioning, ranging from compulsive perfectionism to intentional self-sabotage.

All in the mix

These common features mix together to create pervasive patterns of behavior that differ markedly from the norms of the patient's cultural or ethnic background. (See *Culture and personality disorders.*)

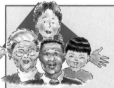

Bridging the gap

Culture and personality disorders

Before concluding that a patient has a personality disorder, always consider his or her cultural, ethnic, and religious background. According to the *Diagnostic and Statistical Manual of Mental Disorders*, 5th Edition (*DSM-5*), the patient's signs and symptoms must deviate markedly from the expectations of his or her culture to qualify for the diagnosis of a personality disorder (APA, 2013).

Stoic versus expressive

Asian and Northern European cultures place a high value on emotional restraint. Thus, stoic behavior in a patient of Japanese descent may be mistaken for avoidant personality disorder.

On the other hand, people from Hispanic, Middle Eastern, and Mediterranean backgrounds tend to be more expressive. Keep that in mind before concluding that an Italian American patient has histrionic personality disorder.

Skirting the stereotypes

At the same time, avoid stereotyping patients. Individuals within a culture—or even within a particular family—may vary widely in personality traits and emotional expression.

Demographic dynamics

Personality disorders are relatively common, affecting an estimated 15% of the U.S. population (APA, 2013). Gender plays a role in their prevalence. For example, antisocial and obsessive-compulsive personality disorders are more common in men, whereas borderline, dependent, and histrionic personality disorders are more prevalent in women.

> More women have borderline and dependent personality disorders, whereas more men have antisocial personality disorder.

Age and intensity

Personality disorders are lifelong conditions with an onset in adolescence or early adulthood. Some personality disorders, such as antisocial and borderline, tend to grow less intense in middle age and late life, whereas other disorders (most notably obsessive-compulsive and schizotypal) tend to become exaggerated.

Causes

No one knows the exact cause of personality disorders. Most likely, they represent a combination of genetic, biological, social, psychological, developmental, and environmental factors.

Chain of influence

Genetic factors influence the biological basis of brain function as well as basic personality structure. In turn, personality structure affects how a person responds to and interacts with life experiences and the social environment. Over time, each person develops distinctive ways of perceiving the world and of feeling, thinking, and behaving.

Out-of-control emotions

Some researchers suspect that poor regulation of the brain circuits that control emotion increases the risk for a personality disorder—when combined with such factors as abuse, neglect, or separation.

For a biologically predisposed person, the major developmental challenges of adolescence and early adulthood (such as separation from the parents, identity, and independence) may trigger a personality disorder. Perhaps this explains why personality disorders usually emerge during those years.

Psychodynamic theories

Psychodynamic theories propose that personality disorders stem from deficiencies in ego and superego development. These deficiencies may relate to mother–child relationships highlighted by unresponsiveness, overprotectiveness, or early separation.

Social theories

According to social theories, personality disorders reflect the responses that a person learns through the processes of reinforcement, modeling, and aversive stimuli. When even low levels of stress occur, chronic trauma or long-term stressors may create new neurochemical pathways. As a result, the person "acts out" old patterns of behaviors.

Evaluation

A patient with a suspected personality disorder should undergo a physical examination to rule out an underlying physical or organic cause for his or her symptoms. (See *Personality changes and physical illness*.)

A psychological evaluation can exclude other psychiatric disorders—or it may suggest additional ones. Psychological tests, such as the Minnesota Multiphasic Personality Inventory-2 (MMPI-2) and the Millon Clinical Multiaxial Inventory-III (MCMI-III), may support or guide the diagnosis. In addition, toxicology screening may be warranted because intoxication with certain substances can mimic the features of a personality disorder.

Personality changes and physical illness

Be aware that a personality change may be the first sign of a serious neurologic, endocrine, or medical illness—which may be reversible if detected early.

For example, a patient with a frontal lobe tumor may show changes in personality and motivation, even though the results of a neurologic assessment are otherwise negative. Such problems should be ruled out before the patient is diagnosed with a personality disorder. The *DSM-5* includes an additional personality disorder: personality change due to another medical condition which is a personality disorder that is directly caused by a medical condition and has physiologic effects, for example frontal lobe injury (APA, 2013).

Diagnostic criteria: General personality disorder

These general criteria from the *DSM-5* apply to all patients with personality disorders. However, each particular disorder has additional criteria that further define and distinguish the disorder.

Criteria

A. An enduring pattern of inner experience and behavior that deviates markedly from the expectations of the individual's culture. This pattern is manifested in two (or more) of the following areas:

    1. Cognition (i.e., way of perceiving and interpreting self, other people, and events)

    2. Affectivity (i.e., the range, intensity, lability, and appropriateness of emotional response)

    3. Interpersonal functioning

    4. Impulse control

B. The enduring pattern is inflexible and pervasive across a broad range of personal and social situations.

C. The enduring pattern leads to clinically significant distress or impairment in social, occupational, or other important areas of functioning.

D. The pattern is stable and of long duration, and its onset can be traced back at least to adolescent or early adulthood.

E. The enduring pattern is not better explained as a manifestation or consequence of another mental disorder.

F. The enduring pattern is not attributable to the physiological effects of a substance (e.g., a drug of abuse, a medication) or another medical condition (e.g., head trauma).

Printed with permission from the American Psychiatric Association. (2013). *Diagnostic and statistical manual of mental disorders* (5th ed.). Arlington, VA: Author. Copyright ©2013. All rights reserved.

Diagnosis

The diagnostic process is virtually the same for all personality disorders. Each disorder has specific criteria determined by the American Psychiatric Association that the patient must meet in order to be diagnosed (APA, 2013). The key to diagnosis is enduring patterns of behavior. In other words, a personality disorder doesn't develop overnight and it isn't diagnosed overnight. Providers are looking for patterns of behavior. Some patients meet the criteria for multiple personality disorders, making diagnosis a particular challenge. As nurses, we frequently see these patients for other health problems. However, the nursing diagnosis will often focus on the underlying behaviors.

Approach to treatment

Personality disorders are among the most challenging psychiatric disorders to treat—partly because, by definition, a personality is an integral part of what defines the individual and his or her self-perceptions. "No sharp division exists between normal and abnormal personality functioning. Instead, personalities are viewed on a continuum from normal at one end to abnormal at the other. Many of the same processes involved in the development of a 'normal' personality are responsible for the development of a personality disorder" (Boyd, 2012, p. 491). Rather than aiming for a cure, treatment typically focuses on enhancing the patient's coping skills, solving short-term problems, and building relationship skills through psychotherapy and education.

The road to rapport

Traditionally, long-term psychotherapy has been the treatment of choice. Effective psychotherapy always requires a trusting relationship with the therapist. Each disorder presents unique challenges in developing a lasting relationship between a patient and a provider.

Adjunctive medication

Today, many patients also receive drugs to relieve associated symptoms, such as acute anxiety or depression. However, drugs should be used only as an adjunct to psychotherapy—not as a cure for the personality disorder.

Paranoid personality disorder

Paranoid personality disorder is marked by a distrust of other people and a constant, unwarranted suspicion that others have sinister motives. Patients with this disorder place excessive trust in their own knowledge and abilities. They search for hidden meanings and hostile intentions in everything that others say and do.

Conspiracy theorists

The paranoid personality is quick to challenge the loyalties of friends and loved ones. Many patients with this disorder seem cold and distant. They shift blame to others and carry long grudges. Because they tend to drive people away, they have few friends—which only bolsters their suspicions of a conspiracy against them.

Prevalence

The prevalence of paranoid personality disorder is estimated at 2.3% to 4.4% of the general population. In clinical samples (and possibly in the general population as well), the disorder is more common in males (APA, 2013).

Causes

The specific cause of paranoid personality disorder is unknown. Its higher incidence in families with a schizophrenic member suggests a possible genetic influence. As children, these individuals are prone to temper outburst and can be difficult to manage. Many times they are perceived as odd by other children and may be teased as a result (APA, 2013; Boyd, 2012).

Signs and symptoms

The hallmarks of paranoid personality disorder are suspicion and distrust of others' motives. Other signs and symptoms include:
- refusal to confide in others
- inability to collaborate with others
- hypersensitivity
- inability to relax (hypervigilance)
- need to be in control
- self-righteousness
- detachment and social isolation
- poor self-image
- sullenness, hostility, coldness, and detachment
- humorlessness
- anger, jealousy, and envy
- bad temper, hyperactivity, and irritability
- lack of social support systems.

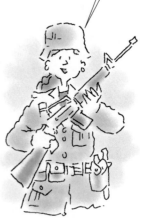

At ease, soldier! Someone with paranoid personality disorder may be unable to relax.

Treatment

Few patients with paranoid personality disorder seek treatment on their own. When they do, health care providers may have difficulty establishing a rapport because of these patients' suspicious, distrustful nature. The challenge is to engage the patient in a collaborative working relationship based on trust.

Psychotherapy

Individual psychotherapy is preferred over group therapy because of the patient's suspicious nature. The most effective psychotherapy for a paranoid patient takes a simple, honest, businesslike approach rather than an insight-oriented approach. It focuses on the current problem that brought the patient to therapy. As therapy progresses, the patient may begin to trust the therapist more and, eventually, start to disclose some of the paranoid ideations.

Pharmacologic therapy

Some health care providers recommend medication for patients with paranoid personality disorder. There is not one drug used to treat paranoid personality disorder. It is important to note that these medications are for symptom control.
- antipsychotic drugs such as olanzapine (Zyprexa) or risperidone (Risperdal) to treat severe agitation or delusional thinking
- antidepressants such as selective serotonin reuptake inhibitors (SSRIs; e.g., fluoxetine [Prozac]) to treat irritability, anger, and obsessional thinking
- antianxiety medications such as benzodiazepines (e.g., alprazolam [Xanax]) to treat severe anxiety that interferes with normal functioning

Doubts about medications

A patient with paranoid personality disorder may distrust medications and, in particular, may resent the suggestion that he or she needs an antipsychotic agent. For this reason, some health care providers delay considering medication until the patient asks about it or until the symptoms warrant the risk of use. Drug therapy should be limited to the briefest course possible. The patient should receive thorough teaching about possible adverse effects so he or she does not get more suspicious if these occur.

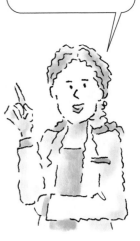

The paranoid patient may distrust medications—especially if they cause adverse effects.

Nursing interventions

These nursing interventions may be appropriate for a patient with paranoid personality disorder:
- Use a straightforward, honest, professional approach rather than a casual or friendly approach.
- Offer persistent, consistent, and flexible care.
- Provide a supportive, nonjudgmental environment in which the patient can safely explore his or her feelings.
- Establish a therapeutic relationship by actively listening and responding.

Don't get too personal

- Avoid inquiring too deeply into his or her life or history unless it's relevant to clinical treatment.

- Don't challenge the patient's paranoid beliefs. Such beliefs are delusional and aren't reality based, so it's useless to argue them from a rational point of view.
- Avoid situations that may threaten the patient's autonomy.
- Be aware that the patient may not respond well to interviewing. (See *Guidelines for an effective interview*.)

You call that funny?

- Use humor cautiously. A paranoid patient may misinterpret a remark that was meant to be humorous.
- Encourage the patient to take part in social interactions. This provides exposure to others' perceptions and realities and helps to promote social skill development.
- Help the patient identify negative behaviors that interfere with relationships so he or she can see how his or her behavior affects others.
- Encourage the expression of feelings, self-analysis of behavior, and accountability for actions.

Advice from the experts

Guidelines for an effective interview

You may have difficulty establishing a rapport with a patient with a personality disorder. These guidelines may be helpful:
- Start the interview with a broad, empathetic statement: "You look distressed. Tell me what's bothering you today."
- Explore normal behaviors before discussing abnormal ones: "What do you think has enabled you to cope with the pressures of your job?"
- Phrase questions sensitively to ease the patient's anxiety: "Things were going well at home and then you became depressed. Tell me about that."
- Ask the patient to clarify vague statements: "Explain to me what you mean when you say, 'They're all after me'."
- If the patient rambles, help him or her focus on the most pressing problem: "You've talked about several problems. Which one bothers you the most?"
- Interrupt a nonstop talker as tactfully as possible: "Thank you for your comments. Now let's move on."
- Express empathy toward a tearful, silent, or confused patient who has trouble describing a problem: "I realize it's difficult for you to talk about this."

Distance yourself

- Recognize the patient's need to be physically and emotionally distant.
- Avoid a defensive attitude and arguments with paranoid patients.
- Assess the patient's coping skills. Teach him or her effective strategies to alleviate stress and reduce anxiety.
- Teach patients about prescribed medications.
- Encourage the patients to continue therapy for optimal therapeutic results.

> Keep your distance—both physically and emotionally—from a paranoid patient.

Schizoid personality disorder

The hallmarks of schizoid personality disorder are detachment, social withdrawal, indifference to others' feelings, and a restricted emotional range in interpersonal settings. People with this disorder are commonly described as loners, with solitary interests and occupations and no close friends. Typically, they maintain a social distance even from family members and seem unconcerned about others' praise or criticism.

They want to be left alone

Most people with this disorder function adequately in everyday life but don't develop many meaningful relationships. Although they fare poorly in groups, they may excel in positions where they have minimal contact with others. (See *What's in a name?*)

Myth busters

What's in a name?

Psychiatric disorders with similar names such as schizophrenia and/or schizotypal don't necessarily share common traits.

Myth: Schizoid personality disorder is similar to schizophrenia.

Reality: People with schizoid personality disorder don't have schizophrenia. (*Schizotypal* personality disorder, on the other hand, does share certain features with schizophrenia.) Unfortunately, because the names sound alike, people with schizoid personality may be misunderstood or even discriminated against.

Prevalence

Schizoid personality disorder affects 3.1% to 4.9% of the general population. More males are affected than females and they also experience higher impairments associated with the disorder (APA, 2013). Some people with schizoid personality disorder also have additional personality disorders, most commonly schizotypal, paranoid, or avoidant personality disorder.

Causes

As with the other personality disorders, the exact cause of schizoid personality disorder is not known. Some researchers think it may be inherited. Other possible causes may include:
- a sustained history of isolation during infancy and childhood
- cold or grossly deficient early parenting
- parental modeling of interpersonal withdrawal, indifference, and detachment.

Signs and symptoms

Assessment of a patient with schizoid personality disorder may reveal:
- emotional detachment
- inability to experience pleasure
- lack of strong emotions and little observable change in mood
- indifference to others' feelings, praise, or criticism
- avoidance of activities that involve significant interpersonal contact
- little desire for or enjoyment of close relationships
- no desire to be part of a family
- strong preference for solitary activities
- little or no interest in sexual experiences with another person
- lack of close friends or confidants other than immediate family members
- shyness, distrust, and discomfort with intimacy
- loneliness
- feelings of utter unworthiness coexisting with feelings of superiority
- self-consciousness and feeling ill at ease with people.

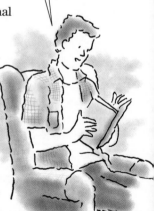

Some people might call me lonely, but I truly prefer solitary activities.

Treatment

For general diagnosis of personality disorders, see page 298. Someone with schizoid personality disorder isn't likely to seek treatment unless he or she is under great stress. Additionally, treatment poses a challenge because of the patient's initial inability or lack of desire to form a relationship with a therapist or other health care professional.

In search of a solitary niche

Treatment goals include:
• helping the patients find the most comfortable solitary niche and cultivate satisfying hobbies that allow them to be on their own
• decreasing their resistance to change
• reducing patients' social isolation and improving their social interaction
• enhancing patients' self-esteem.

Individual psychotherapy

Individual psychotherapy should be short-term, focusing on solving the patient's immediate concerns or problems. Generally, long-term psychotherapy for the schizoid patient has a poor outcome and isn't recommended.

Developing a rapport and trusting therapeutic relationship with this patient is usually a slow, gradual process. To avoid confrontations, the therapist should make every effort to help the patient feel secure and acknowledge the patient's boundaries.

Fears and fantasies

When the patient opens up, he or she may reveal fantasies, imaginary friends, and fears of unbearable dependency. The patient may also fear growing dependent on the therapist and prefer to remain in fantasy and withdrawal. The therapist should bring such feelings into proper focus.

Support, not smothering

Stability and support for the patient are essential—but the therapist must take care not to smother and should expect and tolerate some acting-out behaviors.

Cognitive therapy

Cognitive restructuring may be useful in dealing with illogical thoughts that impede the patient's coping ability and functioning. In this technique, the patient learns to identify his or her own patterns of thought, emotion, and behavior and then works to change his or her own thinking to benefit their overall mental health.

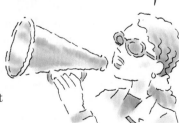

Once more, with some feeling! The therapist should expect some acting out behaviors in a schizoid patient.

Group therapy

Initially, group therapy isn't a good treatment choice because most schizoid patients can't tolerate being in a social group. However, a patient who's graduating from individual therapy with adequate social skills may be able to tolerate group therapy. Supportive group members can help the patient overcome fears of closeness and feelings of isolation.

People who don't need people

In a group therapy session, patients with schizoid personality disorder are usually quiet, seeing little or no reason for social interaction. The group leader should expect this behavior and not pressure them into participating more fully until they are ready. Also, the leader should protect them from criticism by other group members. Eventually, if the group can tolerate their silence, these patients may participate more.

Self-help support groups

Self-help support groups can play an important role in promoting healthier social relationships, enhanced functioning, greater ability to cope with unexpected stressors, and reducing fears of closeness and feelings of isolation. Within the group, the patients can try out new coping skills and learn that social attachments don't have to happen with rejection or fear.

Pharmacologic therapy

Drug therapy isn't warranted if patients are comfortable with their symptoms. However, medications may be prescribed if these patients have an overlapping psychiatric disorder such as major depressive disorder or need relief from other acute symptoms. Patients with psychotic ideations may benefit from low-dose treatment with an antipsychotic, such as olanzapine (Zyprexa) or risperidone (Risperdal). Generally, long-term drug treatment is avoided.

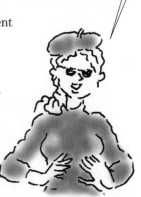

Stay cool, Ladies and Gents. Keep the rhythm slow and steady when trying to build a rapport with a schizoid patient.

Nursing interventions

The following nursing interventions may be appropriate for patients with schizoid personality disorder:
• Respect the patients' need for privacy, and slowly build a trusting therapeutic relationship so that they find more pleasure than fear in relating to you.
• Offer persistent, consistent, and flexible care. Take a direct, involved approach to gain the patients' trust.

No crowding allowed

- Recognize the patient's need for physical and emotional distance.
- Remember that they need close human contact but can become overwhelmed by too much contact.

Time, space, and social skills

- Give the patients plenty of time to express their feelings. Keep in mind that pushing these patients to talk before they are ready may cause them to withdraw.
- Teach the patients social skills, and reinforce appropriate behavior.
- Encourage patients to express their feelings, analyze their own behaviors, and take accountability for their actions.
- Avoid defensive behavior and arguments with schizoid patients.

Schizotypal personality disorder

Schizotypal personality disorder is marked by a pervasive pattern of social and interpersonal deficits, along with acute discomfort with others. People with this disorder have odd thought and behavioral patterns. This disorder is a more advanced form of the schizoid disorder but not as advanced as the diagnosis of schizophrenia (Townsend, 2014).

During times of extreme stress, some patients also have cognitive or perceptual disturbances—although these psychotic symptoms aren't as fully developed as in schizophrenia. Any psychotic episode is short-lived, resolving with the use of an appropriate antipsychotic drug.

Figures of speech

Patients with schizotypal personality disorder commonly exhibit eccentric behaviors and have trouble concentrating for long periods. Their mannerisms and dress may be peculiar and their speech may be unusual—overly elaborate, vague, metaphorical, and hard to follow.

Is there a schizophrenic link?

In the *DSM-5*, "schizotypal disorder is identified as both a personality disorder and the first of the schizophrenia spectrum disorders, which are, in general, listed from least to most severe" (Halter, 2014, p. 459). The patients may have magical thinking, strange fantasies, odd beliefs (such as thinking they have extrasensory abilities), unusual perceptions and bodily illusions, social isolation, and paranoid ideas. However, unlike patients with schizophrenia, people with schizotypal personality disorder are not psychotic. "A major difference between this disorder and schizophrenia is that people with schizotypal personality disorder can be made aware of their misinterpretations of reality. Schizophrenia results in a far stronger grip on delusions" (Halter, 2014, p. 460).

It says here that schizotypal personality disorder is similar to schizophrenia but without the psychotic component.

Party of one

Typically, the patients have severe social anxiety—usually because they are paranoid about others' motivations. They may relate to others in a stiff or inappropriate way or fail to respond to normal interpersonal cues. Although some people with this disorder marry, most have no more than one person they relate to closely.

Prevalence

Schizotypal personality disorder is found in about 3.9% of the general population and 0% to 1.9% in clinical settings. It's slightly more common in men than in women (APA, 2013). "This disorder has a relatively stable course, with only a small proportion of individuals going on to develop schizophrenia or another psychotic disorder" (APA, 2013, p.657). About 30% to 50% of patients with schizotypal personality disorder also have major depression. A large number have an additional personality disorder, especially paranoid, borderline, or avoidant personality disorder.

Causes

Schizotypal personality disorder as part of the schizophrenia spectrum does have a genetic link, as there is a higher incidence of the disorder among first-degree relatives with schizophrenia (APA, 2013; Halter, 2014). Environmental factors (such as severe stress) may determine whether schizotypal personality disorder or schizophrenia manifests.

Dopamine deviance

Some evidence suggests that patients with schizotypal personality disorder have poor regulation of dopamine pathways in the brain.

Psychological and cognitive theories

Psychological and cognitive explanations for schizotypal personality disorder focus on deficits in attention and information processing. These patients perform poorly on tests that assess continuous performance tasks, which require the ability to maintain attention on one object and to look at new stimuli selectively.

Signs and symptoms

Assessment findings in patients with schizotypal personality disorder may include:
- odd or eccentric behavior or appearance
- belief that others are out to get them
- odd beliefs or magical thinking
- unusual perceptual experiences, including bodily illusions
- vague, circumstantial, metaphorical, overly elaborate, or stereotypical speech or thinking
- unfounded suspicion of being followed, talked about, persecuted, or under surveillance
- inappropriate or apathetic affect
- lack of close relationships other than immediate family members
- social isolation
- excessive social anxiety that doesn't go away
- a sense of feeling different and the inability to easily fit in with others.

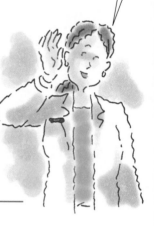

The schizotypal patient may speak in a vague, metaphorical, or elaborate way.

Diagnosis and treatment

General diagnostic parameters for all personality disorders are discussed on page 298. Treatment options for patients with schizotypal personality disorder include individual psychotherapy, family therapy, group therapy, cognitive-behavioral therapy, self-help measures, and medications. The patients may also benefit from social skills training and other behavioral approaches that emphasize the basics of social interactions.

Psychoanalytic intervention focuses on defining ego boundaries. Cognitive-behavioral therapy attempts to help the patients interpret their odd beliefs and teach them valuable coping and interpersonal skills.

Avoid challenges

Initially, individual therapy is usually preferred. A warm, supportive, patient-centered approach helps establish rapport. The therapist should avoid directly challenging the patient's delusional or inappropriate thoughts.

Group prejudice

Group therapy may be considered when these patients make progress in individual therapy. However, patients with this disorder may have trouble tolerating a group because they are mistrustful and suspicious.

Pharmacologic therapy

Antipsychotic agents, such as risperidone (Risperdal), may be used to treat psychotic symptoms; they're usually given in low doses. SSRIs have also been effective in some cases.

Nursing interventions

These nursing interventions may be appropriate for patients with schizotypal personality disorder:
• Offer the patients persistent, consistent, and flexible care. Take a direct, involved approach to promote the patients' trust.
• Know that these patients are easily overwhelmed by stress. Give them plenty of time to make difficult decisions.

The patient likes me, can't stand you

• Be aware that these patients may relate unusually well to certain staff members but not at all to others.
• Recognize the patient's need for physical and emotional distance.

Social skills and self-analysis

• Teach the schizotypal patients social skills, and reinforce appropriate behaviors.
• Encourage the patient's expression of feelings, self-analysis of behaviors, and accountability for actions.
• Avoid defensive behavior and arguments with schizotypal patients.

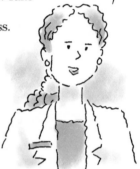

The schizotypal patient may relate well to you but not your colleagues—or vice versa.

Antisocial personality disorder

The highlight of antisocial personality disorder is chronic antisocial behavior that violates others' rights or generally accepted social norms. This disorder predisposes a person toward criminal behavior. This pattern of behavior has been referred to as *psychopathy* or *sociopathy* (APA, 2013).

Other features of this disorder include impulsivity, egocentricity, disregard for the truth, and aggression. The antisocial person can't tolerate boredom and frustration. They are reckless, irritable, and unable to maintain consistent, responsible functioning at work, at school, or as a parent. They lack remorse and exhibit few, if any, feelings. (See *Insight into antisocial personality disorder.*)

Crime and politics

Although individuals with antisocial personality disorder are the most common among people who get into trouble with the

Myth busters

Insight into antisocial personality disorder

Do you think you understand the antisocial personality? Think again.
Myth: Most people with antisocial personality disorder are powerful and are always "out for number 1."
Reality: Patients with antisocial personality disorder see themselves as victims. They seek revenge and don't accept responsibility for their actions.

law, antisocial personality disorder also occurs in milder forms. Examples include the spouse who continually cheats and the con artist who scams others out of their money.

Prevalence

In the general population, the prevalence of antisocial personality disorder is about 0.2% to 3.3%. In prison populations, it may be higher than 70% (APA, 2013). Many of the people with this disorder have a history of arrest and issues with the law.

Antisocial personality disorder affects more males than females. However, there has been some concern that this disorder is underdiagnosed in women because of the "emphasis on aggressive items" in the diagnostic criteria (APA, 2013, p. 662). This diagnosis is not used for children. A conduct disorder in a teenager may lead to an antisocial personality diagnosis after the patient is 18 years old.

Causes

Genetic and biological factors may influence the development of antisocial personality disorder. Biological factors include:

✌ Poor serotonin regulation and low dopamine level can affect impulse control and contribute to aggressive behavior (Boyd, 2012).

✌ Reduced autonomic activity and developmental or acquired abnormalities in the prefrontal brain systems could account for impulsive behavior with aggressive tendency and emotional distance.

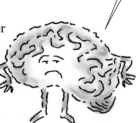

Poor serotonin regulation in certain brain regions may factor into antisocial personality disorder.

Children at risk

Other possible causes or risk factors include attention deficit hyperactivity disorder, large families, and childhood exposure to the following conditions:
- substance abuse
- criminal behavior
- physical or sexual abuse
- neglectful or unstable parenting
- social isolation
- transient friendships
- low socioeconomic status.

Signs and symptoms

Patients with antisocial personality disorder have a long-standing pattern of disregarding the rights of others as well as societal values. Other assessment findings may include:
- repeatedly performing unlawful acts
- reckless disregard for their own safety or the safety of others
- deceitfulness
- lack of remorse
- consistent irresponsibility
- power-seeking behavior
- destructive tendencies
- impulsivity and failure to plan ahead

Memory jogger

Each letter in ANTISOCIAL stands for a feature of antisocial personality disorder.

A Abuses substances (some patients)

N No satisfying interpersonal relationships

T Tends to manipulate others

I Irresponsible and exploitative

S Social norms are disregarded

O Obnoxious toward others (no sense of guilt, shame, or remorse)

C Cold and callous

I Intimidates others

A Argumentative

L Legal problems

- superficial charm
- manipulative nature
- inflated, arrogant self-appraisal
- irritability and aggressiveness
- inability to maintain close personal or sexual relationships
- disconnection between feelings and behaviors
- substance abuse.

Diagnosis

The patient with antisocial personality disorder rarely seeks evaluation or treatment on his or her own. Much more commonly, the patient is mandated by the court or pressured by family members to seek help.

Not all criminals qualify

Because not all criminals have antisocial personality disorder, the health care provider must differentiate this condition from simple criminal activity, adult antisocial behavior, or other behaviors that don't justify the personality disorder as a diagnosis. Formal psychological testing, as with the MMPI-2, may prove invaluable. (See *Personality and projective tests*, page 314.)

The official diagnosis of antisocial personality disorder is confirmed if the patient meets the diagnostic criteria in the *DSM-5*. See general diagnostic information related to all personality disorders on page 298 for more information.

Treatment

Working with patients with antisocial disorder can be challenging because they seem to neither show nor feel emotions, especially guilt after doing something wrong. For therapy to be effective, they need help in drawing the connection between their feelings and behaviors.

Psychotherapy is the usual treatment of choice. Options include individual psychotherapy, group therapy, family therapy, and self-help support groups. If needed, the patients should also undergo drug or alcohol rehabilitation.

Individual psychotherapy

Many patients with antisocial personality disorder are mandated to have therapy, sometimes in a forensic or prison setting.

In a confined setting, therapy should focus on alternative life issues, such as:

- goals the patients can pursue after their release from custody
- improvement in social or family relationships
- learning new coping skills.

Personality and projective tests

Personality and projective tests elicit patient responses that provide insight into mood, personality, or psychopathology. These tests include the Beck Depression Inventory (BDI), draw-a-person test, MMPI-2, sentence completion test, and thematic apperception test.

Beck Depression Inventory

A self-administered, self-scored test, the BDI asks patients to rate how often they experience symptoms of depression, such as poor concentration, suicidal thoughts, guilt feelings, and crying. Questions focus on cognitive symptoms, such as impaired decision making, and physical symptoms such as appetite loss.

The sum of 21 items gives the total, with a maximum possible score of 63. A score of 11 to 16 indicates mild depression; a score above 17 indicates moderate depression.

You may help patients complete the BDI by reading the questions—but be careful not to influence their answers. Instruct patients to choose the answer that describes them most accurately.

If you suspect depression, a BDI score above 17 may provide objective evidence of the need for treatment. To monitor the patient's depression, repeat the BDI during the course of treatment.

Draw-a-person test

In the draw-a-person test, the patient draws a human figure of each sex. The psychologist interprets the drawing systematically and correlates the interpretation with diagnosis. The draw-a-person test also provides an estimate of a child's developmental level.

Minnesota Multiphasic Personality Inventory-2

The MMPI-2 is a structured paper-and-pencil test that provides a practical way to assess personality traits and ego function in adolescents and adults. Most patients who read English need little assistance in completing it. The MMPI—the original version of this test—was developed at the University of Minnesota and introduced in 1942. The MMPI-2 was released in 1989 and subsequently revised in early 2001.

The MMPI-2 has 567 questions and takes 60 to 90 minutes to complete. (A short form consists of the first 370 questions of the long-form version.) Questions are designed to evaluate the thoughts, emotions, attitudes, and behavioral traits that comprise personality.

A psychologist translates the patient's answers into a psychological profile and then combines the profile with data gathered from the interview. Test results shed light on the patient's coping strategies, defenses, personality strengths and weaknesses, sexual identification, and self-esteem. The MMPI-2 may also identify certain personality disturbances or mental deficits caused by neurologic problems.

A patient's test pattern may strongly suggest a diagnostic category. If the results reveal a risk of suicide or violence, monitor the patient's behavior. If they show frequent somatic complaints indicating possible hypochondria, evaluate the patient's physical status. If the complaints lack medical confirmation, help the patient explore how these symptoms may signal emotional distress.

Sentence completion test

In the sentence completion test, the patient completes a series of partial sentences. A sentence might begin, "When I get angry, I . . ." The response may reveal the patient's fantasies, fears, aspirations, or anxieties.

Thematic apperception test

In the thematic apperception test, the patient views a series of pictures depicting ambiguous situations and then tells a story describing each picture. The psychologist evaluates these stories systematically to help analyze the patient's personality, particularly regarding interpersonal relationships and conflicts.

In an outpatient setting, therapy should focus on discussing the patients' antisocial behavior and lack of feelings.

> Judges see the consequences of antisocial personality disorder all too often.

Ultimatums are unwise

Threats are never an appropriate motivating factor for any type of treatment and are least effective in antisocial patients who have been mandated by the courts to have therapy. Instead of threatening to report the patient's lack of motivation to the courts or the prison warden, the therapist should try to help the patients find good reasons to want to work on their problems—for example, avoiding more jail time or further trouble with the law.

Emotional breakthrough

Intensive psychoanalytic approaches aren't indicated for patients with an antisocial personality disorder. Instead, therapy should focus on reinforcing appropriate behaviors, helping patients gain greater access to their feelings, and helping them make connections between their actions and feelings.

These patients may be unfamiliar with their feelings associated with various emotional states, such as depression. Getting them to experience these feelings is crucial. In fact, experiencing intense affect usually is a sign of progress in these patients.

Keeping confidences

A therapeutic relationship can occur only when the patients and the therapists establish a solid rapport and the patients can trust the therapists implicitly. However, fears about confidentiality may pose an obstacle to the patients' trust. (See *Confidentiality in criminal cases*, page 316.)

For example, if the patients were mandated to have therapy, the therapists must report on their progress. Although this can be done in a way that doesn't reveal specific details about the content of the therapy, the patient may be suspicious and distrustful of their therapist—especially at first.

To ease the patient's fear, caregivers should honestly disclose what they'll reveal to the courts. In time, these patients can learn that what they say in therapy won't necessarily become common knowledge.

Consequences, not conscience

If the patient is morally and ethically deficient, dwelling on this problem may bring little progress. A better approach is to try to have the patient face up to the consequences of his or her behavior. Eventually, this may motivate him or her to continue with therapy.

Advice from the experts

Confidentiality in criminal cases

If you're caring for a patient who has been mandated by the courts to have treatment, you may be required by law to disclose confidential patient information to the authorities. Some laws create an exemption to the privilege doctrine in criminal cases, which gives the courts access to all essential information.

Even in states where neither a law nor an exemption to the law exists, the court may find exemption to the privilege doctrine in criminal cases.

Group therapy

After the patient is able to overcome his or her initial fears of joining a group, he or she may find group therapy beneficial. Ideally, the group should consist exclusively of people with antisocial personality disorder. In such a group, the patient has a greater reason to contribute and share. However, the group leader must make sure that the group doesn't become a how-to course in criminal behavior or a forum to brag about criminal exploits. For this disorder, group therapy provides the benefit of allowing others to validate or challenge the patient's view or perspective.

> The group leader must make sure that the group doesn't become a forum for patients to brag about their criminal exploits.

Family therapy

Family therapy can help the family understand the patient's antisocial behavior. Open discussion should be encouraged—especially regarding confusion, guilt, and temptation to make restitution for the patient's criminal acts and the frustrations of being with someone who's ill but resists treatment.

Inpatient care

Although patients with antisocial personality disorder rarely require inpatient hospital care, they may be hospitalized for treatment of a crisis or major depression. Inpatient programs may be intensive and expensive and rarely sought out by patients themselves.

To maintain treatment gains, the patients need to have community follow-up and support by the hospital staff or professionals or possibly, a self-help support group after discharge.

Specialized treatment programs

Specialized treatment programs are available for patients with antisocial personality disorder. For example, a program at Patuxent Institute in Jessup, Maryland uses a strict behavioral approach and is based on treatment progress. Research is ongoing to determine the long-term effectiveness of this radical approach. Anger management is also a beneficial component of therapy for this disorder. Patients with this disorder are impulsive and have aggressive tendencies which can be a difficult combination. Teaching these patients how to express their anger in nonviolent ways is important and for many patients is a priority intervention (Boyd, 2012).

Pharmacologic therapy

Although research doesn't support using medications to treat antisocial personality disorder directly, medications may be given to treat disorganized thinking, stabilize mood swings, or ease the acute symptoms of concurrent psychiatric disorders. "Lithium carbonate and propranolol (Inderal) may be useful for violent episodes observed in clients with antisocial personality disorder" (Townsend, 2014, p. 696).

Nursing interventions

These nursing interventions may be appropriate for a patient with antisocial personality disorder:
- Keep in mind that the patient may seem charming and convincing.
- Using a straightforward, matter-of-fact approach, set limits on acceptable behavior. Encourage and reinforce positive behavior. (See *Setting limits effectively*, page 318.)
- Clearly convey your expectations of the patient as well as the consequences if he or she fails to meet them.

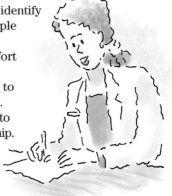

You may have to draw up a behavioral "contract" with a patient who has antisocial personality disorder.

Managing manipulative behavior

- Anticipate manipulative efforts. Help the patients identify such behaviors so that they can learn that other people aren't just extensions of themselves.
- Expect the patient to refuse to cooperate in an effort to gain control.
- Establish a behavioral "contract" to communicate to the patient that other behavior options are available.
- Hold the patient responsible for his or her behavior to promote the development of a collaborative relationship.

No-struggle zone

- Avoid power struggles and confrontations, as this maintain the opportunity for therapeutic communication.
- Avoid defensive behavior and arguments.

Advice from the experts

Setting limits effectively

In a therapeutic setting, placing limits on behavior gives these patients a sense of security and self-control. It also communicates caring on the part of the staff. Limit-setting establishes boundaries, for example, that the patient may not hurt others or destroy property. It also helps the nurse avoid getting angry and frustrated with the patient and increases the effectiveness of the therapeutic relationship. The patients benefits from developing a sense of responsibility for their actions.

To set effective limits, follow these guidelines:

Choosing battles wisely
• Choose your battles wisely by setting limits only as needed.
• Set limits when you first sense that the patient is violating others' rights. Don't tolerate this behavior for several days and then launch an angry tirade.
• Avoid using limits as punishment or retaliation. Don't set limits only when you're angry or under stress because this will hurt your efforts to build a therapeutic relationship.
• Let the patients express their feelings about what the limits mean to them. They may perceive them as a message that you no longer like them or may feel increased anxiety because they are not used to external controls.

Focusing on behavior
• Establish limits strictly for the patient's *behavior*, not their feelings. If the patients overstep the limits, convey that although you don't accept this behavior, you accept them as a person. If instead you focus on such feelings as anger, the patients may sense that their emotions are unacceptable.
• Make sure that the patients know exactly what behavior you expect.
• Apply the rules consistently and, when possible, offer alternatives to unacceptable behavior.

Ensuring consistency
• Inform other staff members of the limits you've set. Otherwise, manipulative patients may try to split between the staff into factions that they can pit against one another.
• Apply the same principles when working with the patients' families. Many patients come from families that have had little success in establishing discipline. Explain to them that rules may be enforced in a way that communicates love, caring, and acceptance.

• When teaching, engage the patient in a discussion and try to guide the discussion to the key points. A lecture approach will not work, as these patients enjoy challenging "rules." Approach learning with a sense of humor and use creative and thought-provoking questions in the discussion (Boyd, 2012).

Anger alert

• Observe the patient for physical and verbal signs of agitation.
• Help the patient manage his or her anger.

- Teach the patient social skills and reinforce appropriate behavior.
- Encourage the patient to express his or her feelings, analyze his or her behavior, and be accountable for his or her actions.

Borderline personality disorder

"The essential feature of borderline personality disorder is a pervasive pattern of instability of interpersonal relationships, self-image, and affects and marked impulsivity that begins by early adulthood and is present in a variety of contexts" (APA, 2013, p. 663). Although people with this disorder may experience it in various ways, most find it hard to distinguish reality from their own misperceptions of the world. Their emotions overwhelm their cognitive functioning, creating many conflicts with others. Alternating extremes of anger, anxiety, depression, and emptiness are common in patients with borderline disorder. However, intense bouts of these emotions typically last only hours or at most a day.

Fluctuations and flip-flops

Distortions in cognition and sense of self can lead to frequent changes in long-term goals, jobs and career plans, friendships, values, and even gender identity.

The patient may see himself or herself as fundamentally bad or unworthy. The patient may feel misunderstood, mistreated, bored, and empty, with little idea of who he or she really is as a person.

People with borderline personality disorder tend to act impulsively without considering the consequences. Impulsive behaviors may include promiscuity, substance abuse, and eating or spending binges. Outbursts of intense anger may lead to violence, which are easily triggered when others criticize or thwart their impulsive acts. Some even have brief psychotic-like experiences.

All or nothing at all

Persons with borderline personality disorder tend to have intense and stormy relationships, alternating between a black and white view of others. Their perceptions of family members and friends may shift suddenly from great admiration and love to intense anger and dislike.

For example, they may adore and idealize another person—but when a slight separation or conflict occurs, they may switch unexpectedly to the other extreme and angrily accuse that person of not caring for them.

Called *splitting*, this tendency to view others as either heroes or villains is a defense mechanism meant to protect these patients from the perception of dangerous anxiety and intense affects. However, instead of offering real protection, splitting leads to destructive behavior and turmoil.

Rejection blues

With borderline personality comes extreme sensitivity to rejection. The patient may react with anger and distress to even mild separations from loved ones, such as vacations, business trips, or a sudden change in plans.

Self-mutilation

To escape from their inner turmoil, they may resort to self-destructive behaviors, such as self-mutilation (cutting or burning themselves), substance abuse, eating disorders, and suicide attempts. These symptoms commonly are triggered by fear of abandonment.

Prevalence

Borderline personality disorder affects 1.6% to 5.9% of the general population, about 10% of psychiatric outpatients, nearly 20% of psychiatric inpatients, and approximately 6% in primary care settings. It is three times more common in females (about 75%) than in males (APA, 2013).

Age and stability

The disorder usually begins in early childhood and peaks in adolescence and early adulthood. It can take a tumultuous course, resulting in the high use of health care resources by patients in their late teens and 20s. However, by their 30s and 40s, up to 60% of patients achieve some stability in their work and personal life (although significant areas of dysfunction usually remain).

Borderline personality disorder commonly overlaps with other personality disorders, as well as bipolar disorder, depression, anxiety disorders, and substance abuse.

Causes

The precise cause of borderline personality disorder is unknown, but several theories are being investigated. Because it's five times more common in first-degree relatives of people who have it, researchers suspect genetics may play a role.

Biological factors may involve:
- dysfunction in the brain's limbic system or frontal lobe
- decreased serotonin activity
- increased activity in alpha-2-noradrenergic receptors.

Early losses and abuse

Prolonged separation from their parents; other major losses early in life; and physical, sexual, or emotional abuse or neglect seem to be more common in patients with this disorder than in the general population.

Signs and symptoms

Major signs and symptoms of borderline personality disorder fall into four main categories: unstable relationships, unstable self-image, unstable emotions, and impulsivity. Symptoms are most acute when the patients feel isolated and without social support, causing them to make frantic efforts to avoid being alone.

Assessment findings may include:
- a pattern of unstable and intense interpersonal relationships
- splitting (viewing others as either extremely good or extremely bad)
- intense fear of abandonment, as displayed by clinging and distancing maneuvers
- rapidly shifting attitudes about friends and loved ones
- desperate attempts to maintain relationships
- unstable perceptions of relationships, with estrangement over ordinary disagreements
- manipulation, as in pitting people against one another
- limited coping skills
- dissociation (separating objects from their emotional significance)
- transient, stress-related paranoid ideation or severe dissociative symptoms
- inability to develop a healthy sense of oneself
- uncertainty about major issues, such as self-image, identity, life goals, sexual orientation, values, career choices, or types of friends
- imitative behavior
- rapid, dramatic mood swings, from euphoria to intense anxiety to rage, within hours or days
- acting out of feelings instead of expressing them appropriately or verbally
- inappropriate, intense anger or difficulty controlling anger
- chronic feelings of emptiness
- unpredictable self-damaging behavior, such as driving dangerously, gambling, sexual promiscuity, overeating, spending, and abusing substances
- self-destructive behaviors, such as physical fights, recurrent accidents, self-mutilation, and suicidal gestures.

Diagnosis and treatment

Standard psychological tests may reveal a high degree of dissociation in a patient with borderline personality disorder. The diagnosis is confirmed if the patient meets the criteria in the *DSM-5*.

Treatment of borderline personality disorder may involve:
- individual psychotherapy
- group therapy

- family therapy
- milieu therapy
- alcohol and drug rehabilitation as indicated.

Psychotherapy

Psychotherapy is usually the treatment of choice for this disorder. Although borderline personality disorder can be hard to treat, individual and group therapy are at least partially effective for many patients.

The patients' unstable relationships and intense anger can cause difficulty in establishing a therapeutic relationship with health care professionals. They may fail to respond to therapeutic efforts and may make considerable demands on the caregiver's emotional resources, especially when suicidal behaviors are prominent.

Sign on the dotted line

Initially, therapists should contract with these patients to decrease the chance of committing suicide or performing self-destructive behavior. Suicidal potential should be carefully assessed and monitored throughout the entire course of treatment. Patients at high risk for suicide may require medications and hospitalization.

Borderlines with boundaries

A structured therapeutic setting is important. The borderline patient may try to test limits, so the therapist must set boundaries for the relationship when therapy begins. Everyone involved in the care should maintain these boundaries consistently. Some patients have had success with a psychosocial treatment called *dialectical behavior therapy*. (See *Dialectical behavior therapy*.)

Other types of psychotherapy

Therapies that focus on social learning theory and conflict resolution may also be used to treat borderline personality disorder. However, these solution-focused therapies may neglect the patient's core problems, such as difficulty expressing appropriate emotions and problems forming emotional attachments to others because of faulty cognitions.

Hospitalization

Long-term care in a hospital setting is rarely appropriate. However, during an episode of acute depression or another crisis, the patient may be seen in a hospital emergency department, an inpatient unit, or a local community health center.

Dialectical behavior therapy

A psychosocial treatment called dialectical behavior therapy (DBT)—developed specifically to treat borderline personality disorder—has proven effective in helping patients cope with the disorder.

In this comprehensive approach, the patients are taught to better control their life and emotions through self-knowledge, emotion regulation, and cognitive restructuring. This approach is now used to treat other disorders as well such as substance use disorders, eating disorders, and posttraumatic stress disorder (Sadock & Sadock, 2007, as cited in Townsend, 2014).

Treatment modes
DBT involves four primary modes of treatment:
- individual therapy
- group skills training
- telephone contact with the therapist
- therapist consultation.

Individual therapy sessions
The main work of therapy occurs in individual therapy sessions. (The therapist may add group therapy and other treatment modes as appropriate.) Between sessions, patients are offered telephone contact with their therapists to give them help and support in applying the skills they are learning to real-life situations and to help them avoid self-injury.

Therapeutic hierarchy
In individual therapy sessions, goals are addressed according to the following hierarchy:
- decreasing suicidal behaviors
- decreasing behaviors that interfere with therapy
- decreasing behaviors that interfere with the quality of life
- increasing behavioral skills
- decreasing behaviors related to posttraumatic stress
- improving self-esteem
- individual goals negotiated with the patient.

Skills training
Skills training is carried out in a group setting. In the group, patients learn:
- core mindfulness skills (meditation-like techniques)
- interpersonal effectiveness skills
- emotion modulation skills (ways of changing distressing emotional states)
- distress tolerance skills (techniques for coping with the emotional states that can't be changed for the time being).

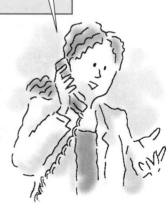

Crisis hotlines and self-help groups are good alternatives to hospitalization for a borderline patient.

Because hospital visits are costly, the patient should be encouraged to find additional social support within the community from such sources as:
- telephone or personal contact with their health care providers
- self-help support groups (including those available through the Internet)
- crisis hotlines.

Partial hospitalization and day treatment programs

Partial hospitalization and day treatment programs provide a safe environment offering support, feedback, and structure for a short time or during the day. Patients usually return home in the evening.

Diminishing dependency

During times of increased stress or difficulty coping, partial hospitalization treatment may be more appropriate than inpatient hospitalization. Also, the patient is less dependent on others to solve problems. Milieu therapy is another option. (See *Milieu therapy*.)

Pharmacologic therapy

There are currently no medications approved by the U.S. Food and Drug Administration (FDA) for the specific treatment of

---

Milieu therapy

Whether it takes place in the hospital or in a community setting, milieu therapy uses the patient's setting or environment to help him or her overcome social anxiety as well as received feedback from peers. If your patient is undergoing this type of therapy, the following guidelines may be helpful.

Patient preparation
Explain the purpose of milieu therapy to the patient. Tell the patient what you expect of him or her, and explain how he or she can participate in the therapeutic community. Orient the patient to the routines of the community, such as the schedule for various activities, and introduce him or her to other patients and staff.

Monitoring and aftercare
Regularly evaluate the patient's symptoms and therapeutic needs. Oversee his or her activities, encouraging him or her to keep a schedule typical of life outside the hospital. Also, encourage the patient to interact with others so that he or she do not become withdrawn or feel secluded. Point out the importance of respecting others and his or her environment.

Home care instructions
If the patient eventually returns to the outside community, encourage him or her to keep follow-up appointments with his or her therapist.

borderline personality disorder. However, the patient may receive drugs to relieve specific symptoms, especially during a crisis. These drugs may include:

• Antidepressants, such as SSRIs (e.g., fluoxetine [Prozac]) or monoamine oxidase inhibitors (MAOIs), can help decrease impulsivity and self-destructive behavior. MAOIs are not used frequently due to the high degree for interaction as well as the extreme risks with overdose (Townsend, 2014).

• Antipsychotic drugs, such as risperidone (Risperdal) or olanzapine (Zyprexa), to ease dissociative symptoms or self-destructive impulses. "The combination of an SSRI and an atypical antipsychotic has been successful in treating dysphoria, mood instability, and impulsivity in clients with borderline personality disorder" (Townsend, 2014, p. 696).

• Opioid receptor antagonist, such as naltrexone (Revia), is used to reduce self-mutilating behaviors.

• Omega-3 supplementation is used for mood and emotional regulation (Halter, 2014).

Overdose alert

Dosages should be kept low and the patients should be under psychosocial intervention. Also, prescriptions must be closely monitored because the patients may overdose impulsively if they have an adequate drug supply.

Nursing interventions

These nursing interventions may be appropriate for patients with borderline personality disorder:

• Encourage the patients to take responsibility. Don't try to rescue them from the consequences of their actions (except suicidal and self-mutilating behaviors).

• Convey empathy and support, but don't try to solve problems they can solve.

• Maintain a consistent approach in all interactions with these patients, and ensure that other team members use the same approach.

• Avoid sympathetic, nurturing responses.

Manipulation and expectation

• Recognize behaviors that patients with borderline personality disorder use to manipulate people so that the nurse can avoid unconsciously reinforcing these behaviors.

• Set appropriate expectations for social interactions and praise the patient when he or she meet these expectations.

• To promote trust, respect the patients' personal space.

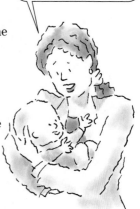

Mothering a baby is appropriate. But mothering a patient with borderline personality disorder does more harm than good.

Staff subjects

- Be aware that the patients may idealize some staff members and devalue others.
- Don't take sides in the patients' disputes with staff members.
- Avoid defensiveness and arguing.
- Try to limit patients' interactions to assigned staff in order to decrease splitting behaviors. Know that using only a few consistent staff members helps maintain consistent treatment.

Cheek checks

- If the patient is taking medications, monitor him or her for "cheeking" (holding medications in the cheek) or hoarding of medications for overdose at a later time.
- Encourage the patients to express their feelings, analyze their behaviors, and be accountable for their actions.

Skills expansion

- Help the patient develop problem-solving skills.
- Review and encourage relaxation techniques.
- Encourage the patients to start an exercise regimen. Exercise promotes stability by decreasing mood swings and aiding the release of anger.

Histrionic personality disorder

Histrionic personality disorder is characterized by a pattern of emotionally driven behaviors and overt attention seeking. People with this disorder are drawn to momentary excitements and fleeting adventures.

Those with histrionic disorder can be charming, dramatic, and expressive. However, they are also easily hurt, vain, demanding, capricious, excitable, self-indulgent, and inconsiderate. The words and feelings they express seem shallow and simulated, not real or deep. As a result, they often come across as manipulative and phony. Despite their emotional responsiveness, their emotions may shift instantly from rage to friendliness.

> With histrionic personality disorder, the drama is always on!

"Look at me!"

Their style of speech is excessively impressionistic, if not downright theatrical, and their gestures are exaggerated. They use grandiose language to describe everyday events and value words more for their emotional content than their factual accuracy.

People with histrionic personality disorder need to be the center of attention at all times. They place great emphasis on physical appearance, often dressing provocatively and behaving seductively. Consumed with superficialities, they devote little time or attention to their internal lives.

Chameleon effect

With limited self-knowledge, they may have no sense of who they are, aside from their identification with others. They may change their attitudes and values depending on the views of significant others. (See *Watching the watchers.*)

Exaggerations and embroidery

People with histrionic personality disorder may exaggerate their illnesses to gain attention, interrupt others so that they can dominate the conversation, and seek constant praise. They exaggerate friendships and relationships, believing that everyone loves them. They consider friendships and relationships to be far more intimate than they are.

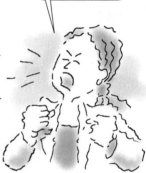

I know I'm being histrionic, but yikes—this chapter is long!!

From fairytale to nightmare

Because they don't view others realistically, people with histrionic personality disorder have trouble developing and sustaining satisfactory relationships. Typically, their relationships start out as ideal and end up as disasters. They idealize the significant other early in the relationship and may see the connection as more intimate than it really is.

If others start to pull back from the incessant demands, the histrionic person becomes dramatic and

---

Watching the watchers

Patients with histrionic personality disorder rarely gain an understanding of others. Instead, they devote their intense observation skills to determining which behaviors, attitudes, or feelings are most likely to win others' admiration and approval. Essentially, they watch other people watch them.

Because of their limited understanding of how others feel, they tend to see their relationships as closer or more significant than they really are. They don't realize when they're being humored or placated by someone who has lost patience with their constant need for attention and their inability to relate in an honest way.

demonstrative in an attempt to bind the other person to the relationship. To avoid rejection, they may resort to crying, coercion, temper tantrums, assault, and suicidal gestures.

Despite their attempts to bind others to them, the individuals with histrionic personality disorder often lack fidelity and loyalty.

Prevalence

Histrionic personality disorder affects an estimated 1.84% of the general population. Although more commonly diagnosed in women, it may be just as common in men (APA, 2013).

Without treatment, the disorder can lead to social, occupational, and functional impairments. However, many people function at a high level and succeed at work (although frequent disruption of intimate relationships is common).

Histrionic personality disorder commonly coexists with somatic symptom disorder, conversion disorder, and major depressive disorder.

Causes

The cause of histrionic personality disorder is not known. "The disorder is more common among first-degree relatives of people with the disorder than in the general population" (Townsend, 2014, p. 676). Learning experiences may also contribute to the disorder. Positive reinforcement, as a child, was only obtained by admired behaviors and may have been inconsistent and contingent on meeting a parent's approval. This may contribute to the excessive need for attention and the attention-seeking behavior (Townsend, 2014).

Signs and symptoms

Assessment of a patient with histrionic personality disorder may reveal:
- constant craving for attention, stimulation, and excitement
- intense affect
- shallow, rapidly shifting expression of emotions
- vanity
- flirting and seductive behavior
- overinvestment in appearance
- exaggerated, vague speech
- self-dramatization
- impulsivity
- exhibitionism
- suggestibility and impressionability
- egocentricity, self-indulgence, and lack of consideration for others

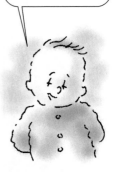

Would you believe I'm the same age as Bob Dylan? Thanks to facelifts and Botox, I plan to stay forever young.

- intolerance of frustration, disappointment, and delayed gratification; impatience
- somatic (physical) preoccupations and symptoms
- angry outbursts and tantrums
- sudden enraged, despairing, or fearful states
- intense anger toward people viewed as withholding
- divisive, manipulative behavior
- intolerance of being alone
- dread of growing old
- demanding and manipulative nature
- use of alcohol or drugs to quickly alter negative feelings
- depression
- suicidal gestures and threats.

Cultural histrionics

When assessing a patient for histrionic personality disorder, keep in mind that the expression of emotion and interpersonal behavior can vary widely across cultures, gender, and age groups (APA, 2013).

Diagnosis and treatment

No specific tests can diagnose histrionic personality disorder; however, personality and projective tests can be helpful. If the patient has somatic complaints, physiologic disorders must be ruled out. The official diagnosis of histrionic personality disorder is confirmed if the patient meets the criteria in the *DSM*-5.

Individuals with histrionic personality disorder rarely seek treatment unless a crisis occurs or a situational factor causes functional impairments and ineffective coping. Psychotherapy is the treatment of choice.

Psychotherapy

Psychotherapy focuses on solving problems in the patients' life rather than producing long-term personality changes. Individual therapy is preferred over group or family therapy because a group environment may trigger the patients' dramatic, attention-seeking behaviors. For this reason, self-help support groups are not recommended.

While establishing a rapport and trust with the patient, therapist must avoid a dependent situation with a needy patient who may see the therapist as their rescuer.

Insight

Insight-oriented and cognitive approaches aren't especially effective because histrionic patients have little capacity or inclination to examine their unconscious motives and thoughts. Instead, therapists should try to help the patients view their interactions objectively and explore and clarify patients' emotions.

Let's get real

Patients with histrionic personality disorder may use mechanisms such as suppression, disavowal, denial, and avoidance to block information that could cause emotional distress. In addition, these patients have difficulty focusing and are easily distracted. Therapists should focus on the issues that the patient is avoiding and work to keep the patient engaged in a reality-based environment.

> A histrionic patient may try to block out distressing information.

Serious about suicide

The patient should be assessed regularly for suicidal potential, and suicidal thoughts and plans should be taken seriously. Some therapists draw up a "suicide contract" that specifies under what conditions the patient may contact the therapist when the patient feels like hurting self. "The actual risk of suicide is not known, but clinical experience suggests that individuals with this disorder are at increased risk for suicidal gestures and threats to get attention and coerce better caregiving" (APA, 2013, p. 668).

Pharmacologic therapy

Medications usually aren't indicated for histrionic personality disorder; however, they may relieve associated symptoms, such as anxiety or depression. In a crisis, the patients may seek drugs for self-destructive or harmful purposes. Also, they may respond to the adverse effects of medications with intense, dramatic overreactions.

Nursing interventions

These nursing interventions may be appropriate for a patient with histrionic personality disorder:
• Give the patient choices in care options, and incorporate his or her wishes into the treatment plan as much as possible. Increasing the patient's sense of self-control may lower his or her anxiety.
• Be aware that the patient will want to "win over" the caregiver and—at least initially—will be responsive and cooperative.

Role modeling

• Teach the patient appropriate social skills and reinforce appropriate behavior.
• Help the patient learn to think more clearly and base his or her reactions on reality.
• Promote the expression of feelings, self-analysis of behavior, and accountability for actions.
• Encourage warmth, genuineness, and empathy.

Crisis management

- Teach stress-reducing techniques, such as deep breathing and an exercise regimen.
- Help them manage crisis situations and feelings.
- Monitor the patient for suicidal thoughts and behavior.

Narcissistic personality disorder

> Sure, I'm a tad self-centered. But with my looks, who wouldn't be?

The hallmarks of narcissistic personality disorder are self-centeredness, self-absorption, and an inability to empathize with the effects of one's behavior on others. A person with this disorder takes advantage of people, using them without regard for their feelings. They have an inflated sense of self and an intense need for admiration.

Image control

The narcissists try to maintain an image of perfection and invincibility to prevent others from discovering their weaknesses and imperfections. However, beneath the image are insecure individuals with low self-esteem.

Superior species?

The narcissists expect to be recognized as superior. Preoccupied with fantasies of brilliance and unlimited success or power, they believe that they are special and entitled to favored treatment. They expect others to comply with their wishes automatically and believe they should associate only with other special or high-status people. Many narcissists are driven and achievement-oriented.

Shattered illusions

The narcissists' illusion of greatness may be shattered by a threat to their ego from:
- physical illness
- loss of a job
- loss of a relationship
- feelings of emptiness and depression despite material wealth and success.

Such threats trigger panic. They feels their world is falling apart and their lives are unraveling.

Prevalence

Narcissistic personality disorder ranges between 0% and 6.2% in the general population. It affects about three times as many males as females (APA, 2013).

Although it develops by early adulthood, this disorder may not be identified until middle age, when the person experiences the sense of a loss of opportunity or faces personal limitations. Many people with narcissistic personality disorder also have histrionic or borderline personality disorder.

Causes

The exact cause of narcissistic personality disorder is unknown. A psychodynamic theory proposes that it arises when a child's basic needs go unmet.

Signs and symptoms

In patients with narcissistic personality disorder, assessment findings may include:

- arrogance or haughtiness
- self-centeredness
- unreasonable expectations of favorable treatment
- grandiose sense of self-importance
- exaggeration of achievements and talents
- preoccupation with fantasies of success, power, beauty, brilliance, or ideal love
- manipulative behavior
- constant desire for attention and admiration
- lack of empathy
- lack of concern for those they offend
- exploiting others to achieve their own goals
- rage, shame, or humiliation in response to criticism.

> A patient with narcissistic disorder thinks the world revolves around him or her.

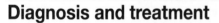

Diagnosis and treatment

The patient should undergo psychological evaluation and personality and projective testing. However, just like most personality disorders, there is not one specific test to diagnose narcissistic personality disorder. Multiple assessments and patterns of behavior are assessed and compared to the diagnostic criteria. The official diagnosis is confirmed if the patient meets the criteria in the *DSM-5*.

Most patients with narcissistic personality disorder seek treatment only in a crisis and terminate it as soon as their symptoms ease. Those who don't terminate treatment may be seeking help for depression or interpersonal difficulties.

Long-term psychotherapy is the treatment of choice because it helps establish a strong alliance between the patient and the therapist. Therapy should focus on making small, not large, changes in personality traits.

Pulling away the pedestal

The goals of therapy include placing the patients' exaggerated self-importance in perspective, helping them develop empathy, and teaching them how to handle slights and rejections without feeling extremely threatened.

Group therapy tends to be ineffective because these patients typically dominate the group. Other participants in the group may tire of hearing about the narcissistic accomplishments and talents. If or when they are being criticized by other participants in the group, they are likely to drop out of the group therapy.

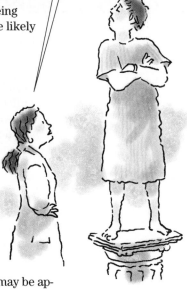

You may have put yourself on a pedestal, but I'm not going to reinforce your grandiosity.

Inpatient therapy

Hospitalization may be necessary for a patient with severe symptoms, such as self-destructive behavior and poor reality testing. However, hospitalization should be brief, with treatment specific to the particular symptoms.

Milieus for weak egos

Patients with little motivation for outpatient treatment, chronic destructive acting out, and chaotic lifestyles may need longer therapy. Inpatient programs can offer intensive milieu therapy, individual psychotherapy, family involvement, or a specialized residential environment. Such treatment may be appropriate for patients with severe ego weakness, helping them to improve their self-concept.

Nursing interventions

The following nursing interventions may be appropriate for patients with narcissistic personality disorder:
• Convey respect and acknowledge the patient's sense of self-importance so that they can reestablish a coherent sense of self. However, don't reinforce their pathologic grandiosity or their weakness.
• Focus on positive traits or on the feelings of pain, loss, or rejection.

Don't play a judge

• If the patient makes unreasonable demands or has unreasonable expectations, tell him or her in a matter-of-fact way that he or she is being unreasonable. However, remain nonjudgmental because a critical attitude may make the patient even more demanding and difficult. Don't avoid the patient, as this could increase his or her maladaptive attention-seeking behaviors.

- Avoid defensive behavior and arguments with patients with narcissistic personality disorder.
- Offer persistent, consistent, and flexible care. Take a direct, involved approach to develop a trusting provider relationship.
- Teach the patients social skills and reinforce appropriate behaviors.

Avoidant personality disorder

Avoidant personality disorder is marked by feelings of inadequacy, extreme social anxiety, social withdrawal, and hypersensitivity to the opinions of others. People with this disorder have low self-esteem and poor self-confidence. They dwell on the negative and have difficulty viewing situations and interactions objectively. To rationalize their avoidance of new situations, they exaggerate the potential difficulties involved. They may create fantasy worlds to substitute for the real one.

Wallflower syndrome

The avoidant person yearns for social interaction but the fear of being rejected or embarrassed in front of others is a daily obstacle. In fact, many times they are not willing to enter into social relationships without the assurance of uncritical acceptance. They even seek out jobs that require little contact with others.

Prevalence

In the adult general population, the prevalence of avoidant personality disorder is estimated at 2.4%, affects males and females equally, and develops by early adulthood (APA, 2013). It is common to see additional psychiatric diagnoses with avoidant personality disorder. One of the more common is dependent personality disorder. When the patient with avoidant personality finds someone whom he or she can trust, he or she may become very attached to the point of dependence (APA, 2013).

> Being belittled as a child makes me want to avoid the world.

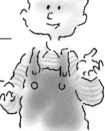

Causes

As with most personality disorder, there is no clear cause of avoidant personality disorder. The disorder most likely results from a combination of genetic, biological, and environmental factors. The primary psychosocial cause seems to center on parental rejection and the feelings of abandonment as a child. These feelings may develop into a low self-worth and because of past abandonment, the world is viewed as dangerous (Townsend, 2014).

Genetic and biological theories

Avoidant personality disorder is closely linked to temperament. Some evidence suggests that a timid temperament in infancy may predispose a person to developing avoidant personality disorder later in life.

Information overload

The inherited tendency to be shy may result from overstimulation or an excess of incoming information. The patient can't cope with the excess information and withdraws in defense. Inability to cope with the information overload may stem from a low autonomic arousal threshold. Research suggests that in people with this disorder, certain structures in the brain's limbic system may have a lower threshold of arousal and a more pronounced response when activated.

Environmental factors

Some experts believe that significant environmental influences during childhood, such as rejection by the parents or peers, leads to the full development of avoidant personality disorder. (See *The rejected child*.)

The rejected child

Normal, healthy infants may encounter varying degrees of parental rejection. In those who subsequently develop avoidant personality disorder, the amount of rejection seems to be particularly intense or frequent.

Particular types of parental rejection can alter a child's attitude and behavior in a way that predisposes him or her to developing avoidant personality disorder later in life. For example, if a parent is aloof or critical when the child expresses positive emotions, the child might learn to spare himself or herself the anguish by keeping positive feelings to himself or herself.

Likewise, if the child is repeatedly told that it's bad to feel angry, he or she might swear off relationships to avoid the intermittent feelings of dissatisfaction or anger that occur in nearly all close relationships.

Peer rejection
Repeated social interactions expose a person to potential rejection over a sustained period. Such rejection can wear down self-esteem. After humiliation and rejection by peers, a person may begin to criticize himself or herself.

Feelings of loneliness and isolation worsen with these harsh self-judgments. Deepening feelings of personal inferiority and self-worthlessness contribute to social withdrawal.

Rejection by peers seems to validate rejection by the parents. When a child can't turn to parents, peers, or even himself or herself for gratification or validation, he or she retreats—and avoidant personality disorder may result.

Memory jogger

For an easy way to remember the signs and symptoms of avoidant personality disorder, think of AVOIDANT.

A Anxious and angry with oneself because of the lack of meaningful relationships

V Very socially withdrawn

O Often feels lonely and unwanted

I Intensely shy

D Desires close relationships but has difficulty developing and sustaining them

A Awkward and uncomfortable in others' company

N No natural optimism or positive regard for oneself

T Terrified by the fear of rejection

Signs and symptoms

Patients with avoidant personality disorder may exhibit or report:
- shyness, timidity, and social withdrawal
- behavior or appearance that is used to drive others away
- reluctance to speak or, conversely, over talkativeness
- constant mistrust or wariness of others
- testing of others' sincerity
- difficulty starting and maintaining relationships
- perfectionism
- rejection of people who don't live up to impossibly high standards
- limited emotional expression
- tenseness and anxiety
- low self-esteem
- feelings of being unworthy of successful relationships
- self-consciousness
- loneliness
- reluctance to take personal risks or to engage in new activities
- frequent escapes into fantasy, such as by excessive reading, watching TV, or daydreaming.

Diagnosis and treatment

No specific tests can diagnose avoidant personality disorder. The patient should undergo a psychological evaluation, along with personality and projective tests. The diagnosis is confirmed if the patient meets the criteria in the *DSM-5*.

People with avoidant personality disorder rarely seek treatment unless something goes wrong in their lives to indicate that they are not coping adequately. High-functioning patients may need psychotherapy only, whereas others benefit from a combination of medication and psychotherapy.

The goals of treatment are to:
- enhance self-esteem
- improve social interaction and increase confidence in interpersonal relationships
- desensitize the reaction to criticism
- decrease resistance to change
- improve coping
- achieve cognitive restructuring
- develop appropriate affect and expression of emotions.

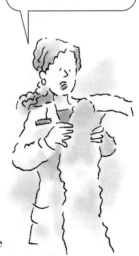

Personality and projective tests can help determine if a patient has avoidant personality disorder.

Psychotherapy

Individual psychotherapy is the preferred treatment. It is the most effective when it is short-term and focused on solving specific life problems. As patients successfully progress through individual therapy, group therapy may be considered.

All's well that ends well

Establishing a solid therapist-patient relationship may be difficult, and the patient may terminate therapy early. However, a successful ending to the relationship is important because it reinforces for the patient the possibility of new relationships.

Self-help support groups

Although self-help support groups can be effective for patients with avoidant personality disorder, such groups may be difficult to find. Additionally, patients with this disorder are likely to avoid groups because of their social anxiety.

Pharmacologic therapy

Medications may be prescribed as an adjunct to psychotherapy when patients have moderate to severe functional impairments. Avoidant personality disorder patients commonly respond well to MAOIs such as phenelzine (Nardil) in particular, which seems to improve confidence and assertiveness in social settings. For individuals who are sensitive to rejection, serotonin-based antidepressants such as sertraline (Zoloft) may be helpful (Sadock & Sadock, 2007). If the patient feels disconnected from his or her emotions, medications may interfere with effective psychotherapeutic management.

Nursing interventions

These nursing interventions may be appropriate for patients with avoidant personality disorder:
• Offer persistent, consistent, and flexible care. Take a direct, involved approach to gain trust.
• Be aware that the patient may become dependent on the few staff members that he or she feel he or she can trust. Monitor for signs of dependency, and encourage self-care.
• Assess the patient for signs of depression because social impairment increases the risk of mood disorders.

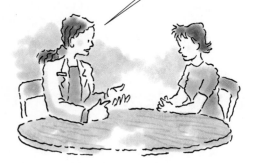

I'm glad you trust me to care for you, but you need to be involved in your care, too.

Advice from the experts

Basic requirements for relaxation

According to Dr. Herbert Benson, the Harvard professor who first described the relaxation response, four basic elements are needed to elicit this response:
• a quiet environment that's free from distraction
• a sound, process, or image to dwell on, such as breathing or a mantra (such as that used in transcendental meditation)
• a passive attitude in which the mind is cleared of thoughts and images
• a comfortable position that can be kept easily for at least 20 minutes.

Advance warning

• Make sure that the patient knows about upcoming procedures in plenty of time to adjust because he or she doesn't handle surprises well.
• Inform the patient when you will and will not be available if he or she needs assistance.

Directives and decisions

• Initially, give the patient explicit directives rather than asking him or her to make decisions. Then gradually encourage him or her to make easy decisions. Continue to provide support and reassurance as his or her decision-making ability improves.
• Avoid actions that foster dependency.
• Encourage the expression of feelings, self-analysis of behavior, and accountability for actions.
• Teach the patient relaxation and stress management techniques to help him or her cope in times of stress and manage his or her anxiety level. (See *Basic requirements for relaxation*.)

A basic requirement for relaxation? I'm thinking a week in Cancun.

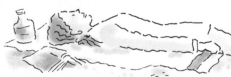

Dependent personality disorder

Dependent personality disorder is characterized by an extreme need to be taken care of, which leads to submissive, clinging behavior and fear of separation or rejection. People with this disorder let others make important decisions for them and have a strong need for constant reassurance and support. To elicit caregiving, they engage in dependent behavior. Feeling helpless and incompetent, they comply passively and transfer responsibility to others. In fact, they seek others to dominate and protect them. Some stay in abusive relationships and are willing to tolerate mistreatment.

Replacement therapy

When the breakup of a romantic relationship is imminent, individuals with dependent personality disorder may become suicidal. After a close relationship ends, they urgently seek another relationship as a source of care and support.

People who need people

These behaviors arise from the perception that they can't function adequately without others. They crave attention and validation and may repeatedly request attention to their complaints. The complaints can be simple or complex in nature such as their overall lifestyle, social relationships, meaning in life, or medical problems.

That worthless feeling

Overly sensitive to disapproval, people with dependent personality disorder often feel helpless and depressed. They belittle their own abilities and are racked with self-doubt. They take criticism and disapproval as proof that they are worthless. They are likely to avoid positions of responsibility. If their job requires independent initiative, they may suffer occupational impairments.

Prevalence

In mental health clinics, dependent personality disorder is among the most frequently reported personality disorders. In the general population, its prevalence is about 0.49% to 0.6%. It affects more females than males but some reports suggest that there is a comparable prevalence between the genders (APA, 2013). Individuals who suffered chronic physical illness in childhood are more prone to develop dependent personality disorder (Sadock & Sadock, 2007).

Many patients with dependent personality disorder have an additional personality disorder—most commonly borderline, histrionic, or avoidant.

Causes

The exact cause of dependent personality disorder is not known. Because it tends to run in families, it may involve a genetic component.

Dictators and coddlers

According to some experts, authoritarian or overprotective parenting may lead to high levels of dependency. These parenting styles may cause these children to believe that they cannot function without others' guidance and protection and that the way to maintain relationships is to give in to others' demands.

Signs and symptoms

Assessment findings in a patient with dependent personality disorder may include:
- submissiveness
- self-effacing, apologetic manner
- low self-esteem
- lack of self-confidence
- lack of initiative
- incompetence and a need for constant assistance
- intense need to be loved in a stable long-term relationship
- anxiety and insecurity, especially when deprived of a significant relationship
- feelings of pessimism, inferiority, and unworthiness
- hypersensitivity to criticism
- in females, little need to overtly control or compete with others
- clinging, demanding behavior
- use of cajolery, bribery, promises to change, and even threats to maintain key relationships
- fear and anxiety over losing a relationship or being alone
- dependence on a number of people, any one of whom could substitute for the other
- difficulty making everyday decisions without advice and reassurance
- avoidance of change and new situations
- exaggerated fear of losing support and approval.

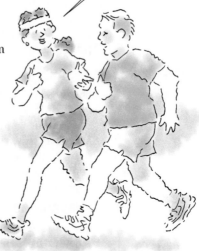

Don't be so self-effacing. You're a hot, handsome hunk!

Somatically speaking . . .

A patient with dependent personality disorder may also present with somatic complaints, such as fatigue and lethargy, as well as tension, anxiety, or depression.

Diagnosis and treatment

The patient should undergo a psychological evaluation and psychological and projective tests, as indicated. If he or she has somatic complaints, he or she should be evaluated medically and, as needed, undergo diagnostic tests to rule out underlying medical conditions. The diagnosis of dependent personality disorder is confirmed if the patient meets the criteria in the *DSM-5*.

Although patients with this disorder frequently attend outpatient mental health clinics, they rarely seek treatment for dependency or help in making decisions. Instead, they typically complain of anxiety, tension, or depression.

Psychotherapy

Psychotherapy is the treatment of choice. Promoting autonomy and self-efficacy are the overriding treatment goals.

Clinging vine

The most effective approach is short-term therapy that focuses on helping the patient solve specific life problems. Long-term therapy is contraindicated because it only reinforces a dependent relationship with the therapist. (However, some degree of dependency is bound to develop no matter the length of therapy.)

Individual and group therapy may be helpful, although the patient may use a group setting to find new dependent relationships.

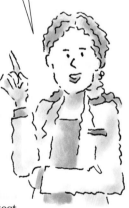

For a dependent patient, long-term therapy only reinforces a dependent relationship with the therapist.

After-hours attention

The patient may be very needy with the therapist and seek tremendous reassurance and attention—especially between therapy sessions. At the start of therapy, the therapist should set boundaries as to how the treatment will be conducted, including such issues as appropriate times to contact the therapist between sessions.

Final endings

Termination of therapy is an important issue because it is a test of how effective the therapy has been. The therapist should set goals for therapy and make it clear to the patient that when he or she attain these goals, therapy will end.

Behavioral approaches

A patient with dependent personality disorder can benefit from such behavioral approaches as assertiveness training. Treatment may include behavior modification using assertiveness techniques.

Self-help support groups

Self-help support groups allow patients with dependent personality disorder to share their experiences and feelings as well as put to use their newly learned skills. However, a support group shouldn't be the sole treatment for this disorder because it may encourage dependent relationships.

Pharmacologic therapy

The doctor may prescribe medications to treat associated symptoms, such as low energy, fatigue, and depression. Some patients respond well to antidepressants. In a crisis, benzodiazepine antianxiety drugs such as alprazolam (Xanax), lorazepam (Ativan), and clonazepam (Klonopin) may be prescribed. However, because the patient may abuse these agents, their use should be limited and monitored.

Nursing interventions

The following nursing interventions may be appropriate for patients with dependent personality disorder:
• Offer persistent, consistent, and flexible care. Take a direct, involved approach to develop a trusting relationship.
• Give the patients as much opportunity to control their treatment as possible. Offer options and allow them to choose, even if they choose all of them.
• Verify the patient's approval before initiating specific treatment.
• Try to limit caregivers to a few consistent staff members to increase the patient's sense of security.

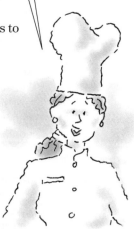

Encourage dependent patients to plan their own meals, balance their own checkbook, and pay bills on their own.

Deter dependency

• Deter actions that promote dependency on caregivers.
• Encourage activities that require decision making (such as balancing a checkbook, planning meals, and paying bills) to promote autonomy.
• Help the patient establish and work toward goals to foster a sense of autonomy.
• If the patient has physical complaints, don't minimize or dismiss him or her—but don't encourage him or her either. Use a simple, matter-of-fact approach.

Aim for assertiveness

• Help the patient express his or her ideas and feelings assertively.
• Be aware that outwardly, the patient may seem compliant, perhaps overly compliant, with suggestions for treatment. However, he or she may fail to make real gains in therapy because his or her compliance is usually superficial.

Monitor medications

- Teach the patient about prescribed medications, including exactly what each medication is prescribed for.
- Emphasize that there are no magical drug effects.
- Monitor the patient to make sure that he or she is not abusing medication. If the patient is receiving benzodiazepines, check for signs and symptoms of psychological dependence.

Obsessive-compulsive personality disorder

Obsessive-compulsive personality disorder is marked by a desire for perfection and order at the expense of openness, flexibility, and efficiency. The person with this disorder sees the world as black and white. Along with perfectionism comes relentless anxiety about not getting things perfect. The patient with obsessive-compulsive personality disorder places a great deal of pressure on himself or herself and those around him or her. Mistakes are viewed as unacceptable and the patient with this disorder may have a constant sense of righteous indignation and feel anger and contempt for anyone who disagrees with him or her.

My way or the highway

Patients with this disorder view their methods as the only right way; all other ways are wrong according to their view. Their inflexibility extends to interpersonal relationships, as well as daily routines. A lifelong pattern of rigid thinking may lead to poor social skills.

Control freak

Those with obsessive-compulsive personality disorder have an overwhelming need to control the environment. They may force themselves and others to follow rigid moral principles and conform to extremely high standards of performance. Conscientious, scrupulous, and inflexible about morality, ethics, and value, they insist on literal compliance with authority and rules.

Indecisive impasse

In their effort to avoid being wrong, they may suffer severe procrastination and indecisiveness because they cannot determine with certainty which choice is correct. They may have trouble even starting a task because of their need to sort

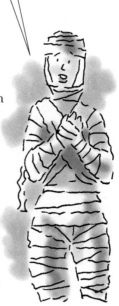

The patient with obsessive-compulsive personality disorder is all bound up in self-imposed rules and regulations.

Myth busters

A confusing similarity

Although the two disorders have almost identical names, obsessive-compulsive personality disorder and obsessive-compulsive disorder share little in common.

Myth: Obsessive-compulsive personality disorder is the same thing as obsessive-compulsive disorder.

Reality: Obsessive-compulsive disorder is an anxiety disorder characterized by obsessions and compulsions.

In contrast, obsessive-compulsive *personality* disorder is marked by a constant striving for perfection and control. Obsessions and compulsions aren't a part of the personality disorder because the patient's preoccupation with orderliness isn't intense enough to be considered an obsession.

out the priorities correctly. Their symptoms may cause extreme distress and interfere with occupational and social functioning. (See *A confusing similarity.*)

Prevalence

Obsessive-compulsive personality disorder affects about 2.1% to 7.9% of the general population. It is one of the most common personality disorders in the general population. About twice as many males as females are diagnosed with this disorder (APA, 2013). Incidence may be higher among the oldest children in a family and among people whose occupations require attention to detail and methodical perseverance.

Causes

Genetic and developmental factors may play a role in the development of this disorder. Twin and adoption studies suggest that it runs in families.

Psychodynamic theories view the patient's needing control as a defense against feelings of powerlessness or shame. Individuals diagnosed with obsessive personality disorder had harsh upbringing discipline (Sadock & Sadock, 2007).

Signs and symptoms

A patient with obsessive-compulsive personality disorder may describe his or her symptoms in a logical way, attaching little emotion to any physical discomfort. Assessment findings commonly include:

* behavioral, emotional, and cognitive rigidity
* perfectionism
* severe self-criticism
* indecisiveness
* controlling manner
* difficulty expressing tender feelings
* poor sense of humor
* cool, distant, formal manner
* solemn, tense demeanor
* emotional constriction
* excessive discipline
* aggression, competitiveness, and impatience
* bouts of intense anger when things stray from the patient's idea of how things "should be"
* difficulty incorporating new information into his or her life
* psychosomatic complaints
* hypochondriasis
* sexual dysfunction
* chronic sense of time pressure and inability to relax
* indirect expression of anger despite an apparent undercurrent of hostility
* hoarding of money and other possessions
* preoccupation with orderliness, neatness, and cleanliness
* scrupulousness about morality, ethics, or values
* signs and symptoms of depression
* physical complaints (commonly stemming from overwork).

A perfectionistic patient simply won't tolerate a poorly made bed.

Diagnosis and treatment

The patient should undergo a psychological evaluation, including personality and projective tests. The diagnosis of obsessive-compulsive personality disorder is confirmed if the patient meets the criteria in the *DSM-5*.

Typically, people with obsessive-compulsive personality disorder seek treatment only if they are depressed, unproductive, or under extreme stress—circumstances that tax their limited coping skills. Treatment usually involves individual psychotherapy, possibly in conjunction with medication.

Psychotherapy

Effective psychotherapeutic treatment centers on short-term symptom relief and support for existing coping mechanisms (with new ones taught as therapy progresses). Long-term work on changing the personality is unrealistic because the inherent nature of obsessive-compulsive personality disorder makes it especially resistant to change.

> A businesslike approach is best if your patient has obsessive-compulsive personality disorder.

Down to business

The therapist should discuss the nature of the disease process and explain typical treatments in a businesslike, factual manner rather than give vague impressions. When patients accept the treatment regimen, they are likely to adhere to it rigorously and strive to be a good patient. They are conscientious, honest, motivated, and hardworking.

Ideally, therapy should replace skills that aren't working with new skill sets, examine social relationships, and identify feeling states. Proper identification and realization of feelings can help produce changes in the patient's life.

Focus on feelings

Because the patients with obsessive-compulsive personality disorder are likely to be out of touch with their emotions, the therapist should lead them away from describing situations, events, and daily happenings. A better approach is to have them express how these events make them feel. Having these patients keep a daily journal of feelings can help them remember how they felt at any given time. Cognitive approaches rarely work with these patients because they are likely to use this type of therapy as a means for verbally attacking the therapist or otherwise taking the focus off himself or herself.

Group therapy

The patients may find group therapy intolerable because of the social contact necessary in healthy group dynamics. In fact, group members may ostracize these patients if they point out their deficits and incorrect ways of doing things.

Pharmacologic therapy

SSRIs are approved by the FDA for use in obsessive-compulsive disorder, which is the more severe form of this disorder. "Drugs such as fluoxetine (Prozac) may help reduce the obsessions, anxiety, and depression associated with this disorder" (Halter, 2014, p. 463).

Nursing interventions

These nursing interventions may be appropriate for patients with obsessive-compulsive personality disorder:
• Offer persistent, consistent, and flexible care. Take a direct, involved approach to gain trust.
• Let the patient control his or her own treatment plan by giving him or her choices whenever possible.
• Maintain a professional attitude. Avoid informality; these patients want strict attention to detail.

Don't get too close

• Recognize the need for physical and emotional distance.

Pay attention!

• Be prepared for long monologues centering on the patient's goals and ambitions and reasons why family members, friends, and work subordinates need to be rigidly controlled. Try to remain attentive.
• Use tolerance and ordinary kindness when dealing with these patients. Remember that they are used to causing exasperation in others but do not fully understand why.
• Avoid defensive behavior and arguments with patients with obsessive-compulsive personality disorder.

No-pressure tactics

• Don't brush aside issues that the patient thinks is important in an effort to get on with affective issues. Pressuring the patient to focus prematurely on emotions will alienate him or her.
• If appropriate, encourage the patient to record his or her feelings in a journal.
• Remember that the patient's defensive structure (which makes him or her seem arrogant and argumentative) is a cover for his or her vulnerability to shame, humiliation, and dread.

Teaching topics

• Teach the patients social skills, and reinforce appropriate behaviors.
• Teach them about prescribed medication.
• Encourage them to continue therapy for optimal results.

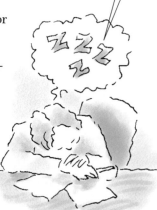

Try to be attentive even if your patient rambles on about others' faults.

References

American Psychiatric Association. (2013). *Diagnostic and statistical manual of mental disorders* (5th ed.). Arlington, VA: Author.

Boyd, M. (2012). *Psychiatric nursing: Contemporary practice* (5th ed.). Philadelphia, PA: Lippincott Williams & Wilkins.

Halter, M. (2014). *Varicolis' foundation of psychiatric mental health nursing: A clinical approach* (7th ed.). St. Louis, MO: Elsevier.

Personality. (n.d.). In *Merriam-Webster's online dictionary.* Retrieved http://www.merriam-webster.com/dictionary/personality

Sadock, B. J., & Sadock, V. A. (2007). *Synopsis of psychiatry* (10th ed.). Philadelphia, PA: Lippincott Williams & Wilkins.

Townsend, M. (2014). *Psychiatric mental health nursing: Concepts of care in evidence-based practice* (8th ed.). Philadelphia, PA: F.A. Davis.

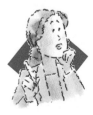

Quick quiz

1. The personality disorder that's characterized primarily by mistrust is:

    A.   paranoid personality disorder.
    B.   antisocial personality disorder.
    C.   dependent personality disorder.
    D.   schizotypal personality disorder.

Answer: A. Paranoid personality disorder is characterized by an extreme distrust of others. Patients with this disorder avoid relationships in which they aren't in control or have the potential of losing control.

2. For patients with most personality disorders, the treatment of choice is:

    A.   group therapy.
    B.   individual psychotherapy.
    C.   self-help support groups.
    D.   inpatient therapy.

Answer: B. Individual psychotherapy is usually the treatment of choice for patients with personality disorders.

3. Ideas of reference and magical thinking may occur in:
   A. borderline personality disorder.
   B. schizotypal personality disorder.
   C. schizoid personality disorder.
   D. histrionic personality disorder.

Answer: B. Schizotypal personality disorder is marked by ideas of reference, odd beliefs, or magical thinking, among other features.

4. The hallmark of borderline personality disorder is:
   A. irresponsibility.
   B. reckless disregard for others.
   C. impulsivity.
   D. unlawful behavior.

Answer: C. Impulsivity is the most prominent characteristic of borderline personality disorder.

5. If a patient with dependent personality disorder reports physical complaints, the nurse should:
   A. overlook the symptoms.
   B. encourage the patient to talk about his or her symptoms.
   C. disregard symptoms until emotional issues have been explored.
   D. explore symptoms in a matter-of-fact way.

Answer: D. The nurse should explore the patient's symptoms in a matter-of-fact way. Although physical complaints should be evaluated promptly, caregivers shouldn't encourage the patient to talk about them.

6. A patient who is preoccupied with details and lists is most likely to have:
   A. histrionic personality disorder.
   B. obsessive-compulsive personality disorder.
   C. schizotypal personality disorder.
   D. narcissistic personality disorder.

Answer: B. Obsessive-compulsive personality disorder is marked by a preoccupation with details, lists, rules, and schedules.

Scoring

✰✰✰ If you answered all six items correctly, take a bow! We won't hold it against you if you're feeling a bit narcissistic right now.

✰✰ If you answered four or five items correctly, you certainly don't need to be rescued. You're right on the borderline between good and excellent.

✰ If you answered fewer than four items correctly, don't get histrionic. Just cling to this chapter a little longer.

10

Eating disorders

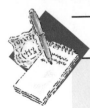

Just the facts

In this chapter, you'll learn:

♦ major features of eating disorders

♦ proposed causes of eating disorders

♦ assessment findings and nursing interventions for patients with eating disorders

♦ recommended treatments for patients with eating disorders.

A look at eating disorders

> People with eating disorders are preoccupied with food, and/or weight, and/or exercise.

Eating disorders are classified as psychological illnesses characterized by persistent abnormal eating patterns and habits. Eating disorders impact health, productivity, and relationships with others. An individual with an eating disorder is preoccupied with thoughts of food and/or weight and exercise to the extent that it disrupts daily life. Serious and life-threatening consequences occur if the condition is left untreated. Several different eating disorders have been identified by the American Psychiatric Association (APA; 2013b) based on presentation of symptoms. Projections indicate up to 30 million individuals in the United States at some time in their lifetime will suffer from a clinically significant eating disorder (Wade, Keski-Rahkonen, & Hudson, 2011). Eating disorders affect both genders, people young to middle age and even into older adults, and from all ethnic groups and backgrounds, yet most frequently appear in adolescence or young adulthood.

Illness inventory

This chapter discusses the three most common psychiatric eating disorders:

- anorexia nervosa
- bulimia nervosa
- binge-eating disorder

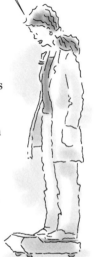

All three of the eating disorders share the common feature: preoccupation with food. Anorexia nervosa and bulimia nervosa share such features as dieting and preoccupation with weight and shape. Additionally, anorexia nervosa and bulimia nervosa can occur simultaneously. Most people diagnosed with these three eating disorders are female (Mayo Clinic, 2014). An eating disorder can be physically and psychologically debilitating. Extreme cases can lead to death from physical complications or suicide. The risk of mortality is especially high if the disorder is long-standing or the patient has comorbid psychiatric problems, such as substance abuse, depression, other mood disorders, and/or obsessive-compulsive disorder (OCD). Eating disorders have the highest rate of mortality than any other psychiatric disorder.

Causes

Currently, the causes of eating disorders are thought to involve a complex interaction of genetics, biological and psychodynamics factors, and social and family influences.

Genetic and biological theories

Eating disorders tend to run in families, with female relatives most often affected. There is a higher rate of eating disorders in monozygotic twins than in dizygotic twins. In addition, an individual whose immediate relative has an eating disorder runs a greater risk of developing the disorder, but this finding also suggests a social influence factor.

Neurochemical factors have also been linked to eating disorders—although it isn't clear if these factors cause, accompany, or follow the development of the eating disorder.

Risk factors

Risk factors or factors that may increase susceptibility for eating disorders include:
- gender—being female
- age—being an adolescent or young adult
- family history—having a parent or sibling with an eating disorder
- mental health—having depression, an anxiety disorder, a mood disorder, and/or OCD
- situation—transitioning in life such as moving, beginning college, or other life changes
- social—being an athlete, actor or performer, dancer, or model (Mayo Clinic, 2012).

Psychological factors

Psychological factors that may play a role in the development of eating disorders include:
- low self-esteem
- conflicts over identity, role development, and body image
- fears concerning sexuality
- chaotic families with few rules or boundaries
- parental overemphasis on, or excessive worry over, the child's weight
- sexual abuse.

Social influences

Society sets unrealistic expectations for appearance, equating thinness with being successful, powerful, and popular. These expectations are conveyed through omnipresent images of thin, beautiful people on television and in films, magazines, and other media.

Anorexia nervosa

Anorexia nervosa is a syndrome in which the affected person relentlessly pursues thinness—sometimes to the point of fatal emaciation—as he or she becomes preoccupied with food and body image. Despite the extreme thinness, these individuals perceive themselves as being fat because they have distorted body image. This syndrome is also characterized by an extreme self-induced starvation and excessive weight loss that result in medical abnormalities. Generally, a person is deemed to have anorexia nervosa when his or her body weight is significantly below expectations for the person's age, height, development, and health. (See *Name games*.)

Disorder subtypes

The APA identifies two anorexia nervosa subtypes in the *Diagnostic and Statistical Manual of Mental Disorders*, 5th Edition (*DSM-5*) (APA, 2013a):
- restricting type, in which the individual loses weight primarily through dieting, fasting, and/or excessive exercise and has not engaged in binging and purging during the last 3 months
- binge-eating or purging type, in which the patient engages in recurring binge-eating or purging behaviors, including self-induced vomiting or abuse of laxatives, diuretics, or enemas during the last 3 months.

Myth busters

Name games

Many people confuse anorexia nervosa with anorexia.

Myth: Anorexia nervosa is the clinical term for anorexia.

Reality: The two conditions aren't the same thing. *Anorexia* refers to loss of appetite. A common symptom of gastrointestinal and endocrine disorders, anorexia may also accompany anxiety, chronic pain, poor oral hygiene, increased body temperature caused by fever or hot weather, and aging-related changes in taste or smell. Some drugs may also cause anorexia.

Anorexia nervosa, on the other hand, is an eating disorder marked by a distorted body image, an extreme fear of gaining weight, and a restricted nutritional intake to maintain a minimally normal body weight. Patients with anorexia nervosa think they're overweight even when they're extremely underweight.

Complications

Serious medical complications can result from the malnutrition, dehydration, and electrolyte imbalances caused by prolonged starvation, vomiting, and laxative abuse. Anorexia nervosa also increases the susceptibility to infection.

Malnutrition may cause hypoalbuminemia and subsequent edema or hypokalemia—possibly leading to ventricular arrhythmias and renal failure. Coupled with laxative abuse, poor nutrition and dehydration produce bowel changes similar to those of chronic inflammatory bowel disease.

Frequent vomiting may cause esophageal erosion, ulcers, tears, and bleeding as well as tooth and gum erosion and dental caries.

Menstrual suspension

Amenorrhea (cessation of menstrual periods) may occur when the patient loses about 25% of normal body weight. Complications of prolonged amenorrhea include estrogen deficiency (which raises the risk of calcium deficiency and osteoporosis) and infertility.

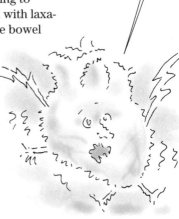

If malnutrition leads to edema or hypokalemia, ventricular arrhythmias may occur.

Disheartening complications

Cardiovascular complications of anorexia nervosa can be life-threatening. They include:

- heart failure
- decreased left ventricular muscle mass and chamber size
- reduced cardiac output
- hypotension
- bradycardia
- electrocardiograph (ECG) changes, such as nonspecific ST intervals, T-wave changes, and prolonged PR intervals
- sudden death, possibly from ventricular arrhythmias.

Prevalence and onset

Precise statistics on the onset and prevalence of anorexia nervosa aren't available. However, by conservative estimates, 0.5% to 1% of females in late adolescence and early adulthood meet the diagnostic criteria. The onset is usually in early to late adolescence with most between 15 and 19 years of age (Lindvall Dahlgren & Rø, 2014). Anorexia nervosa is more common in females than males with the prevalence ratio between females and males of 10:1 respectively (APA, 2013b).

Patient profile

Although more than 90% of those with anorexia nervosa are adolescent and young women, the condition has been diagnosed in males, children as young as age 7, and women up to age 80. (See *Getting past stereotypes*.) Frequently, patients with anorexia nervosa have additional psychiatric disorders, such as anxiety, depression, and obsessive compulsive disorder (APA, 2013b).

Volunteering for help

The prognosis varies but improves if the patient is diagnosed early or seeks help voluntarily. Mortality ranges from 5% to 18% (Sadock & Sadock, 2007).

Causes

No one knows exactly what causes anorexia nervosa.

Genetic causes

Identical twins have a higher risk for anorexia nervosa than fraternal twins, and siblings of those with anorexia nervosa are more likely to suffer from the disorder.

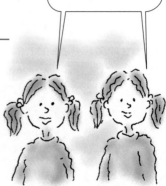

We're identical twins, so if one of us gets anorexia nervosa, the other has an increased risk.

Myth busters

Getting past stereotypes

If you have preconceived notions about who gets anorexia nervosa, you may mistake this disorder for another condition.

Myth: Only young women get anorexia nervosa.

Reality: Although young females are more commonly diagnosed with anorexia nervosa, the disorder is increasingly showing up in males and older women.

Biological causes

In patients with anorexia nervosa, studies have found below-normal levels of the neurotransmitters serotonin and norepinephrine and above-normal levels of cortisol (a "stress" hormone) and vasopressin. These findings suggest that the disorder is linked to inadequate production of norepinephrine and serotonin.

Brain abnormalities are seen in computed tomography (CT) and in positron emission tomography (PET) scans in anorectic individuals during starvation. However, the association of these abnormalities to anorexia is not clear (APA, 2013b).

Behavioral and environmental factors

Because anorexia nervosa occurs mainly in Western and industrialized countries, some experts blame the disorder on societal standards of ideal body shape and the constant pressure to be thin. Additionally, many people first learn about eating disorders from friends and the media. Thus, eating disorders may represent learned behaviors in response to strong social pressures, which are bolstered by society's expectation that individuals stay thin.

Stress may also play a role. As with other psychiatric disorders, stressful events may raise the risk of anorexia nervosa.

Psychological factors

Most experts believe low self-esteem, perfectionism, and a sense of powerlessness underlie anorexia nervosa. Thus, the disorder is both a symptom of and a defense against feelings of inadequacy.

To compensate for the low self-esteem, the patient becomes a perfectionist. In response to failure or rejection, the individual becomes extremely self-critical, which further weakens their fragile self-esteem.

Power and perfection

Because the individuals who suffers from anorexia nervosa doesn't know how to deal with these painful feelings directly, they express them through their eating disorder. Feeling powerless and unable to control their life or environment, they strive for a sense of power and control through caloric restriction. They believe that if they can control their eating, they'll be in control of their world, and that if they achieve the "perfect" body, they'll lead the "perfect" life.

> Restricting calories gives the patient with anorexia nervosa a sense of power and control.

A shield against sexuality

Some psychiatrists see refusal to eat as a subconscious effort to protect oneself from dealing with issues surrounding sexuality.

Family dynamics

According to some authorities, families of patients with anorexia nervosa tend to be chaotic and place a high value on achievement. Family members also have trouble resolving conflict and expressing anger directly. Other family factors that may play a role in the disorder include:
• sexual, physical, or emotional abuse
• one parent who's aggressive and another who's passive
• a mother who's superficially powerful in the family
• a father who's distant and withholds his feelings as the child becomes an adolescent.

Signs and symptoms

The key feature of anorexia nervosa is self-imposed starvation, despite the patient's obvious emaciation. The patient's history usually reveals a significant weight loss with no organic reason, coupled with a morbid fear of being fat and a compulsion to be thin.

Physical findings

Physical findings that suggest anorexia nervosa include:
• emaciated appearance
• skeletal muscle atrophy
• loss of fatty tissue
• breast tissue atrophy
• lanugo (a covering of soft, fine hair) on the face and body

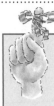

Memory jogger

The word HUNGER is your guidepost to the major features of anorexia nervosa.

H Has an obsession with food and weight

U Underweight or emaciated

N Nutritional needs go unmet

G Gross distortion of body image

E Exercises, vomits, or uses laxatives and diuretics to lose weight

R Refuses to eat

- dryness or loss of scalp hair
- hypotension
- bradycardia and/or irregular heart rhythm
- fatigue
- sleep difficulties
- cold intolerance
- constipation
- bowel distention
- loss of libido
- amenorrhea.

Psychosocial findings

Common psychosocial findings of anorexia nervosa include:
- preoccupation with body size
- distorted body image
- fear of weight gain
- inability to comprehend the severity of the situation
- descriptions of self as "fat"—"fat phobia"
- dissatisfaction with a particular aspect of the appearance
- low self-esteem
- social isolation/withdrawal
- perfectionism
- ritualism
- paradoxical obsession with food such as preparing elaborate meals for others
- feelings of despair, hopelessness, and worthlessness
- suicidal thoughts.

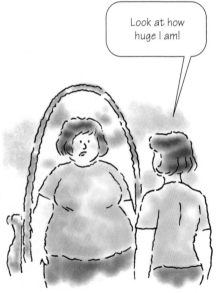

Look at how huge I am!

Behavioral findings

Behavioral signs of anorexia nervosa include:
• wearing of oversized clothing in an effort to disguise body size
• behaviors to prevent weight gain
• layering of clothing or wearing of unseasonably warm clothing to compensate for cold intolerance and loss of adipose tissue
• restless activity and vigor (despite undernourishment)
• avid exercising with no apparent fatigue
• outstanding academic or athletic performance.

Diagnosis

Although anorexia nervosa should be suspected in any young person with weight loss, health care providers often miss the diagnosis because the patient is secretive about his or her symptoms. He or she should undergo a complete physical examination; as indicated, certain laboratory tests should be done.

Laboratory findings

Laboratory tests help rule out endocrine, metabolic, and central nervous system abnormalities; cancer; malabsorption syndrome; and other disorders that cause physical wasting (such as AIDS).

Deviations from the norm

In a patient who has lost more than 30% of their normal weight, findings may include:
• below-normal hemoglobin level, platelet count, and white blood cell count
• prolonged bleeding time (from thrombocytopenia)
• decreased erythrocyte sedimentation rate
• below-normal levels of serum creatinine, blood urea nitrogen, uric acid, cholesterol, total protein, albumin, sodium, potassium, chloride, calcium, and fasting blood glucose (from malnutrition)
• elevated serum amylase levels (unless pancreatitis is present)
• below-normal levels of serum luteinizing hormone and follicle-stimulating hormone
• decreased triiodothyronine level (from a lower basal metabolic rate)
• dilute urine (from the kidney's impaired ability to concentrate urine).
    An ECG may reveal nonspecific changes in ST intervals and T waves, prolonged PR intervals, and ventricular arrhythmias.

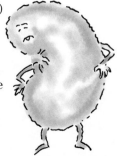

Anorexia nervosa may impair the kidney's ability to concentrate urine.

Exclusion of other medical or psychiatric disorders: Differential diagnosis

Anorexia nervosa must be differentiated from other medical conditions or psychiatric disorders.

Medical conditions include:
- gastrointestinal disease
- hyperthyroidism
- occult malignancies
- AIDS.

Psychiatric disorders include:
- substance abuse (especially with stimulants, such as cocaine and amphetamines)
- anxiety disorders (especially OCD and/or social phobia)
- mood disorders (such as major depression and bipolar disorder)
- personality disorders (especially histrionic, borderline, and narcissistic personality disorders)
- schizophrenia.

The diagnosis of anorexia nervosa is confirmed if the patient meets the criteria in the *DSM-5*. (See *Diagnostic criteria: Anorexia nervosa*.)

Diagnostic criteria: Anorexia nervosa

The diagnosis of anorexia nervosa is confirmed when the patient meets these criteria from the *DSM-5* (APA, 2013a).

- Restriction of energy intake relative to requirements, leading to a significantly low body weight in the context of age, sex, developmental trajectory, and physical health. Significantly low weight is defined as a weight that is less than minimally normal or, for children and adolescents, less than minimally expected.
- Intense fear of gaining weight or of becoming fat or persistent behavior that interferes with weight gain, even though at a significantly low weight.
- Disturbance in the way in which one's body weight or shape is experienced, undue influence of body weight or shape on self-evaluation, or persistent lack of recognition of the seriousness of the current low body weight.

Subtypes of anorexia nervosa
- Restricting type: During the last 3 months, the individual has not engaged in recurrent episodes of binge eating or purging behavior (i.e., self-induced vomiting or the misuse of laxatives, diuretics, or enemas). This subtype describes presentations in which weight loss is accomplished primarily through dieting, fasting, and/or excessive exercise.
- Binge-eating/purging type: During the last 3 months, the individual has engaged in recurrent episodes of binge-eating or purging behaviors (i.e., self-induced vomiting or the misuse of laxatives, diuretics, or enemas).

Treatment

Treatment for anorexia nervosa aims to promote weight gain, correct malnutrition, and resolve the underlying psychological dysfunction. The most effective strategy has been psychotherapy coupled with weight restoration to within 10% of normal. An interdisciplinary team of medical and mental health clinicians and dieticians who have experience in treating anorexia nervosa enhances patient outcomes.

As appropriate, treatment measures may include:
• a reasonable diet, with or without liquid supplements
• vitamin and mineral supplements
• activity curtailment as needed (such as for arrhythmias or other physical reasons)
• group, family, or individual psychotherapy
• behavior modification, with privileges based on weight gain.

Hospitalization

Some patients with anorexia nervosa can be treated successfully as outpatients. However, the patient who exhibits any of the following signs or symptoms requires hospitalization in a medical or psychiatric unit:
• rapid weight loss equal to 15% or more of normal body mass
• persistent bradycardia (heart rate of 50 beats/minute or less)
• systolic blood pressure of 90 mm Hg or lower
• hypothermia (a core body temperature of 97°F [36.1°C] or less)
• medical complications
• persistent sabotage or disruption of outpatient treatment
• denial of the disorder and the need for treatment
• risk for suicide
• nonsuicidal, self-injurious behaviors.

> Hospitalization is warranted if the patient's systolic blood pressure drops to 90 mm Hg or lower.

Two years??

Hospitalization may be as brief as 2 weeks or as long as 2 years or more. Many clinical centers now have inpatient and outpatient programs specifically for managing eating disorders. All too often, however, treatment proves difficult and the results are discouraging.

Psychotherapy

All forms of psychotherapy, from psychoanalysis to hypnotherapy, have been tried in the treatment of anorexia nervosa—with varying success. To be effective, psychotherapy must address the underlying problems of low self-esteem, guilt, anxiety, and depression. Common psychotherapies used for the treatment of anorexia nervosa include:

- cognitive-behavioral therapy (CBT)
- dynamic psychotherapy
- family therapy.

Pharmacotherapy

No definitive medications are identified to improve the symptoms of anorexia nervosa. However, some medications are being used to increase appetite and decrease mood symptoms and anxiety.

Nursing interventions

The following nursing interventions may facilitate recovery for patients with anorexia nervosa:

- During hospitalization, regularly monitor the patients' vital signs, nutritional status, and fluid intake and output.
- Help patients to establish a target weight, and support their efforts to achieve this goal.
- Negotiate an adequate food intake with patient. Make sure that patients understand the importance in compliance with their contract or lose privileges.
- Frequently offer small portions of food or drinks.
- Monitor the patients' for passive or active suicidal potential.

Person to person

- Maintain one-on-one supervision of the patient during meals and for 1 hour afterward to ensure that the patient is complying with the dietary treatment program. Remember that for a hospitalized patient with anorexia nervosa, food is considered a medication.
- Allow the patients to maintain control over the types and amounts of food they eat.
- Teach patients how to keep a food journal, including the types of foods they eat, eating frequency, and feelings associated with eating and exercise.

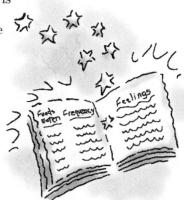

Liquidation strategy

- Be aware that during an acute anorexic episode, nutritionally complete liquids are more acceptable because they don't require the patient to select foods (something patients with anorexia nervosa commonly find difficult).

• If tube feedings or other special feeding measures become necessary, explain these measures to the patient and be ready to discuss patient's fears or reluctance. However, limit the discussion about the food itself.

Pound by pound

• Weigh the patient daily (before breakfast if possible) on the same scale, at the same time, and in the same clothing. Before weighing the patients, observe them to ensure that they did not add objects in their pockets or elsewhere or increase the intake of large amounts of fluids to falsely increase their weight.
• Keep in mind that patients' weight should increase from morning to night.
• Anticipate a weight gain of about 1 lb per week.

Defusing fat fears

• If edema or bloating occurs after the patient resumes normal eating behavior, reassure the patients that this is temporary. Otherwise, they may fear that they are getting fat and may stop complying with the treatment plan.
• Encourage the patient to recognize and assert their feelings freely. If the patients understand that they can be assertive, they gradually may learn that expressing their true feelings won't result in losing control or love.
• Explain to the patient how improved nutrition can reverse the effects of starvation and prevent complications.
• Advise family members to avoid discussing food with the patient.

Preservation tactics

• Remember that patients with anorexia nervosa uses exercise, preoccupation with food, ritualism, manipulation, and lying as mechanisms to preserve the only control they think they have in their life.
• If an outpatient requires hospitalization, maintain contact with the patients' treatment teams to promote a smooth return to the outpatient setting.
• Patients and their families may need therapy to uncover and correct dysfunctional patterns. Refer them to Anorexia Nervosa and Related Eating Disorders, Inc. (*www.anred.com*). This national organization may help them understand what anorexia nervosa is, convince them that they need help, and help them find a psychotherapist or medical doctor who's experienced in treating this disorder.

Memory jogger

Give your patient and family CUES to eating disorders by covering these topics during teaching:

C Causes of eating disorders

U Understanding how to overcome power struggles and issues of separation and autonomy

E Effects of the eating disorder on physical and mental health

S Symptoms of eating disorders and signs of relapse

Bulimia nervosa

Bulimia nervosa is marked by episodes of binge eating. Binge eating is defined as eating in a discrete period of time (usually within 2 hours) a large amount of food, a larger amount than most individuals would eat in a similar period of time and circumstances. During the binge-eating episode, the patient has no control over the eating, the amount of food being eaten, and/or cannot stop eating (APA, 2013b). The binge-eating episode is usually followed by feelings of guilt, humiliation, depression, and self-condemnation. Eating binges may occur up to several times a day.

Many sufferers also use inappropriate measures to prevent weight gain, such as self-induced vomiting, diuretic or laxative use, dieting, or fasting. (See *Erroneous beliefs about eating disorders.*)

Eating to excess

Although males are diagnosed with bulimia nervosa, it is young women of normal or nearly normal weight who typically develop the condition after a history of extended dieting. As dieting continues, the individual may experience a growing impulse to eat restricted foods. Eventually (usually after an anxiety-producing situation), he or she eats to excess, temporarily relieving this impulse. The individual then panics, fearing the food will turn to fat, and induces vomiting or uses diuretics or laxatives (or both) to prevent weight gain.

Myth busters

Erroneous beliefs about eating disorders

What you don't know about eating disorders could prevent you from assessing the condition accurately.

Myth: A patient who binges but doesn't purge doesn't have bulimia nervosa.

Reality: A patient with bulimia nervosa may engage in either the purging or the nonpurging form of this disorder.

Myth: Open conflict and verbal fighting are common among families of adolescents with eating disorders.

Reality: Conflict *avoidance,* not open conflict, is typical in these families.

Catalog of complications

Unless the patient devotes an excessive amount of time to binge-ing and purging, bulimia nervosa seldom is incapacitating.

However, during periods of bingeing, gastric rupture may occur. Repetitive vomiting may lead to such physical problems as dental caries, erosion of tooth enamel, parotitis, and gum infections. Rarely, frequent vomiting leads to esophageal inflammation and rupture. If the patient uses ipecac syrup to induce vomiting, the patient may suffer heart failure.

Deadly imbalances

Dehydration or electrolyte imbalances (including metabolic alkalosis, hypochloremia, and hypokalemia) also may occur, increasing the risk of such serious complications as arrhythmias and sudden death. Laxative abuse may cause chronic irregular bowel movements and constipation.

In addition, patients with bulimia nervosa are at higher risk for suicide and psychoactive substance abuse.

Prevalence and onset

Bulimia nervosa usually begins in adolescence or young adults and peaks in older adolescents and young adulthood. Onset before puberty and after age 40 is uncommon. As in anorexia nervosa, bulimia nervosa also effects both females and males but with a 10:1 female to male ratio (APA, 2013b; Sadock & Sadock, 2007). Approximately 3% of the population meets the diagnostic criteria for bulimia nervosa—but up to 5% to 15% may have some symptoms of the disorder. These numbers may be a gross underestimation because many sufferers are able to hide their symptoms.

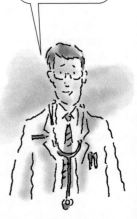

Researchers have linked an area of chromosome 10p to families with a history of bulimia nervosa.

Causes

The exact cause of bulimia nervosa is unknown. As with anorexia nervosa, experts suspect it results from interplay of genetic, biological, behavioral, environmental, family, and psychosocial factors.

Genetic and biological factors

There is an increased incident of bulimia nervosa in first-degree relatives of individuals with the disorder. Although this frequency seems to be related to genetics, family influences may also be important.

Also, researchers have linked a specific area of chromosome 10p to families with a history of bulimia nervosa. This provides strong evidence that genes play a determining role in susceptibility to the disorder.

Some studies suggest that altered serotonin and norepinephrine levels in the brain also play a role in development of the disorder. Feeling good after vomiting may be associated with the increase of endorphins (Sadock & Sadock, 2007).

Other factors

Other factors associated with the development of bulimia nervosa are related to social and psychological influences. Modern society's overemphasis on appearance and thinness is integral in the development of bulimia nervosa. Additional factors include:
- family disturbances or conflict
- sexual abuse
- maladaptive learned behavior
- struggle for self-control or self-identity.

Signs and symptoms

The history of a patient with bulimia nervosa typically includes episodic binge eating within a period of 2 hours, occurring up to several times a day. During bingeing episodes, the individual continues to eat until interrupted by abdominal pain, sleep, or another person's presence. Most patients with bulimia nervosa prefer foods that are sweet, soft, and high in calories and carbohydrates.

Physical findings

Physical findings that suggest bulimia nervosa include:
- thin, normal, or slightly overweight appearance, with frequent weight fluctuations
- weight within the normal range (through the use of diuretics, laxatives, vomiting, and exercise)
- persistent sore throat and heartburn (from vomited stomach acids)
- calluses or scarring on the back of the hands and knuckles (from forcing the hand down the throat to induce vomiting)
- salivary gland swelling, hoarseness, throat lacerations, and dental erosion (from repetitive vomiting)
- tooth staining or discoloration
- abdominal and epigastric pain (from acute gastric dilation)
- amenorrhea.

Memory jogger

Although not all bulimics engage in purging, the term RIDS BODY can help you remember the clinical features of bulimia.

R Recurrent binge-eating episodes

I Intense exercise

D Diuretic, laxative, and enema use

S Self-induced vomiting

B Body image distortion

O Ordinary eating alternating with episodes of bingeing and purging

D Depression and anxiety disorders may be present

Y Yo-yo effect of tension relief and pleasure experienced with bingeing; guilt and depression following purging

Psychosocial findings

Stay alert for these psychosocial features:
- perfectionism
- distorted body image
- exaggerated sense of guilt
- feelings of alienation
- recurrent anxiety
- signs and symptoms of depression
- an image as the "perfect" student, parent, or career professional (a child may be distinguished for participating in competitive activities, such as ballet or gymnastics)
- poor impulse control
- chronic depression
- low tolerance for frustration
- self-consciousness
- difficulty expressing such feelings as anger
- impaired social or occupational adjustment
- history of childhood trauma (especially sexual abuse)
- history of unsatisfactory sexual relationships
- parental obesity
- family dysfunction.

Behavioral findings

Behavioral signs of bulimia nervosa include:
- evidence of binge-eating episodes, such as the disappearance of large amounts of food over short periods or the presence of containers and wrappers (indicating consumption of large amounts of food) in a short period of time (usually within a 2 hour period of time)
- evidence of purging, including frequent trips to the bathroom after meals, sounds and smells of vomiting, and the presence of packages of diuretics and laxatives
- peculiar eating habits or rituals
- excessive, rigid exercise regimen despite poor weather, fatigue, illness, or injury
- a complex schedule (to make time for binge-and-purge sessions)
- withdrawal from friends and usual activities
- hyperactivity
- frequent weighing
- other behaviors suggesting that weight loss, dieting, and control of food are becoming primary concerns.

Diagnosis

The patient should undergo a medical evaluation to rule out an upper gastrointestinal disorder that can cause repeated vomiting. The patient should also undergo a psychological evaluation to identify bulimia nervosa and other comorbid psychiatric disorders. When patients are honest about the length and extent of their behavior, this can help ascertain the seriousness and the severity of their bulimia nervosa disorder.

Eccentric electrolytes

Laboratory tests can determine the presence and severity of complications. For example:
• serum electrolyte studies may reveal above-normal bicarbonate levels and decreased potassium and sodium levels
• blood glucose testing may detect hypoglycemia
• baseline ECG may show cardiac arrhythmias if the patient has severe electrolyte disturbances.

The diagnosis of bulimia nervosa is confirmed if the patient meets the *DSM-5* criteria for this disorder. (See *Diagnostic criteria: Bulimia nervosa*, page 368.)

> The sooner a person gets treatment for bulimia, the greater the chance of a full recovery.

Treatment

Early treatment of bulimia nervosa is crucial because over time, the patient's behavior pattern becomes more deeply ingrained and more resistant to change. Patients treated early in the disorder are more likely to recover fully than those who delay treatment for years. Treatment is most effective when it centers on the issues that cause the behavior, not the behavior itself. Usually, treatment involves individual, group, and family therapy; nutrition counseling; and in many cases, medications.

Spotlight on structure

At all levels of care, treatment requires a high degree of structure and a behavioral treatment plan based on the patient's weight and eating behaviors. Treatment may continue for several years; long-term psychotherapy and medical follow-up are essential.

Psychotherapy

Psychotherapy focuses on breaking the binge–purge cycle and helping patients regain control over their eating behavior. Treatment may take place in an inpatient or outpatient setting.

Diagnostic criteria: Bulimia nervosa

The diagnosis of bulimia nervosa is confirmed when the patient meets these criteria from the *DSM-5*.

• Recurrent episodes of binge eating. An episode of binge eating is characterized by both of the following:

–eating, in a discrete period of time (e.g., within any 2-hour period), an amount of food that is definitely larger than what most individuals would eat in a similar period of time under similar circumstances

–a sense of a lack of control over eating during the episode (e.g., a feeling that one cannot stop eating or control what or how much one is eating).

• Recurrent inappropriate compensatory behaviors in order to prevent weight gain, such as self-induced vomiting; misuse of laxatives, diuretics, enemas, or other medications; fasting; or excessive exercise.

• The binge eating and inappropriate compensatory behaviors both occur, on average, at least once a week for 3 months.

• Self-evaluation is unduly influenced by body shape and weight.

• The disturbance does not occur exclusively during episodes of anorexia nervosa.

It usually includes behavior modification therapy, possibly in highly structured psychoeducational group meetings.

Individual psychotherapy and family therapy address the eating disorder as a symptom of unresolved conflict. This approach may help the patients understand the basis of their behavior and teach them self-control strategies. To supplement psychotherapy, psychotropic medications may be recommended. Antidepressants are effective in treating bulimia nervosa. Selective serotonin reuptake inhibitors (SSRIs) such as fluoxetine (Prozac) increase the serotonin level to decrease binge eating and purging and at the same time treat the depression. Other antidepressants can be effective.

Anonymous help

Patients may benefit from participation in a self-help group such as Overeaters Anonymous or a drug rehabilitation program if they also suffer from a substance abuse problem.

Hospitalization

The patients' physical and mental health determines the degree of control that must be imposed on their eating and total environment. If binge eating and purging have caused serious physical harm, a medical or psychiatric hospitalization may be necessary, with control and around-the-clock observation of all eating and elimination (urinating, bowel movements, and vomiting). As symptoms abate and the eating behaviors and weight stabilize, patients gradually resume control over their eating.

Nursing interventions

The following nursing interventions are recommended for a patient with bulimia nervosa:
- Promote an accepting, nonjudgmental atmosphere. Control your reactions to the patient's behavior and feelings.
- Establish a contract with the patient that specifies the amount and types of food he or she must eat at each meal.
- Supervise the patient during mealtimes and for a specified period afterward (usually 1 to 2 hours).
- Set a time limit for each meal. Provide a pleasant, relaxed eating environment.
- Teach the patient to keep a food journal to monitor their treatment progress.

> When supervising a bulimic patient at mealtimes, set a time limit for the meal.

Prizes for pounds

- Using behavior modification techniques, reward the patient for satisfactory weight gain.
- Encourage patients to recognize and verbalize their feelings about their eating behavior.
- Identify the patient's elimination patterns.
- Encourage the patient to talk about stressful issues, such as achievement, independence, socialization, sexuality, family problems, and control.

Abuse aversion

- Explain to the patient the risks of laxative, emetic, and diuretic abuse.
- Provide patients with assertiveness training to help them gain control over their behavior and achieve a realistic and positive self-image.
- Assess the patient's passive and active suicide potential.

The long haul

- Offer support and encouragement to help the patient stay in treatment.
- Refer the patient and family to the American Anorexia/Bulimia Association or Anorexia Nervosa and Related Eating Disorders, Inc. (*www.anred.com*) for more information and support.

Binge-eating disorder

Binge-eating disorder (BED) involves a regular occurrence of rapidly eating large amounts of food, usually in secret, while feeling out of control of what and how much one is eating. These episodes are followed by guilt, shame, and emotional distress. In many cases, the individual does not engage in compensatory behaviors, such as exercising, thus resulting in being overweight or obese.

Complications

Individuals with BED often have the same health risks that others with clinical obesity have, including:
- high blood pressure
- high cholesterol levels
- heart disease
- non-insulin-dependent diabetes mellitus
- gallbladder disease
- musculoskeletal problems
- obstructive sleep apnea.

Prevalence and Onset

BED is the most common eating disorder in the United States. At some point in their lives, up to 3.5% of females and 2% of males will experience this disorder. BED affects women slightly more than men with the average onset occurring in young adulthood. Individuals with BED are more likely to also have anxiety disorders, mood disorders, and/or substance abuse disorders (Duckworth & Freedman, 2013).

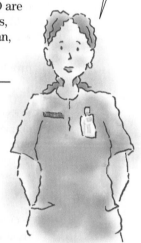

Up to 10% of the U.S. population will suffer from an eating disorder at some point in their life.

Causes

As with bulimia nervosa and anorexia nervosa, BED has been shown to run in families and is believed to have both genetic and environmental influences.

Signs and symptoms

The key feature of BED is bingeing without compensatory behaviors. Other findings include:

Physical findings
- insomnia
- normal or heavier than average weight
- normal or elevated body mass index (BMI).

Psychosocial findings
- constant thoughts of food
- eating in private
- feeling disgusted, guilty, and/or worthless after eating
- feeling powerless to stop eating
- depression, anxiety, and substance abuse are common comorbidities.

Behavioral findings

- feeling out of control when eating
- eating even when uncomfortable
- emotional eating—eating to escape stress or for comfort.

Diagnosis

The patient should undergo a medical evaluation to assess for complications associated with obesity and undergo a psychological evaluation to identify BED and other comorbid psychiatric disorders.

Treatment

Treatment for patients with BED is similar to the treatment for bulimia nervosa. For patients with BED, treatment is aimed at addressing the underlying emotional issues while addressing physical health alterations. Psychotherapy, including cognitive-based therapy and behavioral therapies, has been shown to be the most effective in helping patients identify triggers and thus strategies to interrupt or stop binges. Treatment also should involve nutritional counseling for normal weight management. Pharmacologic therapy, involving an antidepressant, such as citalopram (Celexa), fluoxetine (Prozac), and sertraline (Zoloft), may reduce binging episodes.

Diagnostic criteria: Binge-eating disorder

The diagnosis of bulimia nervosa is confirmed when the patient meets these criteria from the *DSM-5*.

- Recurrent episodes of binge eating. An episode of binge eating is characterized by both of the following:
  - eating, in a discrete period of time (e.g., within any 2-hour period), an amount of food that is definitely larger than what most people would eat in a similar period of time under similar circumstances
  - a sense of lack of control over eating during the episode (e.g., a feeling that one cannot stop eating or control what or how much one is eating).
- The binge-eating episodes are associated with three (or more) of the following:
  - eating much more rapidly than normal
  - eating until feeling uncomfortably full
  - eating large amounts of food when not feeling physically hungry
  - eating alone because of feeling embarrassed by how much one is eating
  - feeling disgusted with oneself, depressed, or very guilty afterward.
- Marked distress regarding binge eating is present.
- The binge eating occurs, on average, at least once a week for 3 months.
- The binge eating is not associated with the recurrent use of inappropriate compensatory behavior as in bulimia nervosa or anorexia nervosa.

Nursing Interventions

The following nursing interventions are recommended for a patient with BED:

Person to person
• Establish a therapeutic nurse–patient relationship.
• Promote an accepting, nonjudgmental atmosphere. Control your reactions to the patient's behavior and feelings.

Setting goals
• Help patients to formulate daily goals and develop a plan to reach the goals.
• Help patients to establish a target weight and support their efforts to achieve this goal.

Maintaining control
• Allow the patient to maintain control over the types and amounts of food they eat.
• Teach patients how to keep a food journal, including the types of foods they eat, eating frequency, and feelings associated with eating.
• Maintain a routine weighing session to help patients assess goal achievement.
• Help patients to learn other coping strategies (other than eating) for dealing with emotions.

Support
• Offer support and encouragement to help the patient stay in treatment.
• Refer patients and their families to Anorexia Nervosa and Related Eating Disorders, Inc. (*www.anred.com*) for information and support for those suffering with binge-eating disorder.

References

American Psychiatric Association. (2013a). *Diagnostic and statistical manual of mental disorders* (5th ed.). Arlington, VA: Author.
American Psychiatric Association. (2013b). *Eating disorders*. Retrieved from http://www.psychiatry.org/eating-disorders
Duckworth, K., & Freedman, J. L. (2013). *Binge eating disorder*. Retrieved from http://www.nami.org/Content/ContentGroups/Helpline1/Binge_Eating_Disorder.htm

Lindvall Dahlgren, C., & Rø, O. (2014). A systematic review of cognitive remediation therapy for anorexia nervosa—development, current state and implications for future research and clinical practice. *Journal of Eating Disorders, 2*(1), 26. doi:10.1186/s40337-014-0026-y

Mayo Clinic. (2012). *Risk factors.* Retrieved from http://www.mayoclinic.org/diseases-conditions/eating-disorders/basics/risk-factors/con-20033575

Mayo Clinic. (2014). *Eating disorders.* Retrieved from http://www.mayoclinic.org/diseases-conditions/eating-disorders/basics/definition/con-20033575

Sadock, B., & Sadock, V. (2007). *Synopsis of psychiatry: Behavioral sciences/clinical psychiatry* (10th ed.). Baltimore, MD: Lippincott Williams & Wilkins.

Wade, T. D., Keski-Rahkonen, A., & Hudson, J. (2011). Epidemiology of eating disorders. In M. Tsuang & M. Tohen (Eds.), *Textbook in psychiatric epidemiology* (3rd ed., pp. 343–360). New York, NY: Wiley.

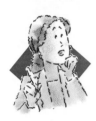

Quick quiz

1. The most serious complication of anorexia nervosa is:
A. high risk of mortality.
B. coexisting depression.
C. poor family relationships.
D. social isolation.

Answer: A. Anorexia nervosa has a mortality rate of 5% to 15%.

2. In caring for a patient with BED, the nurse should perform which of the following actions?
A. Monitor BMI.
B. Prescribe an antidepressant.
C. Provide mental health counseling.
D. Confirm the binge-eating diagnosis.

Answer: A. The patient's BMI indicates the efficacy of treatment. Options B, C, and D are outside the scope of a Bachelor of Science in Nursing–prepared nurse.

3. Purging behavior is usually triggered by:
A. sensations of fullness or bloating.
B. guilt, humiliation, and self-condemnation.
C. fear of being discovered as a binge eater.
D. feelings of nausea.

Answer: B. Guilt, humiliation, and self-condemnation usually trigger the desire to purge. Physical sensations, such as fullness, bloating, or nausea aren't related to this behavior nor is the fear of being discovered.

4. Which medication should the nurse include in the teaching plan for a patient who has bulimia nervosa or BED?

    A.   Clozapine (Clozaril)

    B.   Risperidone (Risperdal)

    C.   Ziprasidone (Geodon)

    D.   Sertraline (Zoloft)

Answer: D. SSRIs such as Paxil, Zoloft, and Prozac are commonly used to treat bulimia nervosa and BED. Clozaril, Risperdal, and Geodon are medications used in treating schizophrenia and are not associated with the treatment of eating disorders.

Scoring

☆☆☆ If you answered all four items correctly, savor the moment! You've satiated yourself on this chapter and fully deserve the success you're now tasting.

☆☆ If you answered two or three items correctly, swell! You've just gained several pounds of knowledge.

☆ If you answered just one item correctly, don't go off on a binge. Just review the chapter again to bulk up on the information.

Substance use disorders

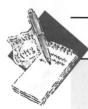

Just the facts

In this chapter, you'll learn:

♦ types of substance use disorders

♦ street names for commonly abused substances

♦ proposed causes of substance use disorders

♦ how to assess for substance use disorders

♦ nursing interventions for patients experiencing substance withdrawal.

A look at substance use disorders

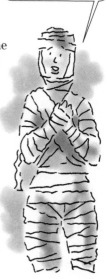

Substance misuse and abuse have been around for centuries. I wonder if King Tut ever got a little tipsy.

NOTE: The *Diagnostic and Statistical Manual of Mental Disorders*, 5th Edition (*DSM-5*), has eliminated the terms *abuse* and *dependence*.

Substance use disorder affects males and females of all ages, cultures, and socioeconomic groups. People have used alcohol and other psychoactive substances—those that affect the central nervous system (CNS)—for centuries to induce changes in perception, mood, cognition, or behavior. These substances produce a state of consciousness that the user deems pleasant, positive, or euphoric.

Substance use disorders commonly coexist with—and complicate the treatment of—other psychiatric disorders. Likewise, many people with emotional disorders or mental illness turn to drugs and alcohol to self-medicate and help them tolerate their feelings.

Suspicious substances

A substance of abuse may be any chemical substance or preparation used therapeutically or recreationally. They are generally

The language of substance abuse

Here are some important definitions you need to know to fully understand this chapter.

• *Addiction:* a primary, chronic disease of brain reward, motivation, memory, and related circuitry. Dysfunction in these circuits leads to characteristic biological, psychological, social, and spiritual manifestations. This is reflected in an individual pathologically pursuing reward and/or relief by substance use and other behaviors.

• *Craving:* an intense desire or urge for the drug that may occur at any time but is more likely when in an environment where the drug previously was obtained or used.

• *Tolerance:* decreased response to a drug that comes with repeated use. A user who develops a tolerance to the rewarding properties of the abused drug must take increasingly higher amounts to get the desired effect.

• *Physical dependence:* an adaptive state that occurs as a normal physiologic response to repeated drug exposure. Physical dependence doesn't necessarily indicate drug abuse or addiction.

• *Withdrawal:* an uncomfortable syndrome that occurs when tissue and blood levels of the abused substance decrease in a person who has used that substance heavily over a prolonged period. Withdrawal symptoms may cause the person to resume taking the substance to relieve the symptoms, thereby contributing to repeated drug use.

• *Intoxication:* a reversible substance-specific syndrome caused by ingestion of or exposure to that substance.

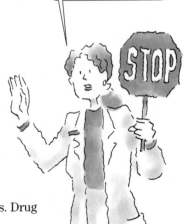

Abusing a single drug is bad enough. Mixing several drugs together is especially dangerous.

substances controlled by the Drug Enforcement Agency (DEA). Commonly abused substances include:

• alcohol
• amphetamines and amphetamine-like drugs
• barbiturates
• cannabis (marijuana)
• cocaine and crack cocaine
• hallucinogens—such as phencyclidine (PCP) and lysergic acid diethylamide (LSD)
• inhalants
• nonbarbiturate sedatives, hypnotics, and anxiolytics (primarily benzodiazepines)
• opioids—heroin, morphine, and oxycodone
• tobacco

Many people abuse a combination of substances. Drug mixing is a very dangerous practice.

Consequences of substance abuse

Substance use disorder commonly leads to physical dependence, psychological dependence, and usually, both. It's often associated with illegal activities and may cause unhealthy lifestyles and behaviors, such as poor diet, sleep problems, and safety issues. Chronic substance use impairs social and occupational functioning, creating personal, professional, and financial problems.

Teenage wasteland

When drug use begins in early adolescence, it may lead to emotional and behavioral problems resulting in the failure to complete school.

Intravenous (I.V.) drug abuse may lead to life-threatening complications. (See *Complications of I.V. drug use.*)

Complications of I.V. drug use

I.V. drug use can lead to numerous complications—even beyond those caused by the drugs themselves.

Using contaminated needles, for example, raises the risk of such infections as HIV, viral hepatitis (especially hepatitis B and C), and bacterial infections. Heroin can cause a nephropathy similar to focal segmental glomerulosclerosis. A condition called *talc granulomatosis* may occur if the drug was adulterated with an inert substance (such as talcum powder).

With chronic I.V. drug abuse, potential complications include:
- skin lesions and abscesses
- thrombophlebitis
- vasculitis
- gangrene
- cardiac and respiratory arrest
- intracranial hemorrhage
- subacute bacterial endocarditis
- septicemia
- pulmonary emboli
- respiratory infections
- malnutrition
- gastrointestinal (GI) disturbances
- musculoskeletal dysfunction
- depression
- psychosis
- increased suicide risk.

Terrible trips

Few people would voluntarily take a drug they expect to cause an unpleasant experience. However, psychoactive substances often produce negative outcomes—among them, problematic behavior, "bad trips," and even long-term psychosis.

Not so street-smart

Illicit street drugs pose added dangers. Materials used to dilute street drugs can cause toxic or allergic reactions. Specific effects of street drugs vary with the substance.

> In the DSM-5, the term *substance-related disorders* encompasses both substance use disorders and substance-induced disorders.

Defining the terms

According to the *DSM-5*, substance-related disorders are divided into two groups: substance use disorders and substance-induced disorders. The essential feature of a substance use disorder is a cluster of cognitive, behavioral, and physiologic symptoms indicating that the individual continues using the substance despite significant substance-related problems.

Defining the problem

Substance abuse is a major public health problem. In 2012, an estimated 23.9 million people in the United States age 12 or older (roughly 9.2% of the total population) were using alcohol or illicit drugs (National Institutes of Health [NIH], n.d.-a). Of this amount:
- 2.8 million were dependent on or abused *both* alcohol and illicit drugs
- 14.9 million were dependent on or abused alcohol but not illicit drugs
- 4.5 million were dependent on or abused illicit drugs but not alcohol.

Alcohol is the most commonly abused substance overall. Among illicit drugs, marijuana ranks first; it's used by approximately 58% of illicit drug users (NIH, n.d.-a).

Teens who toke

Experimentation with drugs commonly begins during adolescence—although recent statistics show a trend toward drug use among preadolescents.

Causes of substance abuse

The exact causes of substance abuse and addiction aren't known but are under intensive investigation. Probable influences include genetic makeup, pharmacologic properties of the particular drug, peer pressure, emotional distress, and environmental factors (Schneider & Levenson, 2008).

Genetic theories

Genetic theories propose that inherited mechanisms cause or predispose a person to drug abuse. Genetic factors have been explored most extensively in alcoholism. For example, studies show that many Asians carry a gene that confers a reduced risk for alcoholism.

Other genetic factors may confer an increased risk for alcoholism. Chromosomes 1 and 7 have been linked to susceptibility to alcohol dependence.

Heredity or environment?

Most likely, both heredity and environment influence whether a person becomes a substance user. Researchers continue to debate which of the two factors is more important, although results of their studies have been confusing (Garmo, 2013).

For example, on the one hand, some alcoholics have no known alcoholic relatives, and many children of alcoholics don't become alcoholic themselves. On the other hand, children of alcoholics who are adopted into nonalcoholic homes at an early age are more likely to become alcoholics than children of nonalcoholics who are adopted into alcoholic homes.

> Some drug addicts may be endorphin-deficient. This makes them more sensitive to pain—and more likely to abuse narcotics.

Neurobiological theories

According to neurobiological theories, chronic exposure to drugs leads to biological and cellular adaptation. Some scientists suspect drug addicts have an inborn deficiency of endorphins—peptide hormones that bind to opiate receptors, reducing the pain sensations and exerting a calming effect. This endorphin deficiency may heighten the sensitivity to pain and confer a greater susceptibility to narcotics abuse.

Endorphins and enzymes

Alternatively, some scientists suspect regular narcotics use reduces the body's natural endorphin production, causing a reliance on the narcotic for ordinary pain relief.

According to another neurobiological theory, enzymes produced by a given gene might influence hormones and neurotransmitters, contributing to the development of a personality that's more sensitive to peer pressure—including the pressure to use illicit drugs (Garmo, 2013).

Psychobiological theories

Introducing a narcotic into the body may cause metabolic adjustments that require continued and increasing dosages to prevent withdrawal. Studies are evaluating cell metabolism changes that are linked to addiction (Garmo, 2013).

Behavioral theories

Behavioral scientists view drug abuse as the result of conditioning or cumulative reinforcement from drug use. Drug use causes a euphoric experience that the user perceives as rewarding, which motivates him to keep taking the drug. The drug, then, serves as a biological reward.

Right on cue

The stimuli and settings associated with drug use may become reinforcing in themselves—or may trigger drug craving that can lead to a relapse. Many recovering addicts change their environment in an effort to eliminate cues that could promote drug use.

Social and psychological theories

According to some social and psychological theories, adolescents and young adults take drugs to preserve childhood and avoid having to deal with adult conflicts and responsibilities. Many users see drugs as a way to cope—however dysfunctionally—with their personal and social needs and changing situational demands. (See *Profile of a drug abuser.*)

Following the crowd

In some cultures, drugs may be more available, or social pressures for drug use may be stronger. Social ritual may also play a role by affecting the meaning and style of drug use adopted by a person in a given setting.

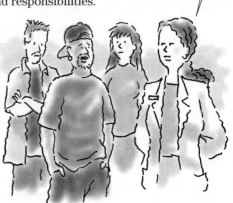

Some people take drugs because of peer pressure or as part of a social ritual.

Profile of a drug abuser

A person who's predisposed to psychoactive drug abuse tends to have low self-esteem, an excessive dependence on others, and a susceptibility to peer pressure. He or she may have inadequate coping skills, few mental or emotional resources against stress, and a low tolerance for frustration.

Tense, lonely, or bored

The typical drug abuser is anxious, angry, or depressed. He or she demands immediate relief of tension or distress, which he or she gets from taking the drug. The drug gives him or her pleasure by relieving tension, abolishing loneliness, inducing a temporarily peaceful or euphoric state, or simply relieving boredom.

Alcohol addiction

Alcohol (ethanol) is a CNS depressant that reduces the activity of neurons in the brain. In the United States, chronic uncontrolled alcohol intake is the largest substance use problem.

Alcohol addiction is characterized by four main symptom clusters—impaired control, social impairment, risky use, and pharmacologic dynamics.

• Impaired control: The individual lacks control of his or her use. This lack of control manifests as:
  • Taking larger amounts or over a longer period of time than intended
  • Repeated but unsuccessful attempts to cut down or stop use
  • Spending a great deal of time obtaining, using, and/or recovering from the substance
  • Having an intense desire or urge for the substance (craving)
• Social impairment: The individual progressively becomes less and less functional by:
  • Failing to fulfill major role obligations at work, school, or home
  • Continuing substance use despite having persistent or recurrent problems caused by the effects of the substance
  • Giving up or reducing important social, occupational, or recreational activities
• Risky use: The individual continues to use:
  • In situations in which it is physically hazardous
  • Despite knowledge of having a persistent or recurrent physical or psychological problem that is likely to have been caused by the substance use
• Pharmacologic dynamics
  • This refers to the presence of tolerance and/or a withdrawal syndrome.

Prevalence

Alcohol use disorder is a common disorder and occurs at all life stages—sometimes starting as early as elementary school age. In the United States, the 12-month prevalence of alcohol use disorder is about 4.6% among 12- to 17-year-olds and 8.5% among adults are 18 years and older (NIH, n.d.-a).

Alcohol use peaks between ages 18 and 29, and males are two to five times more likely than females to abuse alcohol (NIH, n.d.-a).

> Heavy alcohol intake is rough on my buddies, the kidney and the brain and . . . Ooohh . . . it's especially rough on yours truly, the liver!

Health hazards of alcohol abuse

Alcohol abuse decreases the life span by roughly 15 years. It accounts for nearly 25% of premature deaths in men and 15% in women (NIH, n.d.-a). (See *Can alcohol kill?*)

Way beyond blotto

Heavy alcohol intake adversely affects most body tissues, especially the liver, kidney, and brain. Eventually, alcohol abuse can lead to death. (See *Complications of alcohol abuse.*)

Causes

A definite cause of alcoholism hasn't been identified. Most experts believe genetic, biological, psychological, and sociocultural influences are involved (Garmo, 2013).

Myth busters

Can alcohol kill?

Don't assume that alcohol is relatively safe just because it's legal.
Myth: Alcohol intoxication doesn't directly cause death, although it can severely impair a person's functioning level.
Reality: Alcohol intoxication can be fatal if the blood alcohol level exceeds 400 mg/dl.

Complications of alcohol abuse

Alcohol damages body tissues through its direct irritating effects, through changes that occur during its metabolism, by interacting with other drugs, by aggravating existing disease, or through accidents brought on by intoxication. Tissue damage can lead to a host of complications.

Cardiopulmonary complications
• Arrhythmias
• Cardiomyopathy
• Essential hypertension
• Chronic obstructive pulmonary disease
• Pneumonia
• Increased risk of tuberculosis

GI complications
• Chronic diarrhea
• Esophagitis
• Esophageal cancer
• Esophageal varices
• Gastric ulcers
• Gastritis
• GI bleeding
• Malabsorption
• Pancreatitis

Hepatic complications
• Alcoholic hepatitis
• Cirrhosis
• Fatty liver

Neurologic complications
• Alcoholic dementia
• Alcoholic hallucinosis
• Alcohol withdrawal delirium

• Korsakoff syndrome
• Peripheral neuropathy
• Seizure disorders
• Subdural hematoma
• Wernicke encephalopathy

Psychiatric complications
• Amotivational syndrome
• Depression
• Fetal alcohol syndrome
• Impaired social and occupational functioning
• Multiple substance abuse
• Suicide

Other complications
• Beriberi
• Hypoglycemia
• Leg and foot ulcers
• Prostatitis

Genetic factors

These research findings (among others) support a genetic influence in alcoholism:
• Identical twins have a higher risk of alcoholism than fraternal twins do.
• Children of alcoholics have a fourfold increased risk of alcoholism—even if adopted at birth.
• Irish Americans may be up to seven times more likely than Italian Americans to become alcohol-dependent.

Alcoholic markers?

Some researchers believe a genetic marker for vulnerability to alcoholism exists. A follow-up of men originally studied at age 20 found that those with alcoholic fathers had lower response levels to alcohol (including less alcohol-related cognitive and psychomotor impairment and less intense subjective feelings of intoxication). This lower response level was a strong predictor of later alcoholism.

Other genetic influences that may contribute to the risk of alcoholism include such personality traits as higher levels of impulsivity and sensation seeking (Garmo, 2013).

Other factors

Biochemical abnormalities, nutritional deficiencies, endocrine imbalances, and allergic responses may contribute to alcoholism.

Psychological factors include the urge to drink alcohol to reduce anxiety or symptoms of mental illness; the desire to avoid responsibility in family, social, and work relationships; and low self-esteem.

Stress and social attitudes

Sociocultural factors include easy access to alcohol, group or peer pressure to drink, an excessively stressful lifestyle, and social attitudes that approve of frequent alcohol consumption.

Signs and symptoms

Many alcoholics hide or deny their addiction and temporarily manage to maintain a functional life—which can make assessment a challenge. Nonetheless, certain physical and psychosocial symptoms suggest alcoholism.

For example, the patient may have many minor complaints that are alcohol-related—malaise, dyspepsia, mood swings or depression, and an increased incidence of infection. Also check for poor personal hygiene and untreated injuries, such as cigarette burns, fractures, and bruises that he can't fully explain. Note an unusually high tolerance for sedatives and narcotics. Assess for signs of nutritional deficiency, including vitamin and mineral deficiencies (Garmo, 2013).

Watch for secretive behavior, which may be an attempt to hide the disorder or the alcohol supply.

> An alcoholic with no other alcohol source may drink mouthwash, vanilla extract, or sometimes, hand sanitizers.

Desperation tactics

When deprived of the usual supply of alcohol, a patient with alcoholism may consume it in any form available—mouthwash, aftershave lotion, hair spray, and even lighter fluid. Suspect alcoholism in a patient who buys inordinate amounts of aftershave lotion or mouthwash and doesn't use it in the expected way.

Denial, blame, and projection

Characteristically, the patient with alcoholism denies a problem—or rationalizes the problem. The patient also tends to blame others and to rationalize problem areas in life. The patient may project his anger or feelings of guilt or inadequacy onto others to avoid confronting the illness.

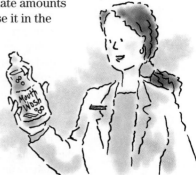

Overt signs and symptoms

Overt indications of excessive alcohol use include:
• episodes of anesthesia or amnesia during intoxication (blackouts)
• violent behavior when intoxicated
• the need for daily or episodic alcohol use to function adequately
• inability to stop or reduce alcohol intake.

Withdrawal symptoms

A heavy drinker who stops drinking or abruptly reduces alcohol intake is likely to go through withdrawal. Symptoms begin shortly after the drinking stops and could possibly last for up to 10 days.

Initially, the patient experiences anorexia, nausea, anxiety, fever, insomnia, diaphoresis, agitation, tremor progressing to severe tremulousness, and, possibly, hallucinations and violent behavior. Major motor seizures (sometimes called *rum fits*) may occur (Garmo, 2013; NIH, n.d.-a).

Deadly delirium

About 5% to 10% of alcoholics experience alcohol withdrawal delirium, also called *delirium tremens* (DTs). A life-threatening complication, this syndrome manifests as delirium accompanied by tremor, severe agitation, and autonomic overactivity—dramatic increases in pulse, respirations, and blood pressure. (See *Assessing for alcohol withdrawal*, page 386.)

Diagnosis

Various laboratory tests may suggest alcoholism and help evaluate for complications such as cirrhosis of the liver.
• A blood alcohol level of 0.10% weight/volume (200 mg/dl) indicates alcohol intoxication. Although this test can't confirm alcoholism, it can reveal how recently the patient has been drinking—and thus when to expect withdrawal symptoms if he or she is a heavy drinker.
• Urine toxicology may uncover the use of others drugs.
• Serum electrolyte analysis may identify electrolyte abnormalities associated with alcohol use.
• Increased plasma ammonia level indicates severe liver disease, as in cirrhosis.
• Liver function studies may point to alcohol-related liver damage.
• Hematologic workup may identify anemia; thrombocytopenia; and increased prothrombin (PT), partial thromboplastin (PTT), and international normalized ratio (INR) times.

Assessing for alcohol withdrawal

Alcohol withdrawal symptoms may vary from mild (morning hangover) to severe (alcohol withdrawal delirium). Formerly known as *delirium tremens* or *DTs*, alcohol withdrawal delirium is marked by acute distress brought on by drinking cessation in a person who's physically dependent on alcohol.

Signs and symptoms	Mild withdrawal	Moderate withdrawal	Severe withdrawal
Motor impairment	Inner tremulousness with hand tremor	Visible tremors; obvious motor restlessness and painful anxiety	Gross, uncontrollable shaking; extreme restlessness and agitation with intense fearfulness
Sleep disturbance	Restless sleep or insomnia	Marked insomnia and nightmares	Total wakefulness
Appetite	Impaired appetite	Marked anorexia	Rejection of all food and fluid except alcohol
GI symptoms	Nausea	Nausea and vomiting	Dry heaves and vomiting
Confusion	None	Variable	Marked confusion and disorientation
Hallucinations	None	Vague, transient visual and auditory hallucinations and illusions (commonly nocturnal)	Visual and, occasionally, auditory hallucinations, usually with fearful or threatening content; misidentification of people and frightening delusions related to hallucinatory experiences
Pulse rate	Tachycardia	Pulse 100 to 120 beats/minute	Pulse 120 to 140 beats/minute
Blood pressure	Normal or slightly elevated systolic	Usually elevated systolic	Elevated systolic and diastolic
Sweating	Slight	Obvious	Marked hyperhidrosis
Seizures	None	Possible	Common

- Echocardiography and electrocardiography may reveal cardiac problems related to alcoholism such as an enlarged heart (cardiomegaly).

Think patterns, not pints

However, the diagnosis of alcohol use disorder centers on a pattern of difficulties associated with alcohol use—*not* on the amount, duration, and frequency of alcohol consumption. The diagnosis of alcohol use disorder or alcohol abuse is confirmed when the patient meets the criteria listed in the *DSM-5*. (See *Diagnostic criteria: Substance use disorder*, page 388.)

Alcoholism can cause an enlarged heart.

Treatment

Acute alcohol intoxication calls for symptomatic treatment, which may involve respiratory support; fluid replacement; I.V. glucose to prevent hypoglycemia; correction of hypothermia or acidosis; and emergency measures for trauma, infection, or GI bleeding, as needed (Garmo, 2013).

Managing acute withdrawal

Because abrupt alcohol withdrawal can cause death, withdrawal should take place in a monitored therapeutic setting. The patient may require I.V. glucose administration and administration of fluids containing thiamin and other B-complex vitamins to correct nutritional deficiencies and aid glucose metabolism.

Other treatment measures may include:
- furosemide to ease overhydration
- magnesium sulfate to reduce CNS irritability
- chlordiazepoxide, diazepam, phenobarbital, anticonvulsants, antiemetics, or antidiarrheals, as needed to ease withdrawal symptoms
- antipsychotics to control hyperactivity and psychosis

Treatment of chronic alcoholism

Alcohol use disorder has no known cure, and total abstinence is the only effective treatment. Management commonly involves:
- medications that deter alcohol use (as in aversion or antagonist therapy) and treat withdrawal symptoms
- measures to relieve associated physical problems
- psychotherapy, usually involving behavior modification, group therapy, and family therapy
- counseling and ongoing support groups to help the patient overcome alcoholism.

Diagnostic criteria: Substance use disorder

The diagnosis of substance dependence is confirmed when the patient meets these criteria from the *DSM-5*.

Problematic pattern

The patient exhibits a problematic pattern of substance use resulting in clinically significant impairment or distress, as indicated by two or more of the following criteria during the same 12-month period:

• taking the substance in larger amounts or over a longer period than intended

• persistent desire or unsuccessful efforts to cut down or control substance use

• significant time spent trying to obtain the substance (e.g., driving long distances or visiting multiple doctors), to use the substance, or to recover from its effects

• craving, such as a strong desire or urge to use the substance

• recurrent substance use which results in a failure to fulfill major role obligations at work, school, or home

• continued substance use even with persistent or recurrent social or interpersonal problems caused or worsened by the effects of the substance

• giving up or cutting back on important social, occupational, or recreational activities because of substance use

• continued use in situations where it is physically hazardous

• continued use of the substance despite knowledge of having a persistent or recurrent physical or psychological problem that's likely to have been caused or worsened by the substance

• tolerance, as defined by either:
  – a need for markedly increased amounts of the substance to reach intoxication or the desired effect
  – markedly decreased effect with continued use of the same amount of the substance

• withdrawal, as manifested by either:
  – a characteristic withdrawal syndrome
  – use of the substance (or a closely related one) to relieve or avoid withdrawal symptoms.

Other features

• Physiologic dependence is *present* if the patient exhibits evidence of tolerance or withdrawal (as defined above).

• Physiologic dependence is *absent* if the patient doesn't exhibit evidence of tolerance or withdrawal.

> You think I look sick? This is nothing compared to what happens when someone takes alcohol and disulfiram together.

Aversion therapy

In aversion therapy, the patient receives a daily oral dose of disulfiram (Antabuse) to prevent compulsive drinking. Disulfiram impedes alcohol metabolism and increases blood acetaldehyde levels. Consuming alcohol within 1 week of taking disulfiram causes an immediate and very unpleasant reaction.

The agonies of Antabuse

Signs and symptoms of a disulfiram reaction include:

• flushing

• throbbing of the neck and head

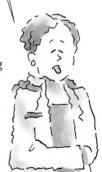

- nausea and vomiting
- headache
- shortness of breath or other respiratory difficulties
- sweating
- thirst
- chest pain
- palpitations
- tachycardia
- hyperventilation
- hypotension
- syncope
- weakness
- vertigo
- blurred vision
- confusion.

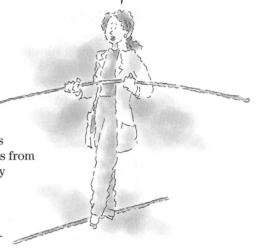

Good thing I never went through aversion therapy. A disulfiram reaction can cause vertigo!

Even small quantities of alcohol, such as the amount in food sauces and cough medicines, or inhaled traces from shaving lotion or furniture varnish may induce these symptoms.

Antagonist therapy

Naltrexone (ReVia), a narcotic antagonist, may reduce alcohol craving and help prevent an alcoholic from relapsing to heavy drinking when it's combined with counseling. Naltrexone blocks the brain's so-called pleasure centers, reducing the urge to drink.

If the patient is also addicted to narcotics or admits using them, the patient must stop taking all narcotics 7 to 10 days before starting naltrexone therapy.

Now there's a long-acting injectable form of naltrexone (Vivitrol). The patient receives a monthly injection which has the same therapeutic effect but usually with the side effects. No need to remember to take a daily tablet—but the patient must remember to get the injection from the health care provider monthly.

Counseling and psychotherapy

For long-term abstinence, supportive programs that offer detoxification, rehabilitation, and aftercare—including continued involvement in Alcoholics Anonymous (AA)—provide the best results. Along with individual, group, or family psychotherapy, these programs improve the patient's ability to cope with stress, anxiety, and frustration and help the individual gain insight into the problems that may have led to abuse alcohol (Alcoholics Anonymous, 2014).

Other types of support

For alcoholics who have lost contact with family and friends and have a long history of unemployment, trouble with the law, or other problems related to alcohol abuse, rehabilitation may involve job training, sheltered workshops, halfway houses, or other supervised facilities.

Nursing interventions

For general nursing interventions during and after an episode of acute alcohol intoxication, see *General interventions for acute drug intoxication*. These interventions may also be appropriate for an alcoholic patient:
• If the patient is taking disulfiram, warn that even a small amount of alcohol (such as the amount in cough medicines, mouthwashes, and liquid vitamins) will induce an adverse reaction. Tell the patient that increasing the length of time the drug is used, the greater the alcohol sensitivity will be. Also inform the patient that paraldehyde, a sedative, is chemically similar to alcohol and may provoke a disulfiram reaction.
• As appropriate, offer to arrange a visit from a concerned religious advisor who can help provide the motivation for a commitment to sobriety.

The A's have it

• Tell the patient about AA, a self-help group with more than a million members worldwide that offers emotional support from others with similar problems. Stress how this organization can provide the support he or she will need to abstain from alcohol. Offer to arrange a visit from an AA member (Alcoholics Anonymous, 2014).
• Inform a female patient that she may prefer a women's AA group, rather than a mixed group where she might hesitate to explore her feelings fully (Alcoholics Anonymous, 2014).
• Teach the patient's family about Al-Anon and Alateen, two other self-help groups. By joining these groups, family members learn to relinquish responsibility for the alcoholic's drinking so that they can live meaningful and productive lives. Point out that family involvement in rehabilitation also reduces family tensions.
• Refer adult children of alcoholics to the National Association for Children of Alcoholics. This organization may provide support in understanding and coping with the past.

Advice from the experts

General interventions for acute drug intoxication

Care for a substance-abusing patient starts with an assessment to determine which substance he's abusing. Signs and symptoms vary with the substance and dosage.

During the acute phase of drug intoxication and detoxification, care focuses on maintaining the patient's vital functions, ensuring his safety, and easing discomfort.

During rehabilitation, caregivers help the patient acknowledge his substance problem and find alternative ways to cope with stress. Health care professionals can play an important role in helping patients achieve recovery and stay drug-free.

These general nursing interventions are appropriate for patients during and after acute intoxication with most types of psychoactive drugs.

During an acute episode

- Continuously monitor the patient's vital signs and urine output. Watch for complications of overdose and withdrawal, such as cardiopulmonary arrest, seizures, and aspiration.
- Maintain a quiet, safe environment. Remove harmful objects from the room. Institute appropriate measures to prevent suicide attempts and assaults, according to facility policy.
- Approach the patient in a nonthreatening way. Limit sustained eye contact, which he may perceive as threatening.
- Institute seizure precautions.
- Administer I.V. fluids to increase circulatory volume.
- Give medications, as ordered; monitor and record their effectiveness.

During drug withdrawal

- Administer medications, as ordered, to decrease withdrawal symptoms. Monitor and record their effectiveness.
- Maintain a quiet, safe environment because excessive noise may agitate the patient.

When the acute episode has resolved

- Carefully monitor and promote adequate nutrition.
- Administer medications carefully to prevent hoarding. Check the patient's mouth to ensure that he has swallowed oral medication. Closely monitor visitors who might supply him with drugs.
- Refer the patient for rehabilitation as appropriate. Give him a list of available resources.
- Encourage family members to seek help regardless of whether the addicted person seeks it. Suggest private therapy or community mental health clinics.
- Develop self-awareness and an understanding and positive attitude toward the patient. Control your reactions to his undesirable behaviors—commonly, psychological dependency, manipulation, anger, frustration, and alienation.
- Set limits when dealing with demanding, manipulative behavior (Garmo, 2013; NIH, n.d.-a; Schneider & Levenson, 2008).

Amphetamine abuse

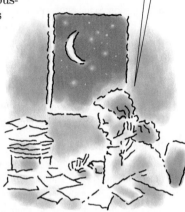

Some people take amphetamines when they have to stay up all night to cram for a test. Not very smart!

Amphetamines increase arousal; reduce fatigue; and can make a person feel stronger, more alert, and more decisive. Although they have a few medical uses (mainly in treating obesity and narcolepsy), most abusers take them for their stimulant or euphoric effects or to counteract the "down" feeling of alcohol or tranquilizers (Garmo, 2013).

The amphetamine group includes amphetamine sulfate, methamphetamine, and dextroamphetamine. On the street, amphetamine sulfate tablets are called *bennies*, *grannies*, or *cartwheels*. Methamphetamine is known as *speed*, *meth*, *crank*, or *crystal*. Made in illegal laboratories, it has a high potential for addiction. Dextroamphetamine sulfate may be referred to as *dexies*, *hearts*, or *oranges*.

Pleasure rush

Amphetamines may be taken orally or by injection, snorting, or smoking. Immediately after methamphetamine is injected or smoked, the user experiences an intensely pleasurable sensation (a "rush") that lasts a few minutes. Snorting produces a longer lasting high rather than a rush, which may last up to half a day (Garmo, 2013; NIH, n.d.-a.).

Users can become addicted quickly, with rapid dose escalation. Higher doses may lead to increasing toxicity and complications.

Prevalence

According to a federal survey, in 2004, an estimated 12 million persons (4.9% of persons aged 12 or older) had used methamphetamine at least once in their lifetime. Use of this drug is highest among native Hawaiian/Pacific Islander males between ages 18 and 25 (Garmo, 2013; NIH, n.d.-b.).

How amphetamines produce their effects

Amphetamines increase the release of the neurotransmitters dopamine, norepinephrine, and serotonin into brain synapses. The "rush" or "high" experienced with these drugs probably results from high levels of dopamine in the brain areas that regulate feelings of pleasure.

Detrimental to dopamine

Amphetamines may also have a neurotoxic effect, damaging brain cells that contain dopamine and serotonin. Studies suggest that over time, methamphetamine reduces dopamine levels, possibly leading to parkinsonian-like symptoms.

Health hazards of amphetamine abuse

Adverse physiologic effects of methamphetamine abuse include headache, poor concentration, poor appetite, abdominal pain, vomiting or diarrhea, sleep difficulties, paranoid or aggressive behavior, and psychosis.

Besides leading to addiction, chronic methamphetamine abuse can inflame the heart lining. Injection may damage blood vessels and cause skin abscesses. Some methamphetamine abusers have episodes of violent behavior, paranoia, anxiety, confusion, and insomnia. With heavy use, progressive social and occupational deterioration may occur.

Running on meth

Users who become drug tolerant must take higher or more frequent doses or change their method of drug intake. In some cases, they forgo food and sleep while indulging in a form of bingeing known as a *run*, injecting as much as 1 g of methamphetamine every 2 to 3 hours over several days until the drug supply runs out or the user becomes too disorganized to continue.

Hallucinations

Chronic methamphetamine abuse may damage the brain's frontal areas and basal ganglia. Some chronic abusers experience a toxic psychosis that resembles paranoid schizophrenia—intense paranoia, rages, auditory hallucinations, mood disturbances, and delusions. For example, some abusers experience formication—the sensation of insects creeping on the skin. Psychotic symptoms may last months or years after drug use ceases.

Causes

As with all types of substance abuse, the exact causes of amphetamine abuse are hard to identify. Some people abuse amphetamines in an effort to relieve fatigue, induce euphoria, or ease depression or other uncomfortable feelings (NIH, n.d.-a).

Signs and symptoms

In a patient under the influence of amphetamines, assessment findings may include:
- euphoria
- hyperactivity and increased alertness
- diaphoresis (sweating)
- shallow respirations

> ### Memory jogger
>
> SPEED helps when assessing a patient for amphetamine use.
>
> **S** Sweating (diaphoresis)
>
> **P** Psychotic behavior
>
> **E** Exhaustion
>
> **E** Everything up (hyperactive tendon reflexes, hypertension, hyperthermia, tachycardia)
>
> **D** Dilated pupils

- dilated pupils
- dry mouth
- exhaustion
- anorexia and weight loss
- nausea or vomiting
- tachycardia
- hypertension
- hyperthermia
- tremors
- seizures
- altered mental status, such as confusion, agitation, or paranoia
- psychotic behavior (with prolonged use).

Findings in amphetamine intoxication

Severe methamphetamine intoxication may cause the signs and symptoms listed earlier plus:
- arrhythmias
- heart failure
- subarachnoid hemorrhage
- stroke
- cerebral hemorrhage
- coma
- death.

Amphetamine withdrawal symptoms

Abrupt amphetamine withdrawal may trigger CNS depression, ranging from lethargy to coma. Some patients experience hallucinations, whereas others show signs of overstimulation, including euphoria and violent behavior. (For additional withdrawal symptoms, see *Assessing for amphetamine withdrawal.*)

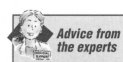

Advice from the experts

Assessing for amphetamine withdrawal

During amphetamine withdrawal, the patient may exhibit or report:
- abdominal tenderness
- muscle aches
- apathy and depression
- disorientation
- irritability
- long periods of sleep
- suicide attempts (with sudden withdrawal).

Diagnosis

Urine drug screening may be performed if amphetamine abuse is suspected. Other diagnostic tests depend on the patient's symptoms. For example, an electrocardiogram (ECG) may be done if he reports chest pain.

The diagnosis of amphetamine abuse or dependence is confirmed if the patient meets the criteria documented in the *DSM-5*. (See *Diagnostic criteria: Substance use disorder*, page 388.)

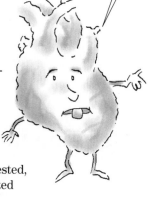

An amphetamine user who reports chest pain may undergo an ECG.

Treatment

A patient with acute amphetamine intoxication may require airway management, fluid replacement, and vigorous cooling measures. Arrhythmias may warrant cardioversion, defibrillation, and antiarrhythmic drugs. Vital signs must be monitored closely. If the drug was ingested, vomiting is induced or gastric lavage is performed; activated charcoal and a saline or magnesium sulfate cathartic may be given.

Other treatments are symptomatic. For example, the patient may require fluid replacement and nutritional and vitamin supplements. Ammonium chloride or ascorbic acid may be added to the I.V. solution to acidify urine to a pH of 5. Mannitol may be given to induce diuresis.

Sedatives may be given to induce sleep, anticholinergics and antidiarrheal agents to relieve GI distress, and antianxiety drugs for severe agitation and symptomatic treatment of complications.

Managing drug addiction

Cognitive-behavioral therapy is commonly used to treat methamphetamine addiction. The goal of this approach is to modify the patient's thinking, expectations, and behaviors and increase his ability to cope with stress.

Post-meth depression

Antidepressants may help combat the depression commonly seen in methamphetamine users who have recently become abstinent.

Rehabilitation

After withdrawal, the patient needs rehabilitation to prevent a relapse of drug abuse. Both inpatient and outpatient rehabilitation programs are available. They usually last a month or longer and may include individual, group, and family psychotherapy.

During and after rehabilitation, participation in a drug-oriented self-help group may be recommended as an adjunct to behavioral interventions and to promote long-term drug-free recovery.

Life after speed

Aftercare means a lifetime of abstinence, usually aided by participation in Narcotics Anonymous (NA) or a similar self-help group.

Nursing interventions

For appropriate nursing interventions during and after an episode of acute amphetamine intoxication, see *General interventions for acute drug intoxication*, page 391.

Caffeine intoxication

A mild CNS stimulant, caffeine may be used to restore mental alertness when a person feels tired, weak, or drowsy. However, when used in excess, caffeine causes uncomfortable symptoms of stimulation. Caffeine intoxication can occur with consumption of more than 250 mg of caffeine (equivalent to about 2½ cups of coffee) (Mayo Clinic, 2014).

Age and body size influence caffeine effects. A child or a small adult may feel the effects more strongly than a large adult. Also, some people are more sensitive to caffeine, feeling the effects at smaller doses.

> Ahhhh, coffee—the quicker picker-upper!

Caffeine habit

Caffeine can be habit forming—most experts agree that some heavy caffeine users may develop caffeine tolerance. Someone who abruptly stops using caffeine may experience symptoms such as headache, fatigue, or drowsiness.

Cupboards full of caffeine

Dietary sources of caffeine include coffee, tea, chocolate, and cola drinks. Caffeine also comes in some prescription and over-the-counter (OTC) drugs. (See *Where's the caffeine?*)

How caffeine produces its effects

Scientists aren't exactly sure how caffeine exerts its effects. A leading theory suggests that caffeine antagonizes adenosine, an inhibitory brain chemical that affects norepinephrine, dopamine, and serotonin activity. This antagonism may increase neurotransmitter levels, causing psychostimulation.

> ## Where's the caffeine?
>
> Common sources of caffeine include:
> - coffee (brewed)—40 to 180 mg per cup
> - coffee (instant)—30 to 120 mg per cup
> - coffee, decaffeinated—3 to 5 mg per cup
> - tea, brewed (American)—20 to 90 mg per cup
> - tea, brewed (imported)—25 to 110 mg per cup
> - tea, instant—28 mg per cup
> - tea, canned iced—22 to 36 mg per 12 ounces
> - cola and other soft drinks—36 to 90 mg per 12 ounces
> - cola and other soft drinks (decaffeinated)—none
> - cocoa—4 mg per cup
> - chocolate milk—3 to 6 mg per ounce
> - chocolate, bittersweet—25 mg per ounce
>
>   OTC preparations that contain caffeine include Caffedrine Caplets, Enerjets, NoDoz Maximum Strength Caplets, and Vivarin. Some pain relievers, such as Excedrin and Midol, also contain caffeine (Mayo Clinic, 2014).

Causes

People consume caffeine for such reasons as preference of beverage, to "get going" in the morning, to relieve fatigue, or to stay awake for a particular purpose.

Risk factors for caffeine overuse or sensitivity to caffeine withdrawal aren't known. Genetic factors, such as differences in the way some people metabolize caffeine or a history of substance abuse or mood disorders, may play a role.

Signs and symptoms

Assessment findings in a patient with caffeine intoxication may include:
- tachycardia
- palpitations
- arrhythmias
- fatigue that worsens during the day
- anxiety, nervousness, irritability, and easy excitability
- exaggerated startle response
- disorganized thoughts and speech
- facial flushing
- dehydration (from caffeine's diuretic effect)

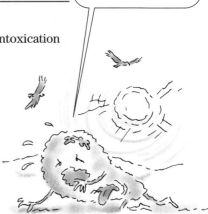

Caffeine has a diuretic effect, which may lead to . . . (gasp) . . . dehydration.

- hyperactivity
- gross muscle tremors
- restless leg syndrome (muscle cramping and twitching)
- sleep disturbances, such as insomnia or decreased sleep quality (with grogginess in the morning caused by withdrawal symptoms occurring overnight).

Caffeine withdrawal symptoms

Caffeine withdrawal symptoms may occur with abrupt caffeine cessation or reduction after a long period of daily use. Withdrawal symptoms tend to be worse in heavy caffeine users (those who consume 500 mg/day or more), although people who consume as little as 100 mg/day (equivalent to one cup of coffee) may also experience discomfort.

Headache from hell

Withdrawal symptoms may start within a few hours after the time of normal caffeine consumption, reach a peak within 1 or 2 days, and persist for up to 2 weeks. They may include:
- headache
- nausea or vomiting
- jitteriness, irritability, and anxiety
- fatigue
- drowsiness
- depression
- poor concentration or poor performance on mental tasks
- caffeine craving.

Diagnosis

Caffeine blood levels have limited use as a screening tool. Urine drug screening can help uncover associated illicit drug use. Thyroid studies can rule out hyperthyroidism.

No other specific tests detect caffeine-induced psychiatric disorders. Cardiac irregularities should be investigated by ECG.

The diagnosis of caffeine intoxication is confirmed if the patient meets the criteria established in the *DSM-5*.

Treatment

Treatment for caffeine intoxication is the avoidance of caffeine in all forms. Symptoms resolve when the caffeine use stops.

The patient should be monitored for caffeine withdrawal. Treatment for withdrawal is symptom based.

Nursing interventions

These nursing interventions may be appropriate for a patient with caffeine intoxication:
• Advise the patient about the expected symptoms of caffeine withdrawal and the duration of those symptoms.
• Reassure him that the symptoms will subside and are benign.
• If discomfort lasts more than 2 weeks, assess the patient for other disorders that cause similar symptoms.

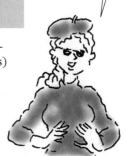

Some people consume cannabis as tea. I'm more of an orange pekoe person myself.

Cannabis abuse

Cannabis is a hemp plant from which marijuana (a tobacco-like substance) and hashish (the plant's resinous secretions) are produced. In the United States and most other Western countries, cannabis is the most widely used illicit drug (Garmo, 2013).

Cannabis may be smoked, consumed as a tea, or mixed into foods. Most users smoke marijuana in hand-rolled cigarettes, although some use pipes or bongs (water pipes) (Garmo, 2013).

Nicknames galore

Common street names for cannabis include *pot, grass, weed, mary jane, mj, roach, reefer, joints, THC, blunt, herb, sinsemilla, smoke, boo, broccoli, ace,* and *Colombian* (Garmo, 2013). The duration of action is 6 to 12 hours, with symptoms most pronounced during the first 1 to 2 hours.

Marijuana as medicine

Medicinal use of cannabis—mainly as an antiemetic in patients undergoing cancer chemotherapy and other types of drug therapy—has been the subject of intense legal and medical debate. Many states have legalized medical marijuana use.

Prevalence

More than 96 million people in the United States age 12 and older (40% of those in this age group) have tried marijuana at least once, according to the 2004 National Household Survey on Drug Abuse. Marijuana is used equally among all races (NIH, n.d.-a).

In surveys of marijuana users, males outnumber females. Although abuse is relatively common in most age groups, adolescents and young adults are the most common abusers.

How cannabis produces its effects

The most powerful psychoactive substance in cannabis is delta-1-tetrahydrocannabinol (delta-1-THC). When marijuana is smoked, delta-1-THC rapidly passes from the lungs into the bloodstream, which carries it to the brain and other organs.

In the brain, delta-1-THC connects to cannabinoid receptors on neurons, influencing their activity. (See *How cannabis affects the brain.*)

Health hazards of cannabis use

Cannabis can be addictive and may cause various adverse physiologic effects.

Respiratory effects

Marijuana smoke can harm the lungs. The smoke contains carcinogens similar to those found in tobacco smoke. Chronic and heavy cannabis use may increase the risk of chronic obstructive lung disease. Also, some studies show that respiratory tumors are more common among habitual marijuana users (Garmo, 2013).

How cannabis affects the brain

When marijuana is smoked, its active ingredient attaches to cannabinoid receptors in the brain. The brain areas with many cannabinoid receptors—including the cerebral cortex, hippocampus, basal ganglia, and cerebellum—influence pleasure, memory, learning, reward, perception, and coordinated movements (Garmo, 2013).

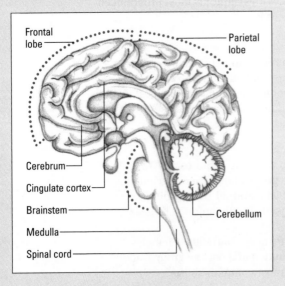

Frontal lobe
Parietal lobe
Cerebrum
Cingulate cortex
Brainstem
Cerebellum
Medulla
Spinal cord

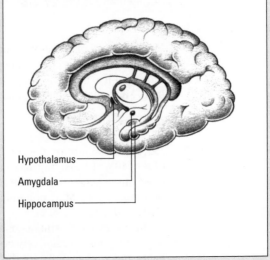

Hypothalamus
Amygdala
Hippocampus

Cardiovascular effects

Acute cannabis intoxication may trigger tachycardia and orthostatic hypotension.

Reproductive effects

In females, cannabis use may increase the number of anovulatory cycles. In males, it may reduce levels of follicle-stimulating hormone, leading to a decrease in testosterone production and, possibly, testicular atrophy.

Although cannabis use has been linked to decreased sperm counts, the drug's effect on fertility remain unclear.

Other health effects

Cannabis may weaken the immune system. In very young teens, it has a profoundly negative effect on development.

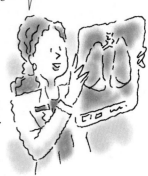

Chronic and heavy cannabis use may raise the risk of chronic obstructive lung disease and respiratory tumors.

Combination drug use

Marijuana may be combined with other substances, such as crack cocaine, PCP, formaldehyde, and codeine cough syrup—sometimes without the user being aware of it. These additional substances compound the risks associated with marijuana use.

Impairments associated with cannabis use

Cannabis use can result in perceptual distortions and impairments in short-term memory, learning ability, judgment, and verbal skills.

Memory and learning impairments

Marijuana's adverse impact on learning and memory can last for days or weeks after the acute drug effects wear off. Therefore, someone who smokes marijuana once a day may be functioning at a reduced intellectual level all of the time.

A study of college students found that among heavy cannabis users, critical skills related to attention, learning, and memory were impaired significantly even after 24 hours of abstinence. These users had more trouble sustaining and shifting their attention and in registering, organizing, and using information (NIH, n.d.-a).

Stoned in school

One study found that 12th graders who smoked marijuana seven or more times weekly had significantly lower scores on standardized tests of verbal and mathematical skills. Also, students who smoke marijuana may be more likely to get lower grades and less likely to graduate from high school.

Wasted at work

Problems at work are more common among marijuana-smoking employees. Several studies have linked marijuana use with increased absences, tardiness, accidents, workers' compensation claims, and job turnover.

Coexisting psychiatric disorders

Marijuana use is associated with anxiety, depression, and personality disturbances. Research shows that marijuana can cause problems in daily life or worsen existing problems.

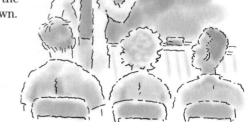

Students who regularly smoke marijuana score lower on standardized verbal and math tests.

Causes

As with other types of substance abuse, the exact causes of cannabis use aren't known. Suggested risk factors include:
• young age
• drug availability (influenced by geographic and cultural factors)
• coexisting alcohol abuse or dependence
• coexisting abuse of other drugs.

Signs and symptoms

Assessment findings in a patient under the influence of cannabis include:
• relaxation
• euphoria
• spontaneous laughter
• feelings of well-being or grandiosity
• visual distortions and other perceptual changes
• subjective sense that time is passing more slowly than normal
• tachycardia
• dry mouth
• conjunctival redness
• drowsiness and sluggishness (or paradoxical hyperalertness)
• decreased muscle strength
• poor coordination
• increased hunger (the "munchies").
    With overdose, you may detect signs or symptoms of pulmonary edema, respiratory depression, aspiration pneumonia, or hypotension.

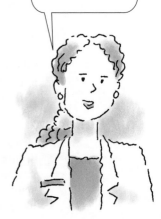

The "munchies" are but one of many telltale signs of cannabis use.

Memory jogger

WEED is a street name for cannabis—and a quick key to assessing a patient for suspected cannabis use.

W Wacky behavior (hallucinations, impaired cognition, paranoia, spontaneous laughter)

E Euphoria

E Elevated heart rate (tachycardia)

D Distorted sense of time and self-perception, decreased muscle tone, dry mouth

Dysphoric effects

In some people, cannabis intoxication causes a dysphoric reaction, which may manifest as:
- panic and disorientation
- paranoia
- mood swings
- altered perceptions (such as illusions or frank hallucinations)
- depersonalization
- psychotic episodes.

Findings in chronic cannabis use

Chronic cannabis users may experience a syndrome marked by appetite changes, lack of ambition and energy, and reduced social and occupational drive (NIH, n.d.-a).

Withdrawal symptoms

Although withdrawal symptoms from cannabis are less severe than from other drugs, some users experience restlessness, irritability, appetite loss, and sleep difficulties (NIH, n.d.-a).

Diagnosis

In a chronic marijuana user, urine screening may reveal cannabis presence for as long as 30 days after use.

The diagnosis of cannabis abuse or dependence is confirmed when the patient meets the criteria in the *DSM-5*. (See *Diagnostic criteria: Substance use disorder*, page 388.)

Treatment

Acute cannabis intoxication usually resolves within 4 to 6 hours. The patient should be moved to a quiet room with minimal stimulation.

Treatment is symptom based. For example, the doctor may prescribe benzodiazepines if the patient has marked anxiety.

Treatment of withdrawal symptoms

To ease cannabis withdrawal symptoms, the patient may receive a short course of sedatives or tranquilizers to manage insomnia, anxiety, and depression. Useful nonpharmacologic measures may include psychotherapy, exercise, relaxation techniques, and nutritional support.

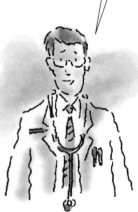

> To stay off marijuana, the user must avoid all drug-related situations.

Treatment of chronic cannabis use

Treatment of cannabis abuse follows the general principles of substance abuse. The goal is total abstinence from all psychoactive substances.

Interventions may include psychiatric evaluation and counseling, individual or group psychotherapy, occupational and family assessment, self-help groups, and lifestyle changes, such as avoiding drug-related situations (NIH, n.d.-a).

Nursing interventions

For general nursing interventions for cannabis intoxication, see *General interventions for acute drug intoxication*, page 391.

Cocaine abuse

A powerfully addictive narcotic and stimulant, cocaine is one of the oldest known drugs. Coca leaves, the source of cocaine, have been ingested for thousands of years. Cocaine hydrochloride, the pure drug, has been abused for more than 100 years. Cocaine use can range from occasional to repeated or compulsive abuse (Garmo, 2013; NIH, n.d.-a).

Cocaine's effects occur almost immediately after a single dose and disappear within a few minutes or hours. Taken in small amounts (up to 100 mg), the drug typically makes the user feel euphoric, energetic, talkative, and mentally alert—especially to sensations of sight, sound, and touch (Garmo, 2013; NIH, n.d.-a).

Cocaine may temporarily reduce the need for food and sleep. Some users find it helps them perform simple physical and intellectual tasks more quickly, although others experience the opposite effect (Garmo, 2013; NIH, n.d.-a).

Crystal or crack

Cocaine exists in two chemical forms:
- Cocaine hydrochloride is a fine, white, crystallized powder. It's generally snorted or dissolved in water and injected, with effects lasting 15 minutes to 2 hours.
- Crack or freebase is a chunky, off-white compound that hasn't been neutralized by an acid. It's smoked after being processed with ammonia or sodium bicarbonate and water and then heated to remove the hydrochloride. Crack produces an immediate euphoric high, followed by a "down" feeling.

> Crack produces an immediate high, followed by a "down" feeling.

By any other name . . .

On the street, cocaine is known as *coke, C, snow, snowball, blow, flake, nose candy, hits, tornado, wicky stick, rock,* or *crank.*

Most street dealers dilute cocaine with inert substances, such as cornstarch, talcum powder, or sugar; some cut it with procaine or amphetamines. Some users combine cocaine powder or crack with heroin known as a "speedball."

Snorting, shooting, and rubbing

When snorted, cocaine is absorbed into the bloodstream through the nasal tissues. When injected, the drug is released directly into the bloodstream, intensifying its effects. When cocaine is smoked, the vapor is inhaled into the lungs, where it's absorbed into the bloodstream as rapidly as by injection. Cocaine also can be rubbed onto mucous membrane tissues.

Medical uses of cocaine

Doctors sometimes have used cocaine for legitimate medical purposes in the past—typically as a local anesthetic for nasal surgeries, to stop nosebleeds, or as a local anesthetic for cuts in children.

Prevalence

Cocaine is the second most commonly used illicit drug in the United States. About 3.6 million U.S. residents are chronic cocaine users. Adults ages 18 to 25 have a higher rate of cocaine use than any other age group. Men have a higher rate than women do (Garmo, 2013; NIH, n.d.-a).

About 10% of U.S. residents over age 12 have tried cocaine at least once; approximately 2% have tried crack.

Health hazards of cocaine use

Cocaine use can have devastating medical consequences. Absorption of toxic amounts may cause:
- sudden death
- acute cardiovascular problems, such as arrhythmias (particularly ventricular fibrillation), tachycardia, myocardial infarction, and chest pain
- stroke
- seizures
- respiratory failure
- bowel gangrene (with cocaine ingestion).

Death-dealing duo

Combining cocaine with alcohol causes the conversion of the two drugs to cocaethylene, which has a longer duration in the brain and is more toxic than either drug alone. In fact, the mixture of cocaine and alcohol is the most common two-drug combination resulting in drug-related death (Garmo, 2013; NIH, n.d.-a).

Binge effects

A cocaine binge (taking the drug repeatedly and at increasingly high doses) may cause increasing irritability, restlessness, and paranoia. The result may be full-blown paranoid psychosis, in which the person loses touch with reality and experiences auditory hallucinations.

> A cocaine binge can bring on paranoid psychosis—complete with auditory hallucinations.

Route-related consequences

Regular cocaine snorting can lead to the loss of the sense of smell, nosebleeds, swallowing difficulty, hoarseness, and nasal septum irritation.

Fatal first use

In rare instances, sudden death can occur on the first use of cocaine or unexpectedly thereafter. Cocaine-related deaths commonly result from cardiac arrest or seizures followed by respiratory arrest.

Impairments associated with cocaine use

Cocaine is powerfully addictive. About 10% of people who try cocaine progress to heavy use. After a person tries it, he or she may have trouble predicting or controlling the extent to which he or she will keep using it.

As cocaine use continues, tolerance commonly develops. The person must take higher doses at more frequent intervals to obtain the same level of pleasure he or she experienced with initial use.

Causes

A family history of substance abuse may be a risk factor for early cocaine use and rapid cocaine dependence. (See *Gathering a history from a drug user*, page 408.)

Some researchers attribute cocaine's addictive properties to the dopamine excess it produces; this excess may be the source of positive reinforcement and addiction. Thus, the drug's dopamine-driven "rush" reinforces repeated use.

Genetic link?

Researchers have identified a brain process that may help explain addiction to cocaine and other drugs of abuse. Studies have found that repeated cocaine exposure causes a genetic change leading to altered levels of a specific brain protein that regulates dopamine's action.

> Euphoria and laughing are common effects of cocaine use . . . or in my case, watching reruns of Seinfeld!

Signs and symptoms

In a patient under the influence of cocaine, general assessment findings may include:
- euphoria
- increased energy
- excitement
- sociability
- reduced hunger
- grandiosity
- sense of increased physical and mental strength
- decreased sensation of pain
- talkativeness or pressured speech
- good humor and laughing
- dilated pupils
- runny nose
- nasal congestion
- nausea and vomiting
- headache
- vertigo.

Something bugging you?

Some users experience more pronounced effects (especially with high doses). These effects include flightiness, emotional instability, restlessness, irritability, apprehension, inability to sit still, teeth grinding, cold sweats, tremors, muscle twitching, seizures, violent or bizarre

Memory jogger

CRACK clues you in to some of the symptoms of cocaine use.

C Cardiotoxicity (tachycardia, ventricular fibrillation, or cardiac arrest)

R Respiratory arrest

A Auditory, visual, and olfactory hallucinations

C Coma and confusion

K Kite-like behavior (excitability, grandiosity, irritability, and psychotic symptoms)

Advice from the experts

Gathering a history from a drug user

If your patient admits to drug use, try to determine the extent to which his or her drug abuse interferes with his or her life. Note whether the patient expresses a desire to overcome his or her addiction.

If possible, obtain a complete drug history. Ask which substances the patient uses, the amount used, frequency of use, and time of his or her last dose.

What to expect
However, you should expect incomplete or inaccurate responses. Drug-induced amnesia, a decreased level of consciousness, or ignorance may distort the patient's recollection of the facts. He may also deliberately fabricate answers to avoid arrest or downplay a suicide attempt. If necessary, interview family members and friends to fill in gaps in the history.

behavior, and hallucinations (cocaine "bugs" or "snow lights" as well as voices, sounds, and smells). A few experience cocaine psychosis, which resembles paranoid schizophrenia.

Cardiovascular and respiratory findings

Cocaine may raise or lower the blood pressure. It may cause chest pain, tachycardia, ventricular fibrillation, or cardiac arrest. Respiratory findings may include tachypnea; deep, rapid, or labored respirations; or respiratory arrest (NIH, n.d.-a).

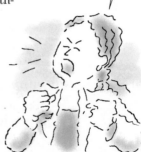

It's not cocaine I'm craving. It's ICE CREAM!

Withdrawal symptoms

Cocaine withdrawal usually isn't as uncomfortable as withdrawal from other drugs. Symptoms may include:
- anxiety, agitation, and irritability
- depression
- fatigue
- angry outbursts
- lack of motivation
- nausea and vomiting
- muscle pain
- sleep disturbances—usually hypersomnia
- intense drug craving
- episodes of ST-segment elevation on ECG.

Diagnosis

The diagnosis of cocaine abuse or dependence is confirmed when the patient meets the criteria documented in the *DSM-5*. (See *Diagnostic criteria: Substance use disorders*, page 388.)

Treatment

A patient with acute cocaine intoxication should receive symptomatic treatment. Cardiopulmonary resuscitation is performed, as indicated, for ventricular fibrillation and cardiac arrest. Vital signs should be monitored closely. Propranolol typically is given for tachycardia. Anticonvulsant medications are given for seizures.

If the patient has ingested cocaine, induced vomiting or gastric lavage may be performed. If he has snorted cocaine, residual drug is removed from the mucous membranes.

Depending on the cocaine dosage and time elapsed before admission, additional treatment may include forced diuresis and, possibly, hemoperfusion or hemodialysis.

Fluids, food, and sleep therapy

Other measures may include fluid replacement therapy and nutritional and vitamin supplements. Sedatives may be given to induce sleep, anticholinergics and antidiarrheal agents to relieve GI distress, and antianxiety drugs for severe agitation.

Withdrawal, detoxification, and rehabilitation

Treatment of cocaine dependence commonly involves detoxification, short- and long-term rehabilitation, and aftercare. The latter means a lifetime of abstinence, usually aided by participation in NA or a similar self-help group.

To ease withdrawal, useful nonpharmacologic measures may include psychotherapy, exercise, relaxation techniques, and nutritional support. Widespread cocaine abuse has led to extensive efforts to develop treatment programs for abusers. Cocaine abuse and addiction must address a variety of problems, including psychobiological, social, and pharmacologic aspects of the patient's drug abuse.

Pharmacologic approaches

Currently, there are several medications used in treating cocaine addiction, for instance, the use of high-dose vitamin preparations containing the amino acid precursors of dopamine, norepinephrine, and serotonin to address the neurotransmitter depletion. Also, the dopamine agonists bromocriptine and amantadine have shown some success.

Antidepressants may be prescribed to treat the mood changes that some patients experience during the early stages of cocaine abstinence. Sedatives and tranquilizers may be given temporarily to help the patient cope with insomnia and anxiety.

> Some cocaine treatment programs give vouchers to patients who have drug-free urine tests.

Behavioral interventions

Many behavioral treatments (both outpatient and residential) have been effective in treating cocaine addiction. The treatment regimen should be tailored to the patient's individual needs, with different components added or removed as indicated.

For many cocaine abusers, a treatment called *contingency management* has had positive results. This voucher-based system gives positive rewards for staying in treatment and remaining cocaine-free. Patients earn vouchers based on drug-free urine tests and can exchange them for items that promote healthy living such as joining a gym.

Cognitive-behavioral therapy

Cognitive-behavioral coping skills therapy is a short-term, focused approach that helps cocaine addicts become abstinent. This approach strives to help patients recognize the situations in which they're most likely to use cocaine, avoid these situations, and cope more effectively with the problems and behaviors associated with drug abuse (Garmo, 2013).

Therapeutic communities

Patients with more severe problems, such as coexisting mental health problems and criminal involvement, may benefit from a therapeutic community—a residential program with 3- to 6-month lengths of stay. These communities focus on resocializing the patient to society; some include on-site job rehabilitation and other supportive services.

Nursing interventions

For nursing interventions that may be appropriate during an acute episode or after the episode has resolved, see *General interventions for acute drug intoxication*, page 391.

Hallucinogen abuse

Hallucinogens (sometimes called *psychedelic drugs*) produce hallucinations or profound distortions in the perception of reality. They may also cause dramatic behavioral changes. Under the influence of hallucinogens, people see images, hear sounds, and feel sensations that seem real but don't actually exist. Some hallucinogens also cause rapid, intense emotional swings (NIH, n.d.-a).

These agents include a wide range of substances, including LSD, ecstasy, ketamine, dextromethorphan, mescaline, and psilocybin. Most are taken orally, but some may be injected (NIH, n.d.-a).

Most hallucinogens have no known medical use; however, naturally occurring hallucinogens have been used in religious rites for centuries. For example, native peoples of Mexico used mushrooms containing psilocybin, and some southwest Native American tribes used peyote.

Timothy Leary's preference

The most potent mood- and perception-altering drug known, LSD is a synthetic substance first developed by a pharmaceutical company in 1938. Its street names include *acid, green* or *red dragon, microdot, sugar,* and *big D.*

LSD is produced in crystalline form. The pure crystal can be crushed to a powder and mixed with binding agents to produce tablets known as *microdots* or thin gelatin squares called *windowpanes.* More commonly, it's dissolved, diluted, and applied to paper (called *blotter acid*).

LSD has dramatic effects on the senses, causing a highly intensified perception of colors, smells, sounds, and other sensations. In some cases, sensory perceptions may blend, causing the person to "see" sounds or "hear" or "feel" colors. Hallucinations also distort or transform shapes and movements and may give rise to the perception that time is moving very slowly or that the user's body is changing shape.

A person who has taken LSD may "see" sounds or "hear" colors.

Some call it ecstasy

Ecstasy, or 3,4-methylenedioxymethamphetamine (MDMA) is a synthetic drug with both stimulant and hallucinogenic properties. Available as capsules or tablets, it's taken orally or, rarely, injected or snorted. On the street, it's called *XTC, clarify, essence,* or *Adam.* The ecstasy experience is sometimes called *rolling.* Ecstasy tablets commonly contain MDMA in addition to other harmful drugs (NIH, n.d.-a).

Previously used mainly at dance clubs and raves, ecstasy is now seen in other social settings. Its effects include distortions in time and perception and an amphetamine-like hyperactivity. Like other stimulants, it seems to have addictive potential. Depending on the dosage, acute drug effects typically last 3 to 6 hours.

Raving over ketamine

Ketamine distorts perceptions of sight and sound and produces dissociative effects—feelings of detachment from the self and the environment. It's increasingly used as a club drug and distributed at raves and parties.

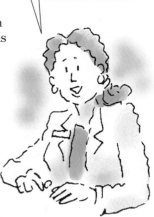

Ketamine induces amnesia and has been used as a date rape drug.

For therapeutic purposes, ketamine is used mainly in veterinary medicine. Most of the ketamine used illicitly is evaporated to form a powder that's snorted, smoked, or compressed into tablets. The liquid form of the drug can be injected I.V. or intramuscularly (I.M.). Street names for ketamine include *K*, *Special K*, *Ket*, *Vitamin K*, *Kit Kat Keller*, *Green*, *Blind Squid*, and *cat Valium* (NIH, n.d.-a).

Odorless and tasteless, ketamine can be added to beverages without being detected; also, it induces amnesia. Because of these properties, the drug sometimes is given to unsuspecting victims to aid in the commission of sexual assault ("drug rape" or date rape).

Dextromethorphan daze

Dextromethorphan, sometimes called *DXM* or *robo*, is a cough-suppressing ingredient found in some OTC cold and cough medications. The most common source of abused dextromethorphan is extra-strength cough syrup.

At low doses, the drug has a mild stimulant effect and causes distorted visual perceptions. At much higher doses, it causes dissociative effects similar to those of ketamine. Effects typically last 6 hours.

Mescaline for mind alteration

Found in several cactus species (most notably, *peyote* and *San Pedro*), mescaline causes hallucinations. Mescaline "buttons" or "discs" are cut, then dried, and usually swallowed. Sometimes, the drug comes in powdered form and is taken by capsule, injection, or smoking.

Mescaline causes visual hallucinations and alters spatial perception. It can produce dizziness, vomiting, tachycardia, increased blood pressure, increased pulse and respiratory rates, sensations of warmth and cold, and headache. Effects last approximately 12 hours.

The 'shrooms of psilocybin

Psilocybin is a compound obtained from the *Psilocybe mexicana* mushroom and some types of European mushrooms. Traditionally, it was used by Mexican healers. Psilocybin can be eaten in the dried mushroom form or consumed as a white powder (NIH, n.d.-a).

Effects resemble those of LSD. Used in small amounts, the drug induces relaxation and a sensation of being detached from the body. Users may also see brilliant arrangements of color and light. Larger doses may cause nausea; anxiety; light-headedness; sweating or chills; and numbness of the mouth, lips, and tongue.

Prevalence

Hallucinogen use is less common than alcohol, amphetamine, and cocaine use. About 12% of people in the United States have tried any hallucinogenic drug (NIH, n.d.-a).

How hallucinogens produce their effects

Hallucinogens disrupt the interaction of nerve cells and affect the functioning of serotonin, a neurotransmitter crucial to the regulation of mood, sleep, pain, emotion, and appetite.

Detecting novelty

LSD, for example, binds to and activates serotonin receptors in the brain. Drug effects are most prominent in two brain regions—the cerebral cortex (involved in mood, cognition, and perception) and the locus ceruleus, which receives sensory signals from all areas of the body and is sometimes called the brain's "novelty detector."

Disrupting serotonin

Mescaline and psilocybin are structurally similar to serotonin and produce their effects by disrupting normal functioning of the serotonin system.

Ecstasy increases levels of at least three neurotransmitters—serotonin, dopamine, and norepinephrine. By causing excess serotonin release and interfering with serotonin synthesis, ecstasy leads to serotonin depletion. A single dose of ecstasy can suppress serotonin levels for up to 2 weeks. At moderate to high doses, users may experience long-term serotonin depletion (which probably accounts for many of the drug's long-lasting behavioral effects).

Health hazards of hallucinogen use

Many hallucinogens cause unpleasant and potentially dangerous flashbacks long after the drug was used. Large doses of hallucinogens may cause seizures, ruptured blood vessels in the brain, and irreversible brain damage.

LSD intoxication may cause seizures and fatal accidents. Ketamine can result in respiratory depression, heart rate abnormalities, heart failure, inability to move the muscles, and insensitivity to pain (which can lead to serious injury) (NIH, n.d.-a).

No ecstasy from these effects

Ecstasy may cause confusion, depression, sleep problems, drug craving, severe anxiety, and paranoia (during and sometimes weeks after taking the drug). Physical symptoms may include muscle tension, involuntary teeth clenching, nausea, blurred vision, rapid eye movements, faintness, and chills or sweating.

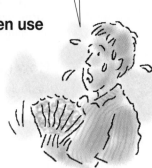

They weren't kidding when they said ecstasy might make you feel hot.

Impairments associated with hallucinogen use

Hallucinogens can cause short-term impairments in cognition, perception, mood, and communication. They may even prevent a person from recognizing reality, sometimes resulting in bizarre or dangerous behavior.

Although hallucinogens are less addictive than most psychoactive drugs, overuse can trigger psychosis in someone with a history of psychosis.

LSD psychosis

Some LSD users experience devastating psychological effects that persist after the trip has ended, producing a long-lasting psychosis-like state. This persistent psychosis—which may include dramatic mood swings from mania to profound depression, visual disturbances, and hallucinations—may last for years.

Bad trips and flashbacks

Many LSD users have "bad trips"—panic attacks at the height of the drug experience characterized by terrifying thoughts and nightmarish feelings of anxiety and despair. The user may perceive real-world sensations as unreal and even frightening.

Some former LSD users report flashbacks—spontaneous, repeated, and sometimes continuous recurrences of the sensory distortions originally produced by LSD. Flashbacks typically consist of visual disturbances, such as seeing false motion on the edges of the field of vision, bright or colored flashes, and halos or trails attached to moving objects.

Flashbacks arise suddenly—commonly without warning—a few days or more than a year after LSD use. They're most common in people who have used hallucinogens chronically or have an underlying personality problem (although otherwise healthy people occasionally have them).

Ecstasy-related impairments

Heavy and prolonged ecstasy use has been linked to confusion, depression, sleep problems, persistent anxiety, aggressive and impulsive behavior, and selective impairment of working memory and attention. Long-term use may damage the brain's serotonin system, leading to various cognitive and behavioral disturbances, including memory impairment.

Ketamine-related impairments

Ketamine may make the user feel disconnected and out of control. Some users report a terrifying feeling of nearly total sensory detachment, described as a near-death experience.

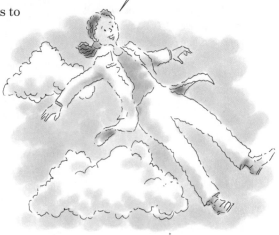

Some hallucinogen users seek to transcend the limits of the body or have a spiritual experience, but not me. I'm high on nursing!

Causes

Some people take hallucinogens to enhance bodily sensations and induce sensory gratification. Under the influence of these drugs, music may sound more clear, colors may seem brighter, and sexual orgasm may feel more intense.

Unlocking the doors of perception?

Other people use hallucinogens to try to transcend the limits of the body and the time-space continuum or to have a spiritual or religious experience.

Signs and symptoms

Signs and symptoms of hallucinogen use vary with the drug used. (See *Assessing for hallucinogen use*, page 416.)

Diagnosis

The diagnosis of hallucinogen abuse or dependence is confirmed when the patient meets the criteria documented in the *DSM-5*. (See *Diagnostic criteria: Substance use disorder*, page 388.)

Advice from the experts

Assessing for hallucinogen use

Suspect hallucinogen use if your patient has these signs and symptoms.

With LSD or mescaline

A patient under the influence of LSD or mescaline may report a sense of depersonalization, grandiosity, hallucinations, illusions, distorted perception of time and space, or mystical experiences.

GI findings include nausea, vomiting, diarrhea, and abdominal cramps. Cardiovascular findings may include arrhythmias, palpitations, tachycardia, and hypertension.

Other signs and symptoms may include:
- chills
- dizziness
- dry mouth
- fever
- sweating
- appetite loss
- hyperpnea
- increased salivation
- muscle aches.

With psilocybin

Signs and symptom of psilocybin use include:
- euphoria
- color distortions
- vivid hallucinations
- "seeing" music or "hearing" color
- dramatic mood swings and personality changes
- increases in blood pressure and body temperature.

With ecstasy

A patient under the influence of ecstasy may report or exhibit:
- distractibility
- heightened alertness
- irritability or confusion
- euphoria
- enhanced emotional and mental clarity
- increased sensitivity to touch
- enhanced sexuality
- increased energy and motor activity.
  Other common findings include:
- increased pulse rate
- elevated blood pressure
- dilated pupils
- perceptual changes
- tightened jaw muscles or jaw grinding or clenching
- increased body temperature, heavy perspiration, and dehydration.

At high doses, ecstasy may cause hallucinations, depression, paranoia, and irrational behavior (including violence).

Ketamine

Ketamine causes dissociative effects and alters visual and auditory perception. At low doses, it causes impairments in attention, learning ability, and memory. At higher doses, it may produce delirium, amnesia, impaired motor function, high blood pressure, depression, and potentially fatal respiratory problems.

Dextromethorphan

Dextromethorphan use may cause euphoria and a floating sensation, along with increased perceptual awareness and altered time perception. The patient may report tactile, auditory, or visual hallucinations. Some users experience paranoia and disorientation.

Memory jogger

When assessing a patient for suspected LSD use, think of the acronym ACID.

A Arrhythmias and abdominal cramps

C Chills

I Illusions and increased salivation

D Diaphoresis, depersonalization, and distortions

Treatment

Treatment measures vary with the patient's status. A patient who's dangerous to himself or others may need to be restrained physically or chemically. Prolonged or excessive physical restraint should be avoided because it can contribute to hyperthermia and rhabdomyolysis and exacerbate paranoia (Garmo, 2013; Schneider & Levenson, 2008).

Cool-down phase

A patient with marked hyperthermia may require aggressive cooling measures. Benzodiazepines typically are given if the patient is anxious or agitated or has hypertension or tachycardia. For severe hypertension or tachycardia, nifedipine or nitroprusside may be indicated. Diazepam is given for seizures.

> You may need to provide aggressive cooling measures if your patient has hyperthermia.

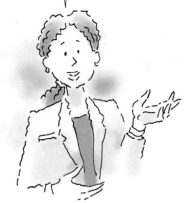

Treatment for LSD flashbacks

No established treatment exists for LSD flashbacks, although antidepressant drugs may ease symptoms. Psychotherapy may help the patient adjust to the visual distraction and ease fears that he or she is suffering from brain damage or a psychiatric disorder.

Nursing interventions

For nursing interventions during an acute episode or when the episode has resolved, see *General interventions for acute drug intoxication*, page 391.

Inhalant abuse

Inhalant abuse, commonly called *huffing* or *bagging*, is the deliberate inhalation of chemical vapors to attain an altered mental or physical state (usually a quick "buzz"). Users inhale vapors from a wide range of substances found in more than 1,000 common household products. Inhalants fall into several general categories. (See *Types of inhalants*, page 418.)

Street names for inhalants include *bang, bolt, boppers, bullet, climax, glading, gluey, hardware, head cleaner, hippie crack, kick, locker room, poor man's pot, poppers, rush,* and *snappers.*

Types of inhalants

Inhalants that are abused for their psychoactive effects include aerosols, gases, nitrites, and volatile solvents.

Aerosols

Aerosol are sprays containing propellants and solvents such as toluene. Common aerosols include whipping cream, paint, deodorant, hair products, cooking sprays, and fabric protector. Silver and gold spray paint are especially popular among inhalant abusers.

Gases

Gases—substances with no definite shape or volume—include refrigerants and medical anesthetics. Abusers may inhale gases found in propane tanks, butane lighters, and air conditioning units as well as those in such medical anesthetics as ether, chloroform, and nitrous oxide (laughing gas). The most commonly abused gas, nitrous oxide, is found in whipped cream dispensers and products that boost octane levels in racing cars. It's also sold at raves or drug paraphernalia stores in the form of balloons or as vials called *whippets*.

Nitrites

Such chemicals as amyl nitrite, butyl nitrite, and cyclohexyl nitrite are taken mainly to enhance sexual experiences. They're available in adult bookstores and shops and over the Internet. Cyclohexyl nitrite is also found in room deodorizers. Amyl nitrite comes in mesh-covered, sealed capsules that are popped or snapped to release the vapors. Butyl nitrite is sold in small bottles.

Volatile solvents

Volatile solvents are liquids that vaporize at room temperature when left in unsealed containers. They're found in paint thinner, gasoline, correction fluid, felt-tip markers, nail polish and nail polish remover, and glue.

By huff or by cuff

Inhalants are breathed in through the nose or mouth in various ways. Users may inhale chemical vapors directly from open containers or may huff fumes from rags soaked in a chemical substance held to the face or stuffed in the mouth.

An aerosol may be sprayed directly into the nose or mouth. Other types of inhalants may be poured onto the collar, sleeves, or cuffs and then sniffed repeatedly.

Prevalence

Inhalant abuse has been increasing steadily. Almost 18 million people in the United States have experimented with inhalants at some time in their lives.

How inhalants produce their effects

Scientists aren't sure how inhalants produce their effects. Some suggest that the inhaled substance changes the solubility of neurons' cell membranes.

Health hazards and impairments associated with inhalants

Inhalants can produce both psychological dependence and physical addiction. Chronic inhalant abuse may lead to serious and possibly irreversible damage to the brain, heart, liver, kidneys, and lungs. Brain damage may cause personality changes, diminished cognitive functioning, memory impairment, and slurred speech. Impaired judgment may lead to fatal injuries from motor vehicle accidents or sudden falls.

Causes

For most users, the goal of inhalant abuse is a rapid euphoric effect similar to alcohol intoxication, along with loss of inhibitions. After the initial excitation, they experience drowsiness, light-headedness, and agitation.

Signs and symptoms

Assessment findings vary with the specific inhalant used. General findings may include:

- loss of muscle control
- slurred speech
- dizziness, drowsiness, or loss of consciousness
- hallucinations and delusions
- belligerence
- apathy
- impaired judgment
- drunk or disoriented demeanor
- double vision
- seizures
- nausea
- appetite loss
- red or runny nose
- watery eyes
- sores or rash around the nose or mouth
- arrhythmias
- seizures.

Strong chemical odors on the breath or clothing as well as paint or other stains on the hands, face, or clothing strongly suggest inhalant use.

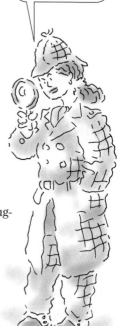

Fetch the scent detector, Watson! Chemical odors may hint at inhalant abuse.

Withdrawal symptoms

A patient undergoing inhalant withdrawal may report or exhibit excessive sweating, headache, rapid pulse, hand tremors, muscle cramps, insomnia, hallucinations, nausea, and vomiting.

Diagnosis

The diagnosis of inhalant abuse or dependence is confirmed when the patient meets the criteria documented in the *DSM-5*. (See *Diagnostic criteria: Substance use disorders*, page 388.)

Treatment

Treatment for acute inhalant intoxication is supportive and symptomatic.

Other measures may include:

- fluid replacement therapy
- sedatives to induce sleep
- anticholinergics and antidiarrheal agents to relieve GI distress
- antianxiety drugs for severe agitation

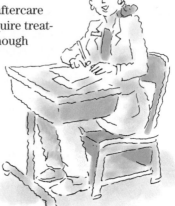

> Inhalant abusers have high relapse rates. Some require up to 2 years of treatment.

Relapse blues

Inhalant abusers have high relapse rates, making aftercare and follow-up extremely important. Some may require treatment in an outpatient or residential program—although few treatment programs exist specifically for inhalant users. For many users, treatment must continue for an extended period—possibly up to 2 years.

Nursing interventions

For nursing interventions during an acute episode or when the episode has resolved, see *General interventions for acute drug intoxication*, page 391.

Nicotine addiction

One of the most frequently used addictive drugs, nicotine is the main psychoactive component found in smoke from tobacco products (cigarettes, cigars, and pipes). Smokeless tobacco products, such as snuff and chewing tobacco, also have a high nicotine content.

Cigarette smoking is the most prevalent form of nicotine dependence in the United States.

Nicotine addiction and withdrawal

Regular nicotine use can result in nicotine addiction.

Most smokers use tobacco regularly because they're addicted to nicotine. Although nearly 35 million smokers make a serious attempt to quit each year, less than 7% who try to quit on their own stay abstinent for more than 1 year. Most of them relapse within a few days of trying to quit.

Drawn-out withdrawal

A nicotine-dependent person who stops using nicotine experiences a withdrawal syndrome that may last a month or more. Some people have intense nicotine cravings for 6 months or longer.

Prevalence

In 2007, an estimated 70.9 million U.S. residents are current cigarette smokers, and 8.1 million use smokeless tobacco. Additionally, the statistics show that 9.7% of teenage girls and 10% of teenage boys smoke (NIH, n.d.-a).

However, smoking has declined dramatically over the years. Currently, about one-half of the U.S. adult population have never smoked, 25% are current smokers, and 25% are ex-smokers. Between 8% and 15% of smokers are occasional or light smokers (NIH, n.d.-a).

How nicotine produces its effects

Absorbed through the skin and mucosal lining of the mouth and nose or by inhalation in the lungs, nicotine activates the brain circuitry that regulates feelings of pleasure (the so-called reward pathways).

Short puffs and long draws

Nicotine can act as both a stimulant and a sedative. Small, rapid doses produce alertness and arousal, whereas long drawn-out doses induce relaxation and sedation (NIH, n.d.-a).

Health hazards of nicotine

Nicotine addiction has a tremendous impact in terms of illness, death, and economic costs to society. Tobacco use is the leading preventable cause of death in the United States. It kills more than 450,000 U.S. residents each year—more than alcohol, cocaine, heroin, homicide, suicide, car accidents, fire, and AIDS combined (NIH, n.d.-a). (See *Nicotine's ugly aftermath*, page 422.)

Nicotine's ugly aftermath

Tobacco use accounts for approximately one-third of all cancers. Cigarette smoking is linked to nearly 90% of all lung cancers—the leading cause of cancer deaths in both men and women. Additionally, it's associated with cancers of the mouth, pharynx, larynx, esophagus, stomach, pancreas, cervix, kidney, ureter, and bladder. Overall death rates from cancer are twice as high among smokers as nonsmokers.

Smoking also causes lung diseases, such as chronic bronchitis and emphysema, and can exacerbate asthma symptoms. It may also heighten the risk for peptic ulcers, GI disorders, maternal and fetal complications, and other disorders.

Cardiovascular disease

Smoking dramatically increases the risk of cardiovascular disease, including coronary artery disease, myocardial infarction, stroke, vascular problems, and aneurysms. Smoking accounts for nearly 20% of deaths from heart disease.

Passive smoking and its consequences

Secondhand smoke (passive smoking) causes approximately 3,000 lung cancer deaths yearly in nonsmokers and contributes to as many as 40,000 deaths from cardiovascular disease (NIH, n.d.-a).

Exposure to tobacco smoke in the home increases the severity of asthma in children and contributes to childhood asthma.

Causes

Scientists suspect that certain genes make some people more susceptible to nicotine addiction and cigarette smoking. Studies involving twins suggest that genes account for 50% to 70% of the risk of becoming a smoker.

Some researchers believe that as many as 50 genes are involved in nicotine addiction. Genetic factors must be distinguished from environmental factors that contribute to smoking.

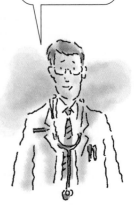

Nicotine addiction may involve as many as 50 genes.

Susceptible teens

Among adolescents, risk factors for cigarette smoking include:

- use of alcohol and other drugs
- attention deficit disorder
- depression
- peer influences
- urge to experiment
- disruptive behavior
- failing to perceive the risks of smoking
- having friends who abuse substances
- having family members who smoke
- divorce or family conflict.

Signs and symptoms

Nicotine withdrawal symptoms may begin within a few hours after the last cigarette—and can quickly drive the smoker back to tobacco use. Usually, symptoms peak within the first few days and subside within a few weeks. For some people, however, increased appetite and nicotine cravings last for months (NIH, n.d.-a).

Nicotine withdrawal symptoms include:
- depressed mood
- insomnia
- irritability, frustration, or anger
- anxiety
- difficulty concentrating
- restlessness
- increased appetite or weight gain
- desire for sweets
- increased coughing
- nicotine craving.

Diagnosis

The diagnosis of nicotine dependence is confirmed when the patient meets the criteria documented in the *DSM-5*.

Treatment

Various behavioral and pharmacologic treatments have proven to be effective in treating nicotine dependence. For patients who are motivated to quit smoking, a combination of behavioral and pharmacologic treatments can double the success rate over placebo treatments (NIH, n.d.-a).

Pharmacologic therapies for smoking cessation include nicotine replacement, antagonist therapy, aversive therapy, nicotine-mimicking agents, and nonnicotine medication. Nonpharmacologic therapies include sensory replacement and acupuncture. To remain abstinent, many patients require behavioral therapy.

Nicotine replacement

Used to relieve withdrawal symptoms and nicotine craving, nicotine replacement products include nicotine gum, transdermal patches, nasal spray, and inhalers.

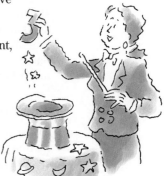

Nicotine replacement therapy isn't magic, but it has helped about 1 million people stop smoking.

Varenicline (Chantix)—the newest nicotine replacement option

Chantix is a medication available by prescription used to stimulate the reward centers in the brain so the person no longer craves cigarettes. So far, it has the highest rate of success for smoking cessation.

Aversive therapy

Aversive therapy typically involves silver acetate, which combines with sulfides in tobacco smoke to produce a bad taste.

Nicotine-mimicking agents

Agents that mimic nicotine's effects include clonidine and anxiolytics (such as diazepam), antidepressants, stimulants, and anorectic agents (such as fenfluramine and phenylpropanolamine, used to suppress appetite and prevent weight gain).

Nonnicotine medication

Bupropion, a prescription antidepressant (marketed as Zyban for smoking cessation), was introduced for nicotine addiction in 1996. It's the first drug approved for smoking cessation that's taken in pill form and the first that doesn't contain nicotine.

Sensory replacement

Sensory replacement agents, such as black pepper extract, capsaicin, denicotinized tobacco, flavorings, and regenerated (denicotinized) smoke can be used to decrease nicotine cravings or withdrawal or to substitute for satisfaction from cigarettes.

Behavioral treatments

Behavioral interventions can play a key role in treating nicotine addiction. Such methods help patients identify high-risk relapse situations, create an aversion to smoking, self-monitor their smoking behavior, and establish alternative coping responses. Identifying and removing environmental cues that influence the patient to smoke (such as cigarettes, lighters, and ashtrays) are crucial.

Adjunctive measures

The single most important factor in nicotine abstinence may be learning and using coping skills that aid both short- and long-term relapse prevention. Social support can also influence the outcome of a smoking cessation program. Ideally, the patient should avoid smokers and smoking environments and receive support from family and friends. (See *Improving the patient's coping skills*.)

Other helpful measures include self-help materials, educational and supportive groups, exercise, hypnosis, 12-step programs, biofeedback, family therapy, interpersonal therapy, and psychodynamic therapies.

Nursing interventions

These nursing interventions may be appropriate for a patient with nicotine dependence:
• Teach the patient about the dangers of smoking and ways to stop.
• Provide emotional support for the patient's attempts to stop smoking.
• Explain how to use nicotine replacement devices, antagonist or aversive medications, or other prescribed drugs.
• As indicated, refer the patient to a smoking cessation program.

Memory jogger

During nicotine withdrawal, a patient NEEDS CARE.

N Nervousness

E Extreme fatigue

E Excited cardiovascular system

D Difficulty concentrating

S Sleep disturbances

C Cravings

A Anxiety

R Restlessness

E Excessive appetite

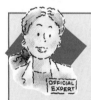

Advice from the experts

Improving the patient's coping skills

Many patients who abuse drugs exhibit ineffective coping and need help in identifying and using available support systems. To enhance your patient's coping skills, use these nursing interventions:
• Spend uninterrupted periods of time with the patient. Encourage expression of feelings; accept what is said.
• Try to identify factors that cause, exacerbate, or reduce the patient's inability to cope, such as the fear of health problems or losing a job.
• Encourage the patient to make decisions about care to increase sense of self-worth and mastery over the current situation.
• Praise the patient for making decisions and performing activities to reinforce coping behaviors.
• Encourage the patient to use support systems that can help with coping.
• Help the patient to evaluate the current situation and coping behaviors to encourage a realistic view of the crisis.
• Encourage the patient to try alternative coping behaviors. A patient in crisis tends to accept interventions and develop new coping behaviors more easily.
• Ask the patient for feedback about behaviors that seem to work. This encourages the patient to evaluate the effect of these behaviors.

Opioid abuse

Opioids are narcotics that can produce euphoria. They have a high potential for addiction. Naturally occurring opioids include morphine and codeine. Partially synthetic morphine derivatives include heroin, oxycodone, hydrocodone, hydromorphone, and oxymorphone. Synthetic opioids include fentanyl, alfentanil, levorphanol, and methadone.

Opioids are used medically as analgesics. Some agents have additional uses. Codeine, for example, is used as an antitussive; opium, as an antidiarrheal.

Opioids produce relaxation with an immediate "rush" but also have initial unpleasant effects, such as restlessness and nausea. With a typical dose, effects last 3 to 6 hours (NIH, n.d.-a).

Codeine and morphine may be ingested, injected, or smoked. Heroin (whose street names include *junk, horse,* and *H*) may be injected, inhaled, or smoked. Opium (known as *O, ope,* or *OP*) may be ingested or smoked (NIH, n.d.-a).

> Opioid drugs stimulate opioid receptors in the brain. Injecting them I.V. causes an initial "rush" of pleasure.

Prevalence

In 2008, 3.8 million U.S. residents reported having used heroin at least once during their lifetime.

The lifetime prevalence of opioid use in people ages 12 to 17 is just over 2%. Lifetime prevalence is slightly higher in people older than the age of 35 (Garmo, 2013; NIH, n.d.-a).

How opioids produce their effects

Opioids stimulate opioid receptors in the CNS and surrounding tissues. CNS effects of opioids include euphoria and sedation, followed by elation, relaxation, and then sedation or sleep.

Causes

Because of their euphoric and anxiolytic effects, opioids are strongly reinforcing agents.

Behavioral theory proposes that basic reward-punishment mechanisms perpetuate addictive behavior. Rapid development of physical dependence and a prolonged withdrawal syndrome can make abstinence difficult.

Genetic, social, and psychological factors also play a role in opioid abuse and dependence (Garmo, 2013; NIH, n.d.-a).

Genetic factors

Some evidence shows that identical twins have similar opioid use patterns. Also, several studies support the theory that genetically transmitted vulnerability predisposes a person to drug dependence (Garmo, 2013; NIH, n.d.-a).

Psychological factors

Opioid abuse sometimes follows the use of prescribed opioids to relieve pain. Some users are motivated by the desire to manage uncomfortable emotions, such as anxiety, guilt, and anger.

Signs and symptoms

A patient who abuses opioids—or other drugs, for that matter—may try to hide drug use from family, friends, coworkers, and health care professionals. However, even if the patient isn't forthcoming, you can check for certain telltale signs. (See *When to suspect drug abuse*, page 428.)

Also check for these signs and symptoms of opioid use:
- constricted pupils, bloodshot eyes, and drooping eyelids
- slurred speech
- sweating
- clammy skin
- anorexia
- respiratory depression
- hypotension
- sweating
- impaired judgment
- euphoria
- drowsiness
- decreased level of consciousness
- sense of tranquility
- detachment from reality
- indifference to pain
- lack of concern
- nystagmus
- seizures
- constipation
- hemorrhoids.

Some patients experience nausea and vomiting, hypotension, and arrhythmia. Severe opioid intoxication can lead to delirium and coma.

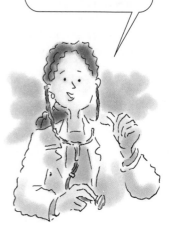

A patient who has taken opioids may have respiratory depression, with slow or shallow breathing.

Tale of the tracks

With I.V. use, the patient may have visible needle marks or tracks, skin lesions or abscesses, soft tissue infection, and thrombosed veins. (See *Identifying I.V. drug abuse*, page 429.)

When to suspect drug abuse

Many patients try to hide their drug abuse—especially if they inject drugs. If you suspect your patient is abusing drugs, carefully review his medical history and perform a physical assessment.

History findings
History findings that suggest drug abuse include:
- use of a fictitious name and address
- reluctance to discuss previous hospitalizations
- seeking treatment at a medical facility across town rather than near his or her own home
- history of a drug overdose
- high tolerance for potentially addictive drugs
- history of hepatitis or HIV infection
- amenorrhea
- complaints of a painful injury or chronic illness—but refusal of a diagnostic workup
- feigned illnesses, such as migraine headache, myocardial infarction, or renal colic, in an attempt to obtain drugs
- claims of an allergy to OTC analgesics
- requests for a specific medication.

Physical findings
Physical findings that hint at drug abuse include:
- fever (from stimulant intoxication, withdrawal, or infection caused by I.V. drug use)
- needle marks or tracks (from I.V. drug use)
- attempts to conceal or disguise injection sites with tattoos
- use of inconspicuous injection sites, such as under the nails or tongue
- cellulitis or abscess from self-injection
- puffy hands (a late sign of thrombophlebitis or of fascial infection caused by self-injection on the hands or arms)
- dental conditions (from poor oral hygiene associated with chronic drug use)
- excoriated skin (from scratching induced by formication, a sensation of bugs crawling on the skin)
- refractory acute-onset hypertension or cardiac arrhythmias (stimulant use)
- liver enlargement, with or without tenderness (from hepatitis caused by sharing contaminated needles).

Behavioral clues
A hospitalized drug abuser is likely to be uncooperative, disruptive, or even violent. He may experience mood swings, anxiety, impaired memory, sleep disturbances, flashbacks, slurred speech, depression, and thought disorders.

To obtain drugs, some patients resort to plays on sympathy, bribery, or threats. They may try to manipulate caregivers by pitting one staff member against another (Garmo, 2013; NIH, n.d.-a).

Findings in opioid withdrawal

Opioid withdrawal can be quite unpleasant. For general findings, see *Evaluating for opioid withdrawal*.

Heroin withdrawal symptoms resemble a bad case of the flu. They generally begin 12 to 14 hours after the last dose, peak within 36 and 72 hours, and may last 7 to 14 days (Garmo, 2013; NIH, n.d.-a).

Opioid overdose

With opioid overdose, auscultation may reveal bilateral crackles and rhonchi caused by opiate overdose. Other cardiopulmonary findings may include pulmonary edema, respiratory depression, aspiration pneumonia, and hypotension.

Advice from the experts

Identifying I.V. drug abuse

Needle marks or tracks are an obvious sign of I.V. drug abuse. Some I.V. drugs abusers try to conceal or disguise injection sites with tattoos or by selecting an inconspicuous injection site such as under the nails.

Be aware that self-injection sometimes causes cellulitis or abscesses, especially in patients who are also chronic alcoholics. Puffy hands may be a late sign of thrombophlebitis or of fascial infection caused by self-injection on the hands or arms.

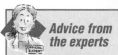

Advice from the experts

Evaluating for opioid withdrawal

Signs and symptoms of opioid withdrawal include:
• abdominal cramps, nausea, or vomiting
• anorexia
• fever or chills
• profuse sweating
• dilated pupils
• hyperactive bowel sounds
• irritability
• nausea
• panic
• piloerection (goose flesh)
• runny nose
• tremors
• watery eyes
• yawning
• bone pain
• diffuse muscle aches
• drug craving.

Diagnosis

A practitioner who suspects opioid addiction may order a urine drug screen. (See *Toxicology screening*, page 430.)

For patients with clinical or historical evidence of I.V. drug abuse, the practitioner may order:
• liver function tests
• rapid plasma reagin test for syphilis
• hepatitis viral testing
• HIV testing
• lung X-rays (to check for pulmonary fibrosis).

The diagnosis of opioid addiction is confirmed if the patient meets the criteria documented in the *DSM-5*. (See *Diagnostic criteria: Substance use disorder*, page 388.)

Treatment

For opioid intoxication or overdose, general supportive measures include ensuring an adequate airway and ventilation (with ventilatory support if needed) and supporting cardiovascular function (Garmo, 2013; NIH, n.d.-a).

Other treatments depend on symptoms, the specific opioid, and administration route. If the drug was ingested, vomiting is induced or gastric lavage is performed.

Toxicology screening

A blood or urine screen may detect drugs that are present in concentrations above 5 μg/ml. Current methods quantitate only drugs detected in the blood.

Toxicology screening commonly is done in the emergency department or on admission. It may require a legal chain of custody in which precautions are taken to prevent anyone from tampering with the specimens.

I.V. fluids and nutritional and vitamin supplements may be given. An opioid antagonist such as naloxone may be administered. (See *Naloxone for opioid reversal.*)

Withdrawal and detoxification

Treatment of withdrawal symptoms may include antidiarrheals, decongestants for runny nose, and nonopioid analgesics for pain.

Substitution strategy

For detoxification, the abused opioid usually is replaced with a drug that has a similar action but a longer duration. Gradual substitution controls withdrawal effects, reducing discomfort and

---

Meds matters

Naloxone for opioid reversal

Naloxone hydrochloride (Narcan) is an opioid antagonist used to reverse the effects of opioids. It works by displacing opioids from their receptors in the CNS.

Naloxone is administered I.V., I.M., or subcutaneously every 2 to 3 minutes, as needed. It rapidly reverses opioid-induced CNS depression and increases the respiratory rate within 1 to 2 minutes. Adverse effects include nausea, vomiting, diaphoresis, tachycardia, CNS excitement, and increased blood pressure.

Relapse and respiratory peril
Because the opioid's duration of action may exceed that of naloxone, the patient may relapse into respiratory depression. Be sure to monitor respiratory rate and depth. Be prepared to provide oxygen, ventilation, and other resuscitation measures.

associated risks. Depending on which drug the patient has abused, detoxification may be managed on an inpatient or outpatient basis.

Maintenance therapy

For maintenance, the patient typically receives an opioid agonist as a substitute for the abused drug. The goal of maintenance is to replace the abused drug with one that's available legally, can be taken orally, and requires only a once-daily dose.

> Buprenorphine, given as a sublingual tablet or strip, is the most common drug used in opioid detox.

Buprenorphine for maintenance

Buprenorphine, in its combination formulation with naloxone (Suboxone), is usually prescribed as a once per day sublingual tablet or strip. It is a partial agonist which does not create the level of euphoria that other opiates may cause but it does neutralize the cravings for other opiates. Treatment with buprenorphine and concurrent psychotherapy has been shown to significantly reduce the risk of relapse and maintain sustained recovery (Garmo, 2013; NIH, n.d.-a).

Psychotherapy

Detoxification alone, without ongoing psychotherapy, isn't sufficient to manage a patient with opioid dependence. To remain abstinent, he or she should receive standard drug counseling along with cognitive-behavioral, dynamic, or group therapy. (Some patients may prefer aversion therapy, in which aversive stimuli are paired with cognitive images of opioid use.)

> An opioid-dependent patient needs psychotherapy in addition to detox.

Cognitive-behavioral therapy focuses on the patient's thoughts and behaviors. It helps him or her learn specific skills for resisting drug abuse as well as coping skills to reduce problems related to drug use.

Dynamic psychotherapy is based on the concept that all symptoms arise from underlying unconscious psychological conflicts. The goal is to make the patient aware of these conflicts and develop better coping mechanisms and healthier ways of resolving intrapsychic conflicts.

Advice from the experts

Reducing impaired social interaction

Impaired social interaction is common among patients who abuse substances. Appropriate nursing interventions can help the patient improve social interaction skills in both one-on-one and group settings.
• If delusions and hallucinations occur, don't focus on them. Instead, provide reality-based information, and reassure the patient of safety.
• Provide additional time with the patient on each shift (besides the time spent on caregiving) to encourage social interaction. Start with one-on-one interaction and increase to group interaction when the patient's social skills indicate readiness.
• Give positive reinforcement for appropriate and effective interaction behaviors (both verbal and nonverbal). This helps the patient recognize progress and enhances feelings of self-worth.
• Assist the patient and family or close friends in progressive participation in care and therapies. This reduces feelings of helplessness and enhances the patient's feeling of control and independence.

Group sobriety

Group therapy targets the social stigma attached to drug abuse. The presence of other group members who acknowledge their abuse problem has a therapeutic effect in helping the patient develop alternative methods of staying sober. (See *Reducing impaired social interaction.*)

Narcotics Anonymous

Established in 1947, NA is based on principles similar to those of AA, including the progression through 12 steps of recovery. Like AA, NA has helped many substance abusers, offering much needed support for those attempting abstinence.

Nursing interventions

These nursing interventions may be appropriate for a patient with acute opioid intoxication:
• Provide extra blankets or a hypothermia blanket for hypothermia.
• Reorient the patient to time, place, and person.
• Monitor breath sounds for evidence of pulmonary edema.
• Frequently monitor vital signs and cardiopulmonary status until opioids have cleared from the system.
• Monitor for withdrawal symptoms.

For other interventions during an acute episode or when the episode has resolved, see *General interventions for acute drug intoxication*, page 391.

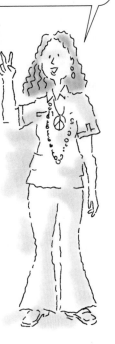

Some people call PCP the peace pill. But from what I hear, taking it is anything but peaceful.

Phencyclidine abuse

A dissociative drug, PCP was developed in the 1950s as an I.V. anesthetic. It was used in veterinary medicine but never approved for human use.

Today, PCP is manufactured illegally in laboratories. On the street, it's available as tablets, capsules, and powders, and it's sold as *angel dust, wack, ozone, love boat, superweed, hog, peace pill, embalming fluid, elephant tranquilizer*, and *rocket fuel*.

PCP can be snorted, smoked, or eaten. For smoking, it's typically applied to a leafy material, such as parsley, oregano, or marijuana. Some users ingest PCP by snorting the powder or by swallowing it in tablet form.

Numb but quarrelsome

PCP makes the user feel disconnected and out of control. It also has a numbing effect on the mind and can cause unpredictable and often violent behavior. Repeated use may result in psychological dependence and craving (NIH, n.d.-a).

Prevalence

PCP use isn't widespread. It's most common in teenagers according to a 2008 survey (NIH, n.d.-a).

How PCP produces its effects

PCP's primary sites of action are glutamate receptors known as *N-methyl-D-aspartate* (NMDA) receptors. PCP acts as an NMDA antagonist, lowering the glutamate levels in the brain.

PCP also increases levels of gamma-aminobutyric acid (GABA), an inhibitory neurotransmitter. Increased GABA levels probably explain the inhibition of pain seen in PCP users. In addition, PCP also alters the action of dopamine, which is responsible for the euphoria and "rush" associated with many psychoactive drugs (NIH, n.d.-a).

Health hazards of PCP

At low to moderate doses, PCP's physiologic effects include increased body temperature, marked rises in blood pressure and pulse, shallow respirations, flushing, and profuse sweating.

At high doses, PCP decreases blood pressure and slows the pulse and respiratory rates. Cardiac arrest, hypertensive crisis, renal failure, and seizures may occur.

Feeling no pain

Other dangerous effects include violent or suicidal behavior, seizures, decreased awareness of pain, coma, and death. (However, death more commonly results from accidental injury or suicide during PCP intoxication).

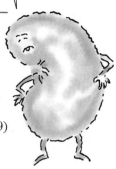

> PCP sometimes causes rhabdomyolysis, a dangerous condition that may lead to kidney failure.

Causes

As with other drugs, the precise causes of PCP abuse aren't known. Some people may use PCP because it provides a feeling of strength, power, and invulnerability.

In young people, drug abuse commonly follows experimentation with drugs stemming from peer pressure. Risk factors for PCP use include male gender and young adulthood (ages 20 to 29) (NIH, n.d.-a, n.d.-b).

Signs and symptoms

A patient under the influence of PCP may report numbness of the arms and legs and may exhibit poor muscle coordination. Psychological effects include changes in body awareness, resembling those caused by alcohol intoxication.

Other physical findings may include:
- sparse, garbled speech
- blurred vision
- blank stare
- drooling
- nausea and vomiting
- loss of balance
- dizziness
- decreased deep tendon reflexes
- fever
- gait ataxia
- nystagmus
- hyperactivity
- increased vital signs
- tachycardia.

Mental status mayhem

Mental status findings may vary greatly—even in the same patient. Your patient may seem normal one moment, then exhibit apparent psychotic symptoms and homicidal or suicidal ideation the next.

Memory jogger

Each letter in ANGEL DUST stands for a sign or symptom of PCP use.

A Amnesia

N Nystagmus

G Gait ataxia

E Euphoria

L Loopiness (poor perception of time and distance)

D Delusions and distortions

U Unpredictable effects

S Sudden behavioral changes

T Tachycardia

Other mental status findings may include:
- euphoria
- amnesia
- delusions and hallucinations
- poor perception of time and distance
- distorted sense of sight, hearing, and touch
- decreased awareness of pain
- distorted body image
- excitation
- panic
- sudden behavioral changes
- violent behavior
- stupor or coma
- paranoia
- disordered thinking.

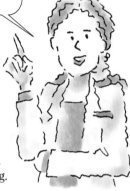

Someone with a history of prolonged PCP use may experience dysphoria and drug craving during withdrawal.

Withdrawal symptoms

Research suggests that with repeated or prolonged PCP use, a withdrawal syndrome may occur when drug use is stopped. Some users experience dysphoria and an intense drug craving.

Diagnosis

The practitioner typically orders a urine drug screen if PCP use is suspected. Because PCP may cause rhabdomyolysis, serum enzyme levels (especially creatine kinase) may be useful.

The diagnosis of PCP abuse or dependence is confirmed when the patient meets the criteria documented in the *DSM-5*. (See *Diagnostic criteria: Substance use disorder*, page 388.)

Treatment

A patient with acute PCP intoxication should be placed in a quiet room with minimal stimulation. If he's violent, restraints may be needed.

Induced vomiting or gastric lavage may be performed, followed by the administration of activated charcoal. Other drug therapy may include:
- benzodiazepines (such as diazepam) to ease seizures, agitation, aggressiveness, psychotic symptoms, hypertension, and tachycardia
- haloperidol for agitation or psychotic behavior
- diuretics to force diuresis
- anticholinergics and antidiarrheal agents to relieve GI distress
- propranolol for hypertension or tachycardia
- nitroprusside for severe hypertensive crisis
- I.V. fluids.

Treatment of PCP-induced psychosis

For a patient with PCP-induced psychosis, treatment must address the high risk of violence. The patient may require seclusion or restraint, and suicide and assault precautions should be instituted.

If psychosis persists, the doctor may prescribe an antipsychotic, such as haloperidol or risperidone. The patient usually needs psychiatric follow-up care and chemical dependency treatment. Most patients with PCP-induced psychosis can be weaned from antipsychotics within 6 months.

Nursing interventions

For appropriate measures, see *General interventions for acute drug intoxication*, page 391.

Sedative, hypnotic, or anxiolytic abuse

> About 100 million benzodiazepine prescriptions are written each year in the United States.

Sedative, hypnotic, and anxiolytic drugs produce sedation, ease anxiety, and relax muscles. Most are classified as benzodiazepines. Typically, benzodiazepines act as hypnotics in high doses, anxiolytics in moderate doses, and sedatives in low doses. Besides the main indications described earlier, they're used to prevent seizures or help patients withdraw from alcohol.

In the United States, benzodiazepines are the most widely prescribed CNS medications, with about 100 million prescriptions written in 1999. Because of their widespread availability, benzodiazepine abuse is common (NIH, n.d.-a). (See *Benzodiazepines from A to T.*)

Forging for drugs

Abusers maintain their drug supply by getting prescriptions from several different prescribers, forging prescriptions, or buying the drugs on the street. Street names for benzodiazepines include *dolls*, *green and whites*, *roaches*, and *yellow jackets*.

Benzodiazepines are ingested or injected. Their duration of action ranges from 4 to 8 hours.

Mixed motives

Some people use benzodiazepines to get intoxicated; others take intentional or accidental overdoses. Heroin users may use benzodiazepines when they can't get heroin, when they want to enhance heroin's effects, or when they're trying to stop using heroin. Amphetamine and ecstasy users may take benzodiazepines when "coming down" from a high or to induce sleep.

Prevalence

In 2008, an estimated 5.7 million U.S. residents used prescription sedatives and tranquilizers nonmedically. Adult males and females have similar rates of nonmedical use of prescription drugs. However, females are almost two times more likely than males to become addicted to sedatives, hypnotics, and anxiolytics (NIH, n.d.-a, n.d.-b).

How benzodiazepines produce their effects

Like alcohol, heroin, and cannabis, benzodiazepines are depressants that slow CNS activity. They work by potentiating the activity of GABA, causing sedation, relaxing muscles, easing anxiety, and have anticonvulsant properties. In the peripheral nervous system, stimulation of GABA receptors may decrease cardiac contractility and enhance perfusion (Garmo, 2013; NIH, n.d.-a, n.d.-b).

Health hazards of benzodiazepines

In addition to causing tolerance and physical dependence, repeated use of large benzodiazepine doses can lead to amnesia, hostility, irritability, and vivid or disturbing dreams. Concurrent use with alcohol or other depressants can be life-threatening.

The risky business of injection

Some people inject benzodiazepines for an enhanced "high" or to increase the effects of other drugs. This practice can lead to severe health effects, such as:

- collapsed veins
- red, swollen, infected skin
- necessity for limb amputation (because of poor circulation)
- stroke
- cardiac and respiratory arrest
- death.

Sharing needles, syringes, and other injecting equipment greatly increases the risk of contracting hepatitis and HIV (Garmo, 2013; NIH, n.d.-a, n.d.-b).

Benzodiazepines from A to T

Benzodiazepines include:

- alprazolam (Xanax)
- chlordiazepoxide (Librium)
- clonazepam (Klonopin)
- diazepam (Valium)
- flurazepam (Dalmane)
- lorazepam (Ativan)
- midazolam (Versed)
- oxazepam (Serax)
- temazepam (Restoril)
- triazolam (Halcion).

Impairments associated with benzodiazepine use

At low to moderate doses, benzodiazepines can produce drowsiness, fatigue, lethargy, dizziness, vertigo, blurred or double vision, slurred speech, stuttering, mild impairment of memory and thought processes, feelings of isolation, and depression.

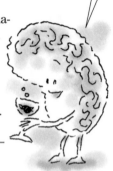

Benzodiazepines and alcohol make for a killer combination.

A booze-like wooziness

At high doses, these drugs may induce oversedation, sleep, or effects similar to alcohol intoxication—confusion, poor coordination, impaired memory and judgment, difficulty thinking clearly, blurred or double vision, and dizziness. Mood swings and aggressive outbursts may also occur. As the high dose wears off, the user may feel jittery and excitable.

Benzodiazepine overdose can cause coma. When combined with alcohol, death may occur (Garmo, 2013; NIH, n.d.-a, n.d.-b).

Causes

Some people may have a genetic tendency toward drug dependence or addiction. Environmental factors also play a significant role. Drug availability and prescriber dispensing practices may contribute to benzodiazepine abuse.

Signs and symptoms

A patient under the influence of benzodiazepine may exhibit:
- ataxia (poor muscle coordination)
- drowsiness
- hypotension
- increased self-confidence
- relaxation
- slurred speech.

Findings in benzodiazepine overdose

Assessment findings in a patient with a benzodiazepine overdose may include:
- dizziness
- altered mental status, ranging from confusion and drowsiness to unresponsiveness or coma
- blurred vision
- anxiety and agitation
- nystagmus
- ataxia
- hallucinations
- slurred speech

- hypotonia (reduced skeletal muscle tone)
- weakness
- impaired cognition
- amnesia
- respiratory depression
- hypotension.

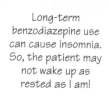

Expect low blood pressure in a patient who has taken a benzodiazepine overdose.

Findings in chronic abuse

Long-term benzodiazepine use (more than several weeks) may result in:
- drowsiness
- lack of motivation
- clouded thinking
- memory loss
- changes in personality and emotional responses
- anxiety
- irritability
- aggression
- insomnia
- disturbing dreams
- nausea
- headache
- skin rash
- menstrual problems
- sexual problems
- increased appetite
- weight gain
- increased risk of accidents (including falls in older adults).

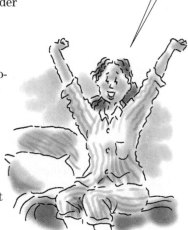

Long-term benzodiazepine use can cause insomnia. So, the patient may not wake up as rested as I am!

Withdrawal symptoms

Benzodiazepine withdrawal resembles that of alcohol withdrawal. It can be severe and may necessitate hospitalization.

Rough withdrawal

Withdrawal symptoms usually develop 3 to 4 days after the drug is stopped; however, they may arise earlier with shorter acting agents or later with longer acting agents. Symptoms can last a few weeks or months; some patients have them for 1 year—or even longer.

Withdrawal symptoms may include:
- headache
- sweating

- confusion
- seizures
- nervousness
- tension
- anxiety and panic attacks
- hypertension
- dizziness
- poor appetite
- nausea, vomiting, and abdominal pain
- inability to sleep properly
- depression
- feelings of isolation and unreality
- delirium and paranoia.

Diagnosis

The diagnosis of benzodiazepine addiction is confirmed if the patient meets the criteria documented in the *DSM-5*. (See *Diagnostic criteria: Substance use disorders*, page 388.)

Treatment

Treatment of benzodiazepine intoxication depends on which drug was taken, how much, and when. The patient may need supportive care and monitoring, including cardiac monitoring, I.V. fluid administration, pulse oximetry, and vital sign monitoring. Respiratory depression may necessitate assisted ventilation. (See *Dealing with drug overdose.*)

Detoxification

For detoxification, single-dose activated charcoal is recommended if the patient ingested the drug within the past 4 hours. Alternatively, gastric lavage may be considered. (Ipecac is contraindicated because of the risk of CNS depression and subsequent aspiration of emesis.)

The only specific benzodiazepine antidote is flumazenil (Romazicon), a GABA antagonist. Given I.V., flumazenil reverses sedation, memory, and psychomotor impairments and respiratory depression produced by benzodiazepines. However, it's usually reserved for severe poisoning because it can cause withdrawal and seizures in chronic benzodiazepine abusers (Garmo, 2013; NIH, n.d.-a, n.d.-b).

Treatment of chronic abuse

Treatment of chronic benzodiazepine abuse usually is done on an outpatient basis or at a drug rehabilitation center. However,

Advice from the experts

Dealing with drug overdose

Whether intentional or accidental, a drug overdose is life-threatening. In very high doses, some drugs cause CNS depression, ranging from lethargy to coma. Others cause CNS stimulation, ranging from euphoria to violent behavior.

Depending on the specific drug and the extent of damage, other symptoms of overdose may include hallucinations, respiratory depression, seizures, abnormal pupil size and response, or nausea and vomiting.

Diagnosing overdose
Arterial blood gas analysis and blood and urine screening tests help detect drug use and guide treatment.

Treatment
A patient with signs of respiratory depression receives oxygen or intubation and mechanical ventilation. He or she is attached to a cardiac monitor, and a 12-lead ECG is taken. Urine, blood, and vomitus specimens are obtained for toxicology screening. Restraints may be applied to prevent him or her from harming himself or others.

Emergency nursing interventions
• Take appropriate steps to stop further drug absorption. If the patient ingested the drug, induce vomiting or use gastric lavage, as ordered. You may administer activated charcoal to help adsorb the substance, and use a saline cathartic to speed its elimination.

• Frequently reassess your patient's airway, breathing, and circulation. Keep oxygen, suction equipment, and emergency airway equipment nearby. Be prepared to perform cardiopulmonary resuscitation, if necessary.
• When possible, find out which drug the patient took, how much, and when. Did he combine several drugs or take a drug along with alcohol? Question the patient's family, friends, or rescue personnel thoroughly.
• Watch for complications. Stay alert for shock, indicated by decreased blood pressure and a faint, rapid pulse. Reassess respiratory rate and depth, and auscultate breath sounds frequently. Know that dyspnea and tachypnea may warn of impending respiratory complications, such as pulmonary edema or aspiration pneumonia. A patient with crackles who's pale, diaphoretic, and gasping for air may have pulmonary edema. A patient with rhonchi or decreased breath sounds probably has aspiration pneumonia.
• Carefully monitor heart rate and rhythm. Because the patient's neurologic status may change as his body metabolizes the drug, frequently assess neurologic function.
• You may detect hypothermia or hyperthermia, so expect to use either extra blankets and a hyperthermia mattress or an antipyretic and a hypothermia mattress, as ordered.
• If the overdose was accidental, recommend a rehabilitation program for substance abuse. If it was intentional, refer the patient to crisis intervention for psychological counseling.

patients who have been using high doses of sedatives or hypnotics, have a history of withdrawal seizures or DTs, or have concurrent medical illnesses should undergo withdrawal in an inpatient setting.

Replacement therapy

The first step involves gradual reduction of the drug to prevent withdrawal and seizures. The benzodiazepine may be replaced gradually with another drug that has a similar action. A long-term benzodiazepine abuser with severe withdrawal symptoms (such as elevated vital signs or delirium) should receive an agent with a rapid onset, in doses sufficient to suppress withdrawal symptoms. I.V. lorazepam or diazepam is commonly given for their immediate results.

When stabilized, the patient is switched to an equivalent dose of a long-acting agent (such as phenobarbital), which causes milder withdrawal symptoms. He or she is tapered off this long-acting agent slowly over 2 to 6 months.

For mild benzodiazepine withdrawal symptoms, anticonvulsants that aren't cross dependent with sedative-hypnotics (such as carbamazepine and valproate) have been used successfully.

Recovery phase

After withdrawal comes a prolonged recovery and rehabilitation phase, in which the patient attempts to stay drug-free. The patient needs social support and involvement of his or her family and friends during this difficult stage.

Rehabilitation programs are available for both inpatients and outpatients. They usually last a month or longer and may include individual, group, and family psychotherapy. During and after rehabilitation, participation in a drug-oriented self-help group may be helpful.

Nursing interventions

Nursing interventions for a patient who abuses benzodiazepine are described in *General interventions for acute drug intoxication*, page 391.

New on the market

Synthetic cannabinoids (cannabicyclohexinol) go the street names of *K2*, *Spice*, and *Kronic*. Their actions are similar to cannabis.

Synthetic stimulants (mephedrone) go by the street names *Plant Food* and *Bath Salts*. These drugs are not the same substance as commercially available plant food or bath salts. They're just called that. They produce effects similar to other stimulants but are more dangerous.

These newer drugs do not show up on common urine drug screens, so always consider the possibility of drug intoxication when the symptoms are present and the urine is negative (Garmo, 2013; NIH, n.d.-a, n.d.-b).

References

Alcoholics Anonymous. (2014). *Alcoholics anonymous.* Retrieved from http://www.aa.org/

Garmo, M. (2013). Substance use disorders. In W. K. Mohr (Ed.), *Psychiatric-mental health nursing: Evidence-based concepts, skills, and practices* (pp. 619–659). Philadelphia, PA: Lippincott Williams & Wilkins.

Mayo Clinic. (2014). *Caffeine content for coffee, tea, soda and more.* Retrieved from http://www.mayoclinic.org/healthy-living/nutrition-and-healthy-eating/in-depth/caffeine/art-20049372

National Institutes of Health. (n.d.-a) *Drug facts.* Retrieved from http://www.drugabuse.gov/publications/finder/t/160/DrugFacts

National Institutes of Health. (n.d.-b). *Trends & statistics.* Retrieved from http://www.drugabuse.gov/related-topics/trends-statistics

Schneider, R. K., & Levenson, J. L. (2008). *Psychiatry essentials for primary care.* Philadelphia, PA: American College of Physicians.

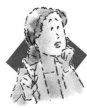

Quick quiz

1. When caring for a patient with alcoholism, the nurse understands that the expected effects of a disulfiram reaction include which of the following?

    A. Chest pain, chills, and hypertension
    B. Slow pulse, chills, and excitation
    C. Slow pulse, slow respiratory rate, and hypertension
    D. Chest pain, headache, and hypotension

Answer: D. A patient who consumes alcohol up to 2 weeks after taking disulfiram will experience a reaction that includes shortness of breath, chest pain, nausea, vomiting, facial flushing, headache, red eyes, blurred vision, sweating, tachycardia, hypotension, and fainting.

2. A patient admits to taking "crystal." The nurse is aware that this is a slang term for which of the following types of drugs?

    A. A depressant
    B. A stimulant
    C. A hallucinogen
    D. An antidepressant

Answer: B. "Crystal" is a street name for methamphetamine, a stimulant. Other amphetamines include amphetamine sulfate and dextroamphetamine.

3. The assessment finding that *most strongly* suggests I.V. drug abuse is which of the following?
- A. Skin lesions
- B. Gastritis
- C. Tachycardia
- D. Tachypnea

Answer: A. Self-injection of drugs can cause skin lesions or abscesses.

4. To treat tachycardia induced by cocaine, the nurse would expect to see which of the following medications ordered?
- A. Buprenorphine
- B. Digoxin
- C. Lidocaine
- D. Propranolol

Answer: D. Propranolol is typically given to treat tachycardia caused by cocaine use.

5. The nurse would expect to observe for the effects of LSD typically for what amount of time?
- A. 4 to 6 hours
- B. 6 to 8 hours
- C. 8 to 12 hours
- D. 14 to 16 hours

Answer: C. The duration of effect of LSD and most other hallucinogens is 8 to 12 hours.

6. When caring for a client with a narcotic overdose, the nurse would expect which antagonist to be ordered?
- A. Disulfiram
- B. Naloxone
- C. Diazepam
- D. Bupropion

Answer: B. Naloxone (Narcan) is a narcotic antagonist that displaces previously administered narcotic analgesics from CNS receptors.

Scoring

✩✩✩   If you answered all six items correctly, mind blowing! Your comprehension of substance abuse has given us quite a rush.

✩✩   If you answered four or five items correctly, far out! One more hit of this chapter may be all you need to achieve euphoria.

✩   If you answered fewer than four items correctly, don't get weirded out! Just abstain from all other activities until you complete a thorough review of this chapter.

12

Sleep disorders

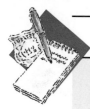

Just the facts

In this chapter, you'll learn:

♦ sleep stages and circadian rhythms

♦ types of sleep disorders and their causes

♦ assessment findings in patients with sleep disorders

♦ special procedures used to diagnose sleep disorders

♦ treatments and nursing interventions for patients with sleep disorders.

A look at sleep disorders

Sleep is a natural state of rest during which muscle movement and awareness of surroundings diminish. Sleep is necessary to restore energy and well-being, allowing us to function optimally the next day. Unlike other states resembling sleep (such as coma), sleep is easily interrupted—or prevented—by noise, light, and other external stimuli. Internal factors, such as stress and anxiety, can also decrease the amount and quality of sleep (Perry, Patil, & Presley-Cantrell, 2013; Silber, Krahn, & Morgenthaler, 2010).

At least 70 million people in the United States suffer from chronic sleeping problems. Nearly one-third of patients seen in primary care settings complain of occasional sleep difficulties (Centers for Disease Control and Prevention [CDC], 2013). Quality sleep is now recognized as a priority in national health as indicated in the sleep quality goals in Healthy People 2020. This chapter discusses the major sleep disorders—breathing-related sleep disorders, circadian rhythm sleep disorders, narcolepsy, hypersomnolence disorder, and insomnia disorder.

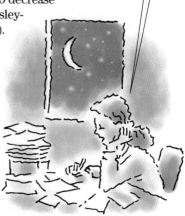

All of this research on sleep disorders is making me sleepy.

Causes

Sleep disorders may be primary or secondary to a medical or psychiatric disorder, substance use, or environmental factors. Medical conditions that can cause sleep disorders include Parkinson disease, Huntington disease, viral encephalitis, brain disease or injury, thyroid disease, and hormonal imbalances (Avidan & Zee, 2011; Reading, 2013).

Psychiatric disorders, such as depression and anxiety, are the most common cause of persistent insomnia. High levels of stress also may contribute to sleep disorders (Pagel & Pandi-Perumal, 2007).

Substances that can disrupt sleep include alcohol, caffeine, and prescription medications—most notably, antihistamines, corticosteroids, and central nervous system (CNS) drugs (Pagel & Pandi-Perumal, 2007).

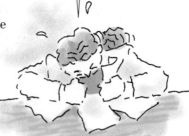

High levels of stress may contribute to sleep disorders. I guess I won't be getting much sleep tonight!

Impact of sleep disorders

Sleep disorders can lead to sleep deprivation, which can seriously interfere with a person's family life, occupation, driving ability, and social activities. In fact, medical costs related to sleep disorders amount to at least $16 billion annually—with even greater indirect costs incurred from such factors as lost productivity (CDC, 2013; Pagel and Pandi-Perumal, 2007).

Chronic sleep deprivation can cause or contribute to accidents, social and marital disruption, and psychiatric disturbances. It's also an independent risk factor for cardiovascular and gastrointestinal (GI) disorders (Pagel & Pandi-Perumal, 2007).

Driving while drowsy

Sleepy drivers and equipment operators cause many accidents. Experts believe sleepy drivers pose an even greater safety threat than alcoholic drivers (CDC, 2013).

At work, someone who isn't well rested can't perform at his best. Poor work performance can lead to corrective action and even job dismissal.

Dangerous deprivation

Sleep-deprived health care professionals are more likely to use poor judgment and make potentially life-threatening mistakes. Sleep-deprived factory workers may cause injury to themselves or others as well as contribute to the manufacture of defective products (CDC, 2012). Major environmental incidents linked to lack of sleep include the near-nuclear disaster of Three Mile Island in 1979, the nuclear meltdown at Chernobyl in 1986, and the oil spill of the Exxon Valdez in 1989.

Fuel for family feuds

Someone who doesn't sleep well is likely to feel tense, unhappy, and even depressed. These feelings can compromise healthy family relationships.

Sleep disturbances can have a direct impact on other family members' sleep patterns. For example, snoring may awaken the patient's spouse or prevent the spouse from falling asleep in the first place.

> Sleep occurs in five stages, growing progressively deeper with each stage.

Sleep stages

Sleep occurs in five stages. With each stage, sleep becomes deeper and brain waves grow progressively larger and slower, as shown by electroencephalography (EEG). Using an EEG to identify disruptions of these stages, through evaluation of the waves, can provide information about potential sleep disorders. (See *Sleep stages and brain waves*, page 448.) Throughout sleep, the person cycles through the different stages over and over again with the first cycle lasting approximately 100 to 120 minutes. Most people will go through five to seven cycles per night (Berry, 2012; Pagel & Pandi-Perumal, 2007).

Stage 1

The lightest stage of sleep, stage 1 occurs as a person falls asleep. The muscles relax and theta waves are produced that are fast and irregular. During this stage, the patient can be easily wakened by sounds, light, and other stimuli. Stage 1 accounts for approximately 5% of an adult's total sleep time and generally lasts around 10 to 15 minutes.

Stage 2

During stage 2, a relatively light stage of sleep, theta waves continue but become interspersed with sleep spindles (sudden increases in wave frequency) and K complexes (sudden increases in wave amplitude). Stage 2 comprises approximately 50% of total sleep time. In this stage, the muscles relax more as the body prepares for deep sleep.

Stages 3 and 4

Stages 3 and 4 are the deepest stages of sleep. Delta waves—large, slow waves of high amplitude and low frequency—appear on the EEG. Stage 3 and stage 4 differ only in the percentage of delta waves seen: During stage 3, delta waves account for less than 50% of brain waves, whereas during stage 4, they account for more than 50%.

Sleep stages and brain waves

Each sleep stage generates distinctive brain waves, as measured by EEG.

During stage 1, which occurs as a person falls asleep, fast, irregular, low-amplitude brain waves called *theta waves* appear on the EEG.

During stage 2, theta waves are interspersed with wave phenomena called *sleep spindles* and *K complexes*.

During stages 3 and 4, the EEG shows large, slow, high-amplitude waves called *delta waves*.

During stage 5, called *rapid eye movement (REM) sleep*, short, rapid brain waves appear.

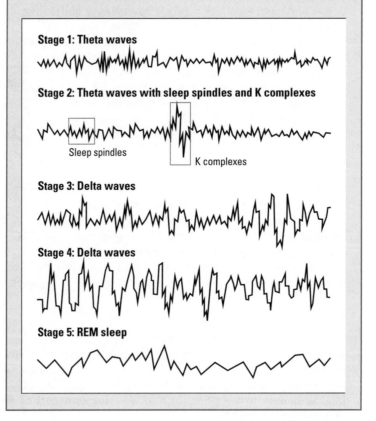

Stage 1: Theta waves

Stage 2: Theta waves with sleep spindles and K complexes

Sleep spindles

K complexes

Stage 3: Delta waves

Stage 4: Delta waves

Stage 5: REM sleep

Conserve as you sleep

Arousing a sleeper from stage 3 or 4 is harder than during any other stage. Because these stages are marked by decreased body temperature and metabolism, researchers believe they function to conserve energy. They account for 10% to 20% of total sleep time. As night fades into morning, stages 3 and 4 get progressively shorter. During the last few cycles of the sleep period, no delta-wave sleep occurs at all.

Stage 5

Stage 5 is a deep sleep called *rapid eye movement sleep*. During this stage, the sleeper shows darting eye movements; muscle twitching; and short, rapid brain waves resembling those seen during the waking state. (See *Sleep stages and brain waves*.)

REM sleep usually begins about 90 minutes after sleep onset. Over the course of the night, REM periods lengthen. Overall, REM sleep accounts for 20% to 25% of total sleep time.

To sleep, perchance to dream

Most story-like dreams take place during REM sleep. People awakened from REM sleep commonly report vivid dreams. In contrast, people awakened during stages 1 through 4 rarely report vivid dreams.

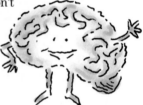

REM is my friend! Scientists think REM sleep may stimulate brain growth.

Functions of REM and NREM sleep

Scientists believe REM and non-rapid eye movement (NREM) sleep serve different biological functions, although they don't know exactly what these functions are. REM sleep may stimulate brain growth or consolidate memory. A person deprived of REM sleep tends to have longer REM cycles during the next sleep episode. These longer REM cycles are more intense, with more eye movements per minute.

Make-up sleep

Similarly, people deprived of NREM sleep have longer NREM sleep during the next sleep period—and the "make-up" NREM sleep produces different EEG patterns than normal NREM sleep.

Neurologic regulation of sleep stages

The various sleep stages are influenced by different parts of the brain. REM sleep is controlled by the pons (a part of the brainstem) and adjacent portions of the midbrain. Chemical stimulation of the pons may induce long periods of REM sleep, whereas damage to the pons may reduce or prevent REM sleep.

Paralysis and the pons

During REM sleep, neurons in the pons and midbrain that control muscle tone show various levels of activity: Some are active, whereas others aren't. Reflecting this variable activity, certain body muscles remain inactive during REM sleep—especially those of the back, neck, arms, and legs. As a result, the sleeper is effectively paralyzed and can't act out dreams. However, if these regulatory neurons malfunction, the sleeper may be more active during dreams, thrashing about or becoming violent.

Baths and the basal forebrain

The basal forebrain, located in front of the hypothalamus, controls NREM sleep. Damage to this region of the brain may cause difficulty falling or staying asleep. Some neurons in the basal forebrain are activated by heat, which may explain the sleep-promoting benefits of taking a warm bath in the evening.

Factors that affect sleep

Factors affecting sleep quality and quantity include the patient's age, lifestyle, sleep environment, and medication use.

Age

Amounts and patterns of sleep differ at each major stage of the life cycle. Both REM and NREM sleep periods decrease with age.

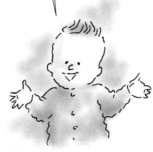

> Newborns need their sleep! On average, they sleep 17 to 18 hours a day.

Newborns and toddlers

Newborns sleep the most, averaging 17 to 18 hours a day, with REM accounting for roughly half of total sleep time.

Go to sleep-y, little baby

At first, a newborn sleeps in episodes of 3 to 4 hours. Gradually, by about age 3 or 4 months, the infant begins to get more sleep at night. A 6-month old typically sleeps 12 hours a night and naps 1 to 2 hours each day.

Toddlers sleep about 11 or 12 hours a night, with a 1- to 2-hour nap after lunch. Nap requirements vary, with some children taking naps up to age 5.

By age 5, children typically sleep 10 to 12 hours a day, with REM sleep accounting for about 20% of the total.

Tweens and teens

Preadolescents need about 10 hours of sleep. Adolescent requirements aren't well defined. Many teenagers get too little sleep because of their busy schedules and academic pressures. Growth spurts can result in an increased need for sleep (George & Davis, 2013).

Young adults

A typical young adult needs about 8 hours of sleep, although the requirement varies widely. Some young adults need as little as 6 or 7 hours, whereas others may need 9 or 10 hours to function

Myth busters

Sleep requirements of elderly adults

Another misconception about elderly adults bites the dust.
Myth: Elderly adults need much less sleep than younger adults.
Reality: Sleep requirements increase in the elderly because they tend
to get decreased amounts of deep sleep and suffer frequent sleep
interruptions.

optimally. Lifestyle choices make this group vulnerable to sleep
disturbances (Vallido, Peters, O'Brien, & Jackson, 2009).

Middle-aged adults

In middle-aged adults, sleep requirements may remain unchanged
from those of the young adult years. Typical sleep disturbances
during middle age may stem from hormonal changes in women,
breathing-related disorders, and insomnia.

Elderly adults

Sleep problems are common among elderly adults
(Pandi-Perumal, Monti, & Monjan, 2010; Valenza et al., 2013).
Besides taking longer to fall asleep, they spend less time in deep
NREM sleep, so their sleep is more easily interrupted or
fragmented. (See *Sleep requirements of elderly adults.*)

Bathroom breaks

Early awakening is also common and may result from an
earlier rise in body temperature. Finally, many seniors have
trouble falling back to sleep after awakening to urinate.

Environment

The sleep environment can greatly affect
sleep quality. Environmental influences
on sleep include noise, bright lights
or sunlight, excessive activity, and an
uncomfortable room temperature. When
these influences are prominent, sleep can
be difficult even for someone who is
sleepy. Removing such stimuli produces
an environment that's more conducive to
sleeping.

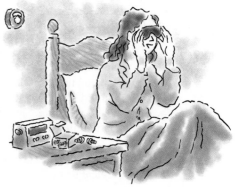

Darkness, silence,
and a comfortable
room temperature
promote sleep.

Lifestyle

Travel, shift work, stress, and anxiety can greatly influence sleep. A person who travels through different time zones may suffer jet lag, which is worse when traveling west to east. A "jet-setter" typically tries to sleep when he or she isn't tired (traveling west to east) and tries to stay awake when it's daylight (traveling east to west).

Night shift blues

Up to 20% of night shift workers experience problems with sleep due to disruption of the body's natural rhythms.

Medications and substances

Medications of any kind may alter sleep patterns. Prescription drugs may cause somnolence (drowsiness) at inappropriate times; some may cause insomnia. Illicit drugs may also disturb established sleep patterns (Kohli, Sarmiento, & Malhotra, 2013).

Alcohol

Although alcohol initially may increase the amount of slow-wave sleep, it later causes sleep disruptions.

Alcohol's effect on sleep varies with the amount and time of consumption. In nonalcoholics, alcohol may have a sedative effect, increasing the amount of slow-wave sleep for the first 4 hours after sleep onset. After alcohol's effects wear off, sleep may be disrupted, with an increased amount of REM sleep and anxiety-causing dreams.

Alcoholics may have trouble falling asleep and staying asleep. Many have REM sleep disturbances.

Withdrawal woes

During alcohol withdrawal, sleep deprivation is common. When sleep occurs, it's usually fragmented and accompanied by nightmares and anxiety-causing dreams.

Approach to assessment

The most important symptoms of sleep disturbances are insomnia at night (the most common symptom) and sleepiness during waking hours. A thorough medical and psychological history should be obtained from a patient who complains of sleep problems. The family may also need to be questioned because the patient may be unaware of sleep behavior.

Sometimes, a physical examination is also warranted. Because sleep disorders are commonly linked to mood disorders, psychological tests may be administered as well.

Breathing-related sleep disorders

Breathing-related sleep disorders are marked by abnormal breathing during sleep. Obstructive sleep apnea hypopnea syndrome (OSAHS) is the most common breathing-related sleep disorder. Other disorders in this category include central sleep apnea syndrome and central alveolar hypoventilation syndrome (McCabe & Hardinge, 2011).

Breathing blockade

In OSAHS, the upper airway becomes blocked during sleep, impeding airflow. Reduced airway muscle tone and the pull of gravity in the supine position further limit airway size during sleep. As tissue collapse worsens, the airway may become completely obstructed. (See *Airway obstruction during sleep apnea*, page 454.)

With either partial or complete airway obstruction, the patient struggles to breathe. Blockage of airflow lasts 10 seconds to 1 minute and arouses the patient from sleep as the brain responds to decreased blood oxygen levels. (However, arousal is commonly partial and goes unrecognized by the patient.)

I hear a symphony . . . of snoring. That patient needs to be checked for sleep apnea.

Snoring, then silence

This pattern causes disturbed and fragmented sleep, with periods of loud snoring or gasping when the airway is partly open alternating with silence when the airway is blocked. (However, not everyone who snores has OSAHS.)

With arousal, the muscle tone of the tongue and airway tissues increases, causing the patient to awaken just enough to tighten the upper airway muscles and open the windpipe. However, when falling back to sleep, the tongue and soft tissue relax again—and the cycle begins anew. This cycle may repeat hundreds of times each night (McCabe & Hardinge, 2011).

Complications

Repetitive cycles of snoring, airway collapse, and arousal may lead to cardiovascular problems—high blood pressure, arrhythmias, and even myocardial infarction or stroke. In some high-risk patients, sleep apnea may lead to sudden death from respiratory arrest during sleep (Kohli, Sarmiento, & Malhotra, 2013).

Drowsy, irritable, and indifferent

Frequent awakenings leave the patient sleepy during the day and can cause irritability or depression. The patient may suffer morning headaches, decreased mental functioning, and a reduced sex drive.

Airway obstruction during sleep apnea

In a patient with obstructive sleep apnea, the airway is blocked by increased tissue of the soft palate or tongue, increased amounts of fat around the pharynx, or a small or receding jaw that leaves too little room for the tongue.

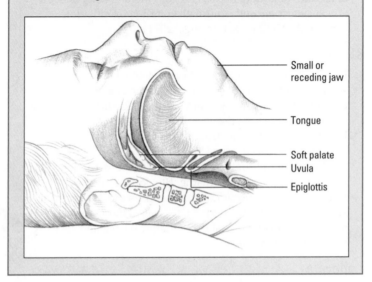

Small or receding jaw

Tongue

Soft palate
Uvula
Epiglottis

People with severe, untreated sleep apnea have two or three times the risk of motor vehicle accidents.

Exhibit A: Note the short, thick neck and fat around the pharynx. These features contribute to sleep apnea.

Prevalence

OSAHS affects approximately 2% to 3% of the population. Incidence rises with age—especially after age 50. It's most common in overweight, middle-aged men but can affect females and males of any age. In women, menopause is a significant precipitating factor (McCabe & Hardinge, 2011).

Causes

Most patients with OSAHS are overweight with a short, thick neck and fat infiltration around the pharynx that increases the risk of airway blockage. Some have an unusually large soft palate and tongue.

Apnea and anatomy

In people who aren't overweight, OSAHS typically results from a small or receding jaw that leaves insufficient room for the tongue. Other structural causes of OSAHS include malformations of the oropharynx or jaw and tumors and other growths that narrow the airway. Among elderly adults, loss of muscle tone may contribute to the condition (McCabe & Hardinge, 2011).

Rotational forces

People with rotating work schedules may be at higher risk for OSAHS. The use of alcohol or sedatives may increase the frequency and length of apneic periods.

Signs and symptoms

Patient with OSAHS typically report chronic daytime sleepiness. Some also report snoring, which may be pronounced enough to disturb the sleep of other household members. In fact, the patient may not be aware of heavy snoring and nocturnal arousals, so the nurse may need to question family members about these symptoms (American Academy of Sleep Medicine, 2001; McCabe & Hardinge, 2011).

Other symptoms in a patient with OSAHS include:
- frequent headaches
- general feeling of tiredness and fatigue
- frequent daytime naps (which usually aren't effective in restoring energy)
- irritability
- difficulty paying attention
- learning or memory problems
- depression
- excessive urination at night
- impotence
- heartburn or acid indigestion (suggesting esophageal reflux).

Body reconnaissance

During the physical examination, stay alert for:
- obesity
- hypertension
- jaw malformation
- signs and symptoms of tumors or other tissue abnormalities
- reduced chest excursion (from obesity)
- indications of cardiovascular and cerebrovascular conditions.

Diagnosis

Polysomnography, a sleep study performed in a sleep laboratory, is the gold standard for diagnosing OSAHS.

> Polysomnography is a sleep study used to evaluate patients for sleep disorders.

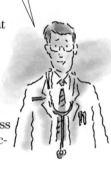

Treatment

Treatments for OSAHS include lifestyle changes, continuous positive airway pressure (CPAP) therapy, and dental devices that modify tongue or jaw position.

Lifestyle changes

Lifestyle changes—especially weight loss—are the simplest treatments for OSAHS. Weight loss reduces the amount of excess tissue in and around the airway. Decreasing the body mass index to 30 or less significantly reduces the frequency of obstructive sleep episodes. However, even small weight reductions can improve the patient's condition.

Supine is not sublime

Sleeping on the side rather than in a supine (back-lying) position may reduce apneic episodes. Avoiding alcohol and sleeping pills can decrease the number and duration of these episodes.

> If you hear snoring during a nap, make way for CPAP!

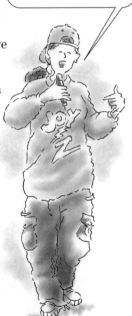

Continuous positive airway pressure

CPAP therapy during sleep is the most common and effective treatment for OSAHS. Positive pressure splints the airway open, preventing its collapse. The desired level of pressure varies with the type of CPAP device used. The patient wears either a full facial mask or a nasal mask.

Dental devices

Oral appliances worn during sleep may help to relieve airway obstruction. However, they may be uncomfortable for some patients and may cause excessive salivation.

Surgery

Surgical procedures used to correct OSAHS include:
• tonsil and adenoid removal, which increases the size of the pharynx
• removal of any growths or nasal polyps obstructing the airway
• correction of jaw abnormalities
• uvulopalatopharyngoplasty—surgical revision of the uvula, tonsils, soft palate, and soft tissues of the oropharynx

Polysomnography: It knows when you're asleep

Polysomnography is an overnight sleep study, performed in a special laboratory or a sleep center that measures various physiologic functions related to sleep and wakefulness. Sensor leads and other detectors are placed on the patient to gather the following information:

• Brain wave activity, recorded by EEG. The EEG reveals the stage of sleep that the patient is in during any given period.

• Eye movements, recorded by electrooculography (EOG). EOG determines when the patient is experiencing REM sleep. Along with the EEG, it also helps determine how long it takes the patient to fall asleep, total sleep time, time spent in each sleep stage, and the number of arousals from sleep.

• Muscle movements, measured by electromyography (EMG). The EMG recording helps document wakeful periods, arousal, or spastic movements.

• Respiratory effort, which determines chest and abdominal excursion during breathing. Velcro bands are placed around the patient's chest and around the abdomen and connected to a transducer. The force of chest and abdominal expansion on the bands stretches the transducer and alters the signal to a recorder.

• Oxygen saturation, recorded by a pulse oximeter probe placed on the finger, earlobe, or other appropriate site, to determine oxygen starvation during an apneic episode.

• Electrocardiography (ECG), which can reveal whether low oxygen saturation during apneic episodes leads to arrhythmias. The ECG also alerts the technician to any emergency condition.

• Airflow, recorded by a thermistor secured to the patient's nose. The thermistor detects the amount of air moving into and out of the airways, thus revealing apneic or hypopneic (inadequate breathing) episodes.

• Blood pressure, to detect dangerous blood pressure elevations (sometimes causes by apneic episodes).

Optional monitoring includes core body temperature, penile tumescence, and the pressure and pH at various esophageal levels. Information gathered from all the leads and sensors is fed into a computer and transformed into a series of waveform tracings.

Smile for the camera

The patient may be videotaped so the technician can determine whether any abnormal waveforms were caused by an actual arousal, a period of wakefulness, or normal movement in bed. Sound recordings may be made to evaluate snoring.

Sleep latency testing

The day after polysomnography, the patient may undergo multiple sleep latency testing (MSLT) to evaluate excessive daytime sleepiness or narcolepsy. MSLT records sleep patterns (including napping) throughout the day.

MSLT usually involves five testing periods spaced about 2 hours apart. For each testing period, the patient is taken to a "sleeping" room, where electrodes are attached to the face and scalp to record eye movements, muscle tone, and brain waves.

Then the lights are turned off and the patient is asked to sleep for 15 to 20 minutes, during which recordings are taken. The technician awakens the patient after the testing period. Even if the patient can't sleep during the test, the information can be useful. All told, MSLT takes about 8 hours.

Nursing interventions

These nursing interventions may be appropriate for a patient with OSAHS:

• Remember the patient is likely to be tired and irritable. Be helpful and supportive.

• If the patient reports associated symptoms, such as esophageal reflux, nocturia, or impotence, refer for appropriate treatment.

• Assist the patient in a weight loss program, if indicated.

• Urge the patient to stop smoking, if indicated.

• Encourage the patient to avoid alcohol and illicit drug use.

• Help family members deal with issues related to the patient's snoring.

Circadian rhythm sleep disorder

In circadian rhythm sleep disorder, the patient's internal sleep-wake pattern is out of synch with the demands of work schedule, travel requirements, or social activities. The result is insomnia and sleepiness.

Circadian lullaby

Circadian refers to biological rhythms with a cycle of about 24 hours. (*Circadian* comes from the Latin phrase "circa diem," meaning "about a day.") The circadian rhythm functions as the body's internal "clock," regulating the 24-hour sleep-wake cycle and other body functions, such as body temperature, hormones, and heart rate. (See *Tick tock, it's the body clock.*)

The body's internal clock can reset itself to help a person adjust to such disturbances as seasonal changes, transitions to or from daylight savings time, or the start of a new workweek. However, it can't always overcome longer lasting disruptions resulting from shift work or jet lag (air travel across time zones).

The body's internal clock governs the sleep-wake cycles and many other body functions.

Weirded-out rhythms

Disruption of circadian rhythms may cause sleep difficulties, fatigue, a short attention span, impaired cognitive abilities (such as poor judgment and decision making), and even GI disorders (Elder, Wetherell, Barclay, & Ellis, 2013).

Tick tock, it's the body clock

The human body has an internal "clock" that follows a 24-hour cycle of wakefulness and sleepiness. This clock runs on circadian rhythms, which are linked to nature's cycle of light and darkness.

Critical organs, such as the heart, liver, and kidneys, have their own "clocks" that work in a coordinated fashion with the body's master clock. Researchers know, for example, that certain cardiac events, such as heart attacks and sudden cardiac death, occur more often during specific times of the circadian cycle.

Lark versus owl

The body's clock keeps us alert during daylight hours and makes us sleepy when night falls. All of our physiologic functions are geared toward being active during the day and resting at night. The desire to sleep is strongest between 12 and 6 a.m.

Nonetheless, individual patterns of alertness vary, explaining why some people are relatively more alert during the day ("larks"), whereas others are more alert at night ("night owls").

Mighty melatonin

The body's internal clock is regulated by melatonin, a hormone that causes sleepiness. Melatonin is secreted by the pineal gland, a structure located in the roof of the brain's third ventricle. Influenced by light, the pineal gland slows melatonin production during daylight hours to promote alertness and increases production when darkness falls, causing sleepiness.

With age, the body produces less melatonin. Not surprisingly, many elderly adults suffer from sleep disorders. Some pharmacologic therapies try to increase the level of melatonin or enhance its effectiveness to try and readjust the internal clock.

Types of circadian rhythm sleep-wake disorders

The main types of circadian rhythm sleep-wake disorders include the delayed sleep phase, advanced sleep phase, irregular sleep-wake, non-24-hour sleep-wake, and shift work type (American Psychiatric Association [APA], 2013).

Delayed sleep phase

In delayed sleep phase sleep disorder, the patient sleeps according to a delayed clock time, relative to the light-dark cycle and social, economic, and family demands. Typically, there is trouble falling asleep until the early hours of morning and the patient ends up sleeping through much of the day. This disorder often begins in childhood and is relatively common among adolescents. These patients may consider themselves "night owls."

Advanced sleep phase

With advanced sleep phase sleep disorder, the patient is unable to stay awake in the evening and consistently awakens very early. These patients may consider themselves "early birds or larks."

Non-24-hour sleep-wake

In the non-24-hour sleep-wake pattern disorder, the patient will experience a sleep-wake cycle that does not correlate with a typical 24-hour environment. For these patients, sleep is characterized by a daily drift towards later sleep and wake times (APA, 2013).

Shift work

In the shift work sleep disorder, night shift work or frequently changing shift work causes insomnia during the major sleep period or excessive sleepiness during the major awake period. The patient typically suffers chronic sleep disruption.

Asleep on the job

Few, if any, night workers regularly get restful restorative day sleep. An estimated 10% to 20% of night workers report falling asleep on the job, usually during the second half of the shift. Twenty percent of the U.S. workforce is engaged in shift work, placing them at risk for circadian rhythm disorders (Boyd, 2012).

Prevalence

The prevalence of circadian rhythm sleep disorders is unclear. However, there are estimates associated with night shift workers that range from 5% to 10%. Prevalence is also indicated to increase with age (APA, 2013).

Causes

A circadian rhythm sleep disorder results from intrinsic factors such as delayed sleep phases or extrinsic factors such as jet lag or shift work.

Signs and symptoms

Assessment findings vary with the type of circadian rhythm sleep disorder.

Symptoms in delayed sleep phase type

Patients with delayed sleep phase may report:
- inability to fall asleep before 2 a.m. to 6 a.m.
- difficulty awakening in the morning
- feeling of being sleep deprived
- significant social or work impairment
- need for multiple means to awaken (several alarm clocks, other persons, telephone wake-up calls, or a combination of these).

Symptoms in shift work type

Patients with shift work type commonly report:
- sleepiness while performing their jobs, especially if working nights
- insufficient daytime sleep because of family or social demands or environmental disturbances
- significant social or work impairment.

Diagnosis

The patient's history may suggest a circadian rhythm sleep disorder. A sleep diary or wrist-worn motion/sleep detector may be used to assist in diagnosis. The diagnosis is confirmed through comparison of the history with a set of established diagnostic criteria (APA, 2013).

Treatment

Various treatments have been used for circadian rhythm disorders.

Chronotherapy

Chronotherapy involves manipulating the patient's sleep schedule by progressively delaying bedtime by one or more hours each night until the patient can go to sleep and wake up at appropriate times. Chronotherapy is most commonly used to treat delayed sleep phase sleep.

Luminotherapy

Luminotherapy is the use of bright light to manipulate the circadian system. Typically administered with light boxes, it's safe and effective when used according to recommendations.

The value of nursing assessment

Many times, the nurse is the first to identify that a sleep disorder may be an issue for a patient. Over time, patients become used to living in a constant state of feeling "tired." In addition, because lack of sleep isn't often recognized as a problem, patients will minimize feeling tired and chalk it up to lifestyle or life demands. When asked appropriate questions, the data emerge that can show trends in sleeping patterns.

Sleep disorder assessment questions:
1. Do you have difficulty falling asleep?
2. Do you feel tired when you wake up?
3. Do you take medication to help you sleep or stay awake?
4. What is your caffeine intake on a normal day?
5. Do you feel sleepy at "normal" sleep times?
6. When do you prefer to sleep and does this coincide with your work and social schedule?

Here comes the sun

For patients with delayed sleep phase–type sleep-wake disorder, some doctors recommend exposure to bright light on awakening. Sunlight exposure for night shift workers or jet travelers at their destination may help reset the circadian clock to environmental time.

> Sunlight exposure can help a night shift worker or jet-setter adjust the body clock.

Chronopharmacotherapy

Chronopharmacotherapy involves the use of drugs to induce sleep or promote wakefulness when desired. Short-acting sedative-hypnotic drugs may be used to promote sleep, especially when associated with jet lag.

Many night shift workers use caffeine to keep themselves awake on the job. However, some become tolerant to caffeine's effects over time.

Mellowing out with melatonin

Supplemental melatonin therapy has been studied recently as a treatment for circadian rhythm sleep disorders. Data is limited regarding effectiveness of melatonin therapy. However, recent research into prolonged use of melatonin has shown some promise (Halter & Varcarolis, 2014).

Bypassing jet lag

To prevent jet lag, some experts suggest travelers try to reach their destination by early evening and go to sleep around 10 p.m. local time. To prepare their bodies for the change, they should go to sleep at the new bedtime for a few days before the trip. Avoiding alcohol and caffeine in-flight may help minimize jet lag.

Nursing interventions

These nursing interventions may be appropriate for a patient with a circadian rhythm sleep disorder:
• Be sure to include a thorough assessment that includes sleep pattern and wake pattern assessment.
• To promote compliance with sleep interventions, review the required procedures with the patient. Assess understanding of these procedures.
• If the patient is using chronotherapy, ensure patient knows how to adjust bedtime correctly.
• Teach the patient about purpose, administration, and adverse effects of prescribed drugs such as sedative-hypnotics. Monitor for adverse effects.
• If the patient is taking a herbal supplement such as melatonin, reinforce this product isn't always manufactured under quality-controlled conditions.

Narcolepsy

Narcolepsy is characterized by sudden, uncontrollable attacks of deep sleep lasting up to 20 minutes. These "sleep attacks" come on without warning and may be accompanied by paralysis and hallucinations. Although the brief sleep is refreshing, the urge to sleep soon returns.

Sleep paralysis and hallucinations typically occur during sleep onset (hypnagogic hallucinations) or during the transition from sleep to wakefulness (hypnopompic hallucinations). Mostly visual, these hallucinations are intense, dreamlike images commonly involving the immediate environment.

A confounding cataplexy

About 70% of patients with narcolepsy experience attacks of cataplexy—sudden loss of muscle tone and strength. (In more subtle forms of cataplexy, the patient's head may drop or jaw may slacken.)

Cataplexy is commonly triggered by emotions—for example, the knees may buckle after the patient laughs, gets angry, or feels elated or surprised. Cataplexy typically lasts just a few seconds, and the patient remains alert during the episode. However, in severe cases, the patient falls down and becomes completely paralyzed for up to several minutes.

Complications

Narcoleptic sleep attacks may occur at any time of day. All too often, they occur during activities that call for undivided attention, such as driving.

Image problems

Besides causing accidents, narcolepsy can be disabling, impairing work performance and disrupting leisure activities and interpersonal relationships. Coworkers may perceive the patient as lazy; an employer may suspect illegal drug use.

Jeers from their peers

In children, narcolepsy impairs school performance and social relationships and invites ridicule from peers. Teenagers with the disorder are at increased risk for automobile accidents.

Prevalence and onset

Narcolepsy is not rare, as it is estimated to occur in 1 out of every 3,000 people. However, it is also believed to be underrecognized and underdiagnosed (National Institute of Neurological Disorders and Stroke, 2014).

Narcolepsy is the second leading cause of daytime sleepiness diagnosed in sleep centers. (OSAHS is the most common.) The disorder affects males and females equally. The usual onset is during young adulthood and can be abrupt or progressive in nature (APA, 2013).

Causes

The exact cause of narcolepsy is unknown. However, most patients with narcolepsy have a deficit in the neurotransmitter hypocretin, which helps people stay awake (National Institute of Neurological Disorders and Stroke, 2014). Narcolepsy isn't related to the amount of sleep a person gets.

> If someone you know is a narcoleptic, you might see him with his arm raised like this after suffering from an episode of sleep paralysis.

Signs and symptoms

Assessment findings in narcolepsy include:
- excessive daytime sleepiness, even during active states, such as eating and talking
- cataplexy
- brief episodes of sleep paralysis (inability to move or speak when falling asleep or waking up)
- dreamlike hallucinations at sleep onset or when awakening from sleep
- disturbed nighttime sleep, such as tossing and turning, leg jerks, nightmares, frequent awakenings, and abnormal REM sleep.

Diagnosis

A history of excessive daytime sleepiness, uncontrollable sleep, and observed cataplexy strongly suggests narcolepsy. However, other possible causes of excessive daytime sleepiness—heart disease, brain tumors, anemia, and depression, to name a few—must be ruled out.

Napping on demand

Overnight polysomnography and an MSLT may be performed. After these naps, the time required to fall asleep (sleep latency) is averaged. In narcolepsy, sleep latency is less than 8 minutes. Diagnosis is confirmed by using the diagnostic criteria in the *Diagnostic and Statistical Manual of Mental Disorders*, 5th Edition (*DSM-5*), and can be further classified as mild, moderate, or severe (APA, 2013).

Treatment

Although no cure exists for narcolepsy, symptoms can be controlled with behavioral and pharmacologic interventions. Behavioral interventions include lifestyle adjustments, such as regulating sleep schedules and taking daytime naps.

A stimulating strategy

Symptomatic treatment is focused on excessive somnolence and cataplexy. CNS stimulants may be prescribed (such as methylphenidate [Concerta] or modafinil [Provigil]) to decrease daytime sleepiness and antidepressants (such as imipramine [Tofranil] or fluoxetine [Prozac]) to reduce cataplectic attacks. (See *Modafinil: Narcolepsy treatment.*) The disturbance doesn't result from direct physiologic effects of a substance or another general medical condition.

Nursing interventions

These interventions may be appropriate for a patient with narcolepsy:
- Review recommended lifestyle changes.
- Help the patient plan and maintain a regular sleep schedule.

Meds matters

Modafinil: Narcolepsy treatment

A CNS stimulant that promotes wakefulness and alertness, modafinil (Provigil) is used to prevent excessive daytime sleepiness in patients with narcolepsy. When taken as directed, it doesn't interfere with nighttime sleep.

Modafinil seems to be safe, effective, and well tolerated. It's less likely than traditional stimulants (such as amphetamines and methylphenidate) to cause jitteriness, anxiety, excessive motor activity, or a rebound effect. The drug may cause mild psychological dependence.

How it works
Modafinil is a central alpha-1 adrenergic agonist that induces wakefulness partly through its action in the brain's hypothalamus. It acts selectively through the brain's sleep-wake center, stimulating the patient only when stimulation is required and avoiding the highs and lows caused by other stimulants such as amphetamine.

How it's given
The standard dosage is 200 mg/day, given as a single dose in the morning. Adverse effects typically are mild and may include headache, anxiety, nervousness, insomnia, nausea, and infection.

Nursing considerations
- Teach the patient about the drug, including the dosage, purpose, administration, and adverse effects.
- Monitor the patient for adverse effects.
- Instruct the patient not to drive or operate other complex machinery until understanding how the drug affects ability to function.
- Advise patient to avoid alcohol while using this drug.
- Tell patient to call the prescriber if the following develop: skin rash, hives, or an allergic reaction.
- Know that patients with severe hepatic impairment should receive one-half of the standard dosage.
- Be aware that elderly patients may need a decreased dosage.
- Don't give this drug to patients who have a history of cardiovascular disease or are taking oral contraceptives, cyclosporine, theophylline, diazepam, phenytoin, warfarin, or propranolol.

- Discuss the need for ample sleep opportunity with the patient.
- Teach about the purpose, administration, and adverse effects of prescribed drugs.
- Monitor for adverse effects.

> Even after 12 hours of sleep, a patient with hypersomnia may feel drowsy during the day.

Hypersomnolence disorder

Hypersomnia is a condition of excessive sleepiness characterized by either prolonged sleep periods at night or daytime sleep episodes occurring nearly every day. During long periods of drowsiness, the patient may exhibit automatic behavior, acting in a semicontrolled fashion. There may be trouble meeting morning obligations, frequently arriving late (Gulyani, Salas, & Gamaldo, 2013). The diagnosis of hypersomnolence disorder is reserved for those patients who have no other direct cause of daytime sleepiness such as OSAHS or narcolepsy (Boyd, 2012, p. 632).

Signs and symptoms

The primary symptom associated with hypersomnolence disorder is feeling tired to the point where the feeling interferes with the activities of daily living. Patients may report extended sleep periods at night or the desire to sleep or nap frequently during the day. In some cases, morning behavior can resemble "drunkenness" in the manifestation of confusion, disorientation, poor motor coordination, and slowness on awakening (Boyd, 2012; Gulyani et al., 2013).

Prevalence

The prevalence of hypersomnolence disorder in the general population isn't known. In sleep disorder clinics, an estimated 5% to 10% of patients are diagnosed with this disorder.

"Hypersomnolence fully manifests in most cases in late adolescence or early adulthood, with a mean age at onset of 17 to 24 years. Individuals with hypersomnolence disorders are diagnosed, on average, 10 to 15 years AFTER the appearance of the first symptoms" (APA, 2013, p. 370).

Causes

Based on the underlying cause of the disorder, experts have identified two possible risk and prognostic factors.

Environmental

Alcohol use and psychological stress can lead to increased hypersomnolence on a temporary basis. In addition, viral infections such as HIV pneumonia, mononucleosis, and Guillain-Barré syndrome can also lead to hypersomnolence (APA, 2013). Even after the infectious process resolves, these patients continue to need significantly more nighttime sleep and feel very tired.

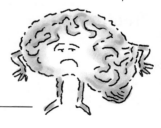

A viral infection with neurologic symptoms has been linked to some cases of hypersomnia.

Genetic and Physiologic

There may be a genetic modality associated with hypersomnolence, as there are familial patterns inherited (APA, 2013).

Signs and symptoms

In patients with hypersomnolence disorder, assessment findings typically include:
- excessive sleepiness on a daily basis
- daytime napping without feeling refreshed
- long nighttime sleeping (8 to 12 hours)
- difficulty awakening in the morning.

Many patients also complain of irritability, mild depression, memory loss, headache, poor concentration, impaired performance, fainting episodes, and dizziness on standing (from orthostatic hypotension). A few report hypnagogic hallucinations and sleep paralysis.

Diagnosis

Physical examination, a complete blood cell count, and thyroid-stimulating hormone tests may rule out other possible causes of excessive sleepiness or prolonged nocturnal sleep, including:
- OSAHS
- circadian rhythm sleep-wake disorders
- narcolepsy
- thyroid abnormalities
- chronic pain
- CNS disorders, damage, or malfunction
- viral infection
- primary depression
- medication withdrawal
- adverse drug effects.

Out like a light

Polysomnography typically reveals short sleep latency, long sleep duration, and a normal sleep pattern.

Diagnosis is confirmed by using the diagnostic criteria in the *DSM-5* and can be further classified as acute, subacute, or persistent. The level of severity can also be determined as mild, moderate, or severe (APA, 2013).

Treatment

Treatment focuses on relieving symptoms and may include behavioral approaches, sleep hygiene techniques, and pharmacologic interventions.

Awake and wired

Drugs used to treat hypersomnolence disorder include antidepressants and stimulants (such as modafinil [Provigil], methylphenidate [Concerta], and dextroamphetamine [Dextrostat]). Stimulants are the only effective agents, although they often bring partial relief. Typically, the patient is maintained on daily stimulants, with the dosage titrated so the patient can stay alert during the day (Gulyani, Salas, & Gamaldo, 2013). These medications, in the stimulant category, are controlled substances and abuse of these medications can occur and should be assessed.

> Many patients with hypersomnia rely on caffeine to keep them perky.

Java jolt therapy

Self-medicating with caffeine is probably the most commonly tried treatment. Caffeine temporarily improves psychomotor performance and increases alertness.

- Teach patient about prescribed drugs; include purpose, administration, and adverse effects.
- Caution the patient about driving or using dangerous machinery when drowsy. Help develop an alternate plan, such as taking public transportation or carpooling.
- Inform the patient that excessive caffeine may cause anxiety, irritability, jitteriness, and tolerance.
- Provide information on the causative ties between excessive caffeine intake and angina.

Insomnia Disorder

The most common sleep disorder of insomnia encompasses many types of problems—difficulty falling asleep, sleeping too lightly, frequent awakenings during the night, inability to fall back to sleep once awakened, and waking up in the early morning and being unable to fall back to sleep.

Obsessing over insomnia

Insomnia can be episodic, persistent, or recurrent. With persistent insomnia, the person may become preoccupied with getting enough sleep. The more the patient tries to sleep, the greater the sense of frustration and distress—and the more elusive sleep becomes.

Consequences

Insomnia commonly leads to daytime drowsiness that causes poor concentration, memory impairments, difficulty coping with minor problems, and reduced ability to enjoy family and social relationships.

You snooze, you lose

Insomniacs are more than twice as likely as the general population to have a fatigue-related motor vehicle accident. Those who sleep less than 5 hours per night may have a higher death rate, too.

Prevalence

Insomnia disorder occurring over 1 month is found in approximately 6% to 10% of the population. Prevalence increases with age and is greater in women. Insomnia can be a symptom, its own disorder, or most commonly, observed as a comorbid condition with another medical or mental disorder (APA, 2013).

Causes

Episodic insomnia often stems from a specific event—a physical or emotional stressor (such as illness), a significant life change (such as divorce), or an environmental disturbance that makes sleep difficult (such as noise, unwanted light, or an uncomfortable room temperature).

> Alcohol, caffeine, and anxiety are the main culprits in persistent insomnia.

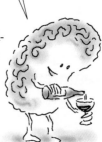

You booze, you may not snooze

Persistent insomnia may result from either a single factor or multiple factors. Everyday stress and anxiety, caffeine consumption, and alcohol use are the biggest culprits.

Risk factors for developing persistent insomnia include:
• history of being a light sleeper
• tendency toward easy arousal at night
• inability to fall asleep or stay asleep after an initial stressful situation is resolved
• conversion of feelings into physical symptoms rather than expressing them outright or dealing with them constructively.

Signs and symptoms

A patient with insomnia disorder may report or exhibit:

- difficulty falling asleep
- difficulty staying asleep
- waking up too early in the morning
- inability to fall back to sleep once awakened
- nonrestorative sleep
- daytime fatigue and lack of energy
- haggard appearance
- irritability
- short attention span
- poor concentration
- anxious concern over his or her health
- interpersonal, social, or occupational problems stemming from anxiety over sleeplessness
- inappropriate use of sedative-hypnotic drugs, alcohol, or caffeine.

(See *Key questions to ask when assessing for insomnia.*)

Memory jogger

Typical findings in patients with INSOMNIA

I Intermittent wakefulness

N Not able to fall asleep easily

S Stressed by the inability to fall asleep

O Overly concerned with the consequences of not sleeping

M May medicate with inappropriate drugs

N Needs frequent daytime naps

I Irritable

A Attention and concentration problems

Diagnosis

Insomnia disorder may be diagnosed from the patient history and physical findings. Polysomnography can rule out other sleep disorders such as OSAHS. Polysomnography usually shows increased stage 1 sleep and decreased slow-wave sleep.

Sleep scribblings

To aid diagnosis, the doctor may ask the patient to keep a sleep diary for 1 to 2 weeks. (See *Dear Sleep Diary*, pages 472 and 473.) In the acute care setting, sleep-wake logs are a common technique.

Diagnosis of insomnia disorder is confirmed by using the diagnostic criteria in the *DSM-5* and can be further classified as episodic, persistent, or recurrent (APA, 2013).

Recording bedtimes, awakening times, and other sleep-related information can help the doctor diagnose a patient with insomnia.

Treatment

Treatment for insomnia disorder may involve relaxation techniques, improved sleep hygiene, behavioral interventions, cognitive therapy, alternative and complementary measures, or pharmacologic options.

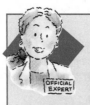

Advice from the experts

Key questions to ask when assessing for insomnia

When assessing a patient who complains of insomnia, ask the following questions:
• When did the problem begin?
• Do you have a medical or psychiatric illness that might affect your ability to sleep?
• What's your sleep environment like? Is it dark? Quiet? Bright? Noisy? Does it have a comfortable room temperature?
• Do you use your bedroom for things other than sleep or sexual activity (such as watching television, eating, or working)?
• What time do you usually go to bed?
• What time do you usually get up in the morning on weekdays? On weekends?
• Do you drink alcohol or smoke? Are you taking prescribed medications? Nonprescription preparations? Street drugs?
• What's your typical work schedule?
• How do you feel the day after a poor night's sleep?

Family inquiries
If possible, ask the patient's spouse or other family members if the patient snores or has unusual limb movements when sleeping.

Nipping it in the bud

With episodic insomnia, the need for treatment is based on the severity of daytime symptoms and duration of the episode. A patient who suffers brief episodes of insomnia should be monitored for prolonged negative effects because untreated episodic insomnia can lead to a chronic condition.

Relaxation techniques

Because many insomniacs display high levels of physiologic and cognitive arousal (both at night and during the day), relaxation-based interventions may provide relief. Techniques that help deactivate the arousal system include progressive muscle relaxation, abdominal or deep breathing, biofeedback, and imagery training (Gilsenan, 2012).

(Text continues on page 474.)

Dear Sleep Diary

A sleep diary, like the one shown here, can aid the diagnosis and treatment of insomnia disorder. The diary provides a night-by-night account of the patient's sleep schedule and perception of sleep. The sleep diary serves as a baseline for monitoring treatment efficacy. In the diary, the patient records information such as:

- bedtime of the previous night
- total sleep time
- time elapsed before sleep onset
- number of awakenings
- morning awakening time
- total time awake
- use of sleep medications
- subjective rating of sleep quality and daytime symptoms.

Sample sleep diary

Name _Willa Selby_

		Date	Mon 5/12	Tues 5/13
Complete in AM		**Bedtime (previous night)**	11:00 pm	10:45 pm
		Awakening time	7:30 am	7:45 am
		Estimated time to sleep onset (previous night)	45 minutes	1 hour
		Estimated number of awakenings and total time awake (previous night)	6 times/total of 3 hours	5 times/total of 4 hours
		Estimated amount of sleep obtained (previous night)	4 1/2 hours	5 hours
Complete in PM		**Naps (time and duration)**	4:00 pm for 30 minutes	4:30 pm for 30 minutes
		Alcoholic drinks (number and time)	2 drinks at 8:00 pm	1 drink at 9:00 pm
		Stresses experienced today	Car wouldn't start, argued with boss	none
		Rate how you felt today 1—Very tired/sleepy 2—Somewhat tired/sleepy 3—Fairly alert 4—Wide awake	1	2
		Irritability 1—Not at all 5—Very	5 (very)	3
		Medications	Benadryl	Benadryl

Encourage the patient to complete the diary each morning using estimates rather than exact times to make the process less disruptive to sleep.

Wed 5/14	Thu 5/15	Fri 5/16
11:00 pm		
7:30 am		
30 minutes		
6 times/total of 3 hours		
4 1/2 hours		
4:00 pm for 45 minutes		
2 drinks at 8:00 pm		
argued with a friend		
1		
4		
Benadryl		

Sleep hygiene

For some patients, insomnia responds well to lifestyle changes, referred to as *sleep hygiene* (Gilsenan, 2012). Such changes include going to bed at the same time every night, optimizing sleeping conditions, and avoiding naps during the day. (See *Getting hygienic about sleep.*)

Behavioral interventions

Behavioral interventions aim to change maladaptive sleep habits, reduce autonomic arousal, and alter dysfunctional beliefs and attitudes. A wide range of behavioral techniques may be used to

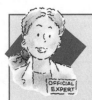

Advice from the experts

Getting hygienic about sleep

For most patients with insomnia, lifestyle measures—termed *sleep hygiene*—are used first. When teaching your patient about sleep hygiene, cover the following do's and don't's.

Sleep-promoting measures
• Use the bed only for sleep and sex—not for reading, watching television, or working.
• Establish a regular bedtime and a regular time for getting up in the morning. Stick to these times even on weekends and on vacations.
• Exercise in the evening. Energy levels bottom out a few hours after exercise, promoting sleep at that time.
• Take a hot bath 90 minutes to 2 hours before bedtime. This alters core body temperature and helps you fall asleep more easily.
• During the 30 minutes before bedtime, do something relaxing, such as reading, meditating, or taking a leisurely walk.
• Keep the bedroom quiet, dark, relatively cool, and well ventilated.
• Eat dinner 4 to 5 hours before bedtime. At bedtime, a light snack (low in sugar and calories) may promote sleep.
• Spend 30 minutes in the sun each day. (However, be sure to take precautions against overexposure.)
• If you don't fall asleep after 15 or 20 minutes, get up and go into another room. Read or perform a quiet activity, using dim lighting, until you feel sleepy.

• If your bed partner distracts you, consider moving to another bedroom or the sofa for a few nights.

What not to do
• Don't use the bedroom for work, reading, or watching television.
• Avoid large meals before bedtime.
• Don't look at the clock. Obsessing over time makes it harder to sleep.
• Avoid naps, especially in the evening.
• Don't drink a large amount of fluid after dinner, or the need to urinate may disturb your sleep.
• Avoid exercising close to bedtime because this may make you more alert.
• Avoid alcohol and caffeine in the evening.
• Don't take a bath just before bedtime because this could increase your alertness.
• Don't engage in highly stimulating activities before bed, such as watching a frightening movie or playing competitive computer games.
• Don't smoke because nicotine's effects may contribute to sleep loss.
• Don't toss and turn in bed. Instead, get up and read or listen to relaxing music. However, don't watch television because it emits too bright of a light.

treat persistent insomnia (Gilsenan, 2012). Stimulus control is a behavioral intervention that connects behavior associated with sleep hygiene to sleep behavior. For example, with behavioral intervention, patients are instructed to go to bed only when sleepy and make the behavioral choice to get out of bed when realizing that sleep is not naturally occurring (Halter & Varcarolis, 2014).

Stimulus control centers on the theory that insomnia represents a learned response to bedtime and bedroom cues.

Bedroom behavior

Give your patient these instructions:
• Go to bed only when sleepy. See *Getting hygienic about sleep*.
• Use the bed and bedroom only for sleep (or sex).
• If you can't fall asleep or stay asleep, get out of bed and go to another room. Return to bed only when you feel sleepy.
• Awaken and get out of bed at the same time every morning regardless of how much sleep you got.
• Avoid naps.

Paradoxical intention

In paradoxical intention, the patient does the opposite of what is wanted, sometimes taking it to an extreme. For instance, instead of going through activities that promote sleep, the patient prepares to stay awake and might be doing something energetic. If worry is a factor in insomnia, it may intensify.

Biofeedback

In biofeedback, the patient is connected to a device that measures brain waves and other body functions. Then the patient is given feedback to help learn to recognize certain states of tension or sleep stages—and either avoid or repeat these states voluntarily.

Sleep restriction

Sleep restriction creates a mild state of sleep deprivation, which may promote more rapid sleep onset and more "efficient" sleep. The patient limits the amount of time spent in bed so as to increase the percentage of time spent asleep.

Bedtime amendments

To maintain a consistent sleep-wake pattern, the patient usually alters bedtime rather than rising time. However, time in bed shouldn't be reduced to less than 5 hours a day. Naps aren't allowed (except in elderly adults).

Cognitive therapy

Cognitive therapy helps the patient identify dysfunctional beliefs and attitudes about sleep (such as "I'll never fall asleep") and replace them with positive ones. Changing beliefs and attitudes can decrease the anticipatory anxiety that interferes with sleep. Cognitive therapy also focuses on actions intended to change behavior.

Alternative and complementary therapies

Alternative and complementary therapies that may be used to treat insomnia include acupressure, acupuncture, aromatherapy, massage, biofeedback, chiropractic, homeopathy, light and dark therapy, meditation, reflexology, visualization, and yoga (Reading, 2013).

Supplements to sleep by

Some patients use herbal preparations (such as St. John's wort and chamomile), nutritional substances, and other nonprescription preparations to treat insomnia. However, few of such products have been demonstrated to be safe and effective. An additional consideration is the lack of any standardized dosing or purity among nutritional supplements. Therefore, potency and actual dosage can vary based on the manufacturer.

Dietary supplements sometimes recommended for insomnia relief include vitamins B_6, B_{12}, and D. Some practitioners also recommend calcium and magnesium. Tryptophan may relieve insomnia in some patients, but the patient must be monitored for adverse effects.

Melatonin is a hormone that is released from the pineal gland and can help regulate sleep-wake cycles. Melatonin is also found in a number of plants including Saint John's Wort, along with a number of fruits such as grapes and cherries. It is believed to bind to melatonin receptors in the body leading to their activation (agonist). Activation of these receptors is then believed to help restore the sleep-wake cycle. Few side effects have been found, primarily drowsiness and a worsening of orthostatic hypertension.

Valerian is a perennial flowering plant native to Europe commonly used in the treatment of anxiety and insomnia. It is believed to have a pharmacologic mechanism similar to benzodiazepines, in which an effect is exerted on an inhibitory neurotransmitter (gamma-aminobutyric acid [GABA]). Evidence is mixed as to whether or not this can be an effective treatment for sleep disorders. It can result in stomach upset and nausea. Additional side effects are a sense of asthenia (lack of energy) and allergic reactions.

Memory jogger

Help your patient DISCOVER ways to overcome sleep disorders.

D Define what may be causing the problem.

I Identify changes in the patient's sleep pattern.

S State an understanding of "good" sleep.

C Calculate how many hours of sleep needed.

O Offer assistance on ways to promote sleep.

V Venting feelings about sleep problems can be therapeutic.

E Educate the patient about how sleep patterns change throughout life.

R Review the negative effects of stress on sleep.

Pharmacologic options

If insomnia persists despite other measures, the prescribing health provider may recommend drug therapy (Proctor & Bianchi, 2012). The most commonly prescribed drugs are short-acting sedative-hypnotics (primarily benzodiazepines), antidepressants, and antihistamines. (See *Pharmacologic therapy for sleep disorders*, page 478.)

Sleep aids

Sedative-hypnotics—usually temazepam (Restoril) and zolpidem (Ambien)—are commonly prescribed for short-term management of insomnia. Benzodiazepines such as temazepam (Restoril) help maintain sleep, whereas nonbenzodiazepines such as zolpidem (Ambien) help the patient fall asleep. Recently, zolpidem (Ambien) has developed a controlled release (CR) form labeled Ambien CR that helps the patient also stay asleep longer. Newer sedative-hypnotics such as zaleplon (Sonata) and ramelteon (Rozerem) are also used according to the symptoms the patient describes that interrupt the sleep-wake cycle (Boyd, 2012).

Both prescription and nonprescription antihistamines can be used for short-term management of insomnia particularly with adolescents and the elderly. The most common over-the-counter agents are doxylamine (Unisom) and diphenhydramine (Benadryl). Adverse effects include daytime sedation, cognitive impairment, and anticholinergic effects (e.g., dry mouth, constipation, or urinary retention). Tolerance or reliance may also occur.

Antidepressants may be given in low dosages—especially if the patient has related psychiatric disorders or a history of substance abuse. These medications can also be effective in the treatment of chronic pain. However, some antidepressants can exacerbate other disorders, such as mania or restless leg syndrome, so the patient should be monitored closely (Proctor & Bianchi, 2012).

Nursing interventions

These nursing interventions may be appropriate for a patient with insomnia disorder:
• Provide teaching about prescribed medications, including drug purpose, administration, and adverse effects. Inform the patient that taking these drugs for more than a few weeks may lead to tolerance and withdrawal, making it even more difficult to sleep when the medication is stopped.

Memory jogger

Cover these basic TEACHING points to help your patient get better sleep.

T Take prescribed sleep medications appropriately.

E Eliminate caffeine, alcohol, and nicotine at least 4 hours before bedtime.

A Attend to adequate sleep hygiene.

C Consider the effects of foods and fluids on sleep.

H Have a consistent bedtime routine.

I Initiate relaxation strategies before bedtime.

N Nightmares and dreams that disrupt sleep must be addressed.

G Get family support, as needed.

Meds matters

Pharmacologic therapy for sleep disorders

Several different medications are used to treat sleep disorders. A patient with insomnia may receive a benzodiazepine, a nonbenzodiazepine hypnotic, an antidepressant, or a medication that influences melatonin. All of these therapies can lead to drowsiness and should not be taken in combination with other sedating medication or alcohol (Proctor & Bianchi, 2012).

Drug	Adverse effects	Contraindications	Nursing interventions
Antihistamines			
Diphenhydramine hydrochloride (Benadryl)	Drowsiness Dry mouth Possible increase in heart rate	Should not be used in acute asthma Use of monoamine oxidase inhibitors	Avoid alcohol and other sedating agents. Be cautious when operating heavy machinery after taking medication. Recommend hard candies to aid in alleviating dry mouth if experienced.
Benzodiazepines			
Temazepam (Restoril) Triazolam (Halcion)	Dizziness Drowsiness Lethargy Orthostatic hypotension	Pregnancy and breast-feeding Triazolam should not be taken at the same time as ketoconazole, itraconazole, or nefazodone therapy.	Teach the patient about drug action, dosage, and adverse effects. Caution the patient not to drink alcohol, drive a motor vehicle, or operate machinery while under the influence of this drug. Advise the patient to change position slowly to avoid dizziness. Inform the patient of potential for physical and psychological dependence.
Nonbenzodiazepines			
Eszopiclone (Lunesta) Zaleplon (Sonata) Zolpidem (Ambien)	Amnesia Dizziness Fugue states (sleep-walking and performing other activities such as driving while appearing asleep)	Pregnancy and breast-feeding Hepatic impairment	Teach the patient about drug action, dosage, and adverse effects. Avoid alcohol and other sedating agents. Be cautious when operating heavy machinery after taking medication.

Pharmacologic therapy for sleep disorders *(continued)*

Drug	Adverse effects	Contraindications	Nursing interventions
Melatonin receptor agonists			
Ramelteon (Rozerem)	Dizziness Fatigue Headache Nausea	Angioedema Hepatic impairment Should not be taken at the same time as fluvoxamine	Teach the patient about drug action, dosage, and adverse effects. Avoid alcohol and other sedating agents. Be cautious when operating heavy machinery after taking medication.
Antidepressants			
Amitriptyline (Elavil) Doxepin (Silenor) Trazodone (Desyrel)	Blood dyscrasias Ataxia Blurred vision Dry mouth Increased heart rate Palpitation	Certain cardiovascular disorders, particularly those associated with prolonged QT interval Trazodone should not be given at same time as serotonergic drugs.	Monitor for a compromised immune system. Assess for changes in mood and potential suicidal ideation. Avoid alcohol and other sedating agents. Be cautious when operating heavy machinery after taking medication. Can increase liver function test results

- Monitor the patient for adverse drug effects.
- Instruct the patient in good sleep hygiene, such as maintaining a regular bedtime and awakening times; avoiding naps; and eliminating caffeine, alcohol, and nicotine.
- Encourage the practice of relaxation routines, such as progressive muscle relaxation or meditation.
- Caution about the possible dangers of using unproven therapies.
- Advise the patient to move the alarm clock away from the bed if it's distracting.

References

American Academy of Sleep Medicine. (2001). *International classification of sleep disorders, revised: Diagnostic and coding manual.* Chicago, IL: Author.

American Psychiatric Association. (2013). *Diagnostic and statistical manual of mental disorders* (5th ed.). Washington, DC: American Psychiatric Publishing.

Avidan, A. Y., & Zee, P. C. (2011). *Handbook of sleep medicine* (2nd ed.). Philadelphia, PA: Lippincott Williams & Wilkins.

Berry, R. B. (2012). *Fundamentals of sleep medicine*. Philadelphia, PA: Elsevier.

Boyd, M. (2012). *Psychiatric nursing: Contemporary practice* (5th ed.). Philadelphia, PA: Lippincott Williams & Wilkins.

Centers for Disease Control and Prevention. (2012). Short sleep duration among workers—United States, 2010. *Morbidity and Mortality Weekly Report, 61*(16), 281–285.

Centers for Disease Control and Prevention. (2013). Drowsy driving—19 states and the District of Columbia, 2009–2010. *Morbidity and Mortality Weekly Report, 61*(51–52), 1033–1037.

Elder, G. J., Wetherell, M. A., Barclay, N. L., & Ellis, J. G. (2013). The cortisol awakening response—Applications and implications for sleep medicine. *Sleep Medicine Reviews, 18*(3), 215–224. doi:10.1016/j.smrv.2013.05.001

George, N. M., & Davis, J. E. (2013). Assessing sleep in adolescents through a better understanding of sleep physiology. *American Journal of Nursing, 113*(6), 26–32.

Gilsenan, I. (2012). Nursing intervention to alleviate insomnia. *Nursing Older People, 24*(4), 14–18.

Gulyani, S., Salas, R. E., & Gamaldo, C. E. (2013). Sleep medicine pharmacotherapeutics overview: Today, tomorrow, and the future (part 2: Hypersomnia, parasomnia, and movement disorders). *Chest, 143*(1), 242–251. doi:10.1378/chest.12-0561

Halter, M., & Varcarolis, E. (2014). *Varcarolis' foundation of psychiatric mental health nursing: A clinical approach* (7th ed.). St. Louis, MO: Elsevier.

Kohli, P., Sarmiento, K., & Malhotra, A. (2013). Update in sleep medicine 2012. *American Journal of Respiratory and Critical Care Medicine, 187*(10), 1056–1060. doi:10.1164/rccm.201302-0315UP

McCabe, C., & Hardinge, M. (2011). Obstructive sleep apnoea. *Practice Nurse, 41*(10), 36–41.

National Institute of Neurological Disorders and Stroke. (2014). *Narcolepsy fact sheet*. Retrieved from http://www.ninds.nih.gov/disorders/narcolepsy/detail_narcolepsy.htm

Pagel, J. F., & Pandi-Perumal, S. R. (2007). *Primary care sleep medicine: A practical guide*. Totowa, NJ: Humana Press.

Pandi-Perumal, S. R., Monti, J. M., & Monjan, A. A. (2010). *Principles and practice of geriatric sleep medicine*. Cambridge, United Kingdom: Cambridge University Press.

Perry, G. S., Patil, S. P., & Presley-Cantrell, L. R. (2013). Raising awareness of sleep as a healthy behavior. *Preventing Chronic Disease, 10*, E133. doi:10.58888/pcd10.130081

Proctor, A., & Bianchi, M. T. (2012). Clinical pharmacology in sleep medicine. *ISRN Pharmacology, 2012*, 914168. doi:10.5402/2012/914168

Reading, P. (2013). *ABC of sleep medicine*. Chichester, United Kingdom: John Wiley & Sons.

Silber, M. H., Krahn, L. E., & Morgenthaler, T. I. (2010). *Sleep medicine in clinical practice* (2nd ed.). New York, NY: Informa.

Valenza, M. C., Cabrera-Martos, I., Martín-Martín, L., Pérez-Garzón, V. M., Velarde, C., & Valenza-Demet, G. (2013). Nursing homes: Impact of sleep disturbances on functionality. *Archives of Gerontology & Geriatrics, 56*(3), 432–436. doi:10.1016/j.archger.2012.11.011

Vallido, T., Peters, K., O'Brien, L., & Jackson, D. (2009). Sleep in adolescence: A review of issues for nursing practice. *Journal of Clinical Nursing, 18*(13), 1819–1826. doi:10.1111/j.1365-2702.2009.02812.x

Internet-Based Resources

American Sleep Apnea Association—http://sleepapnea.org/
American Sleep Association—http://www.sleepassociation.org/index.php
American Academy of Sleep Medicine—http://www.aasmnet.org/practiceguidelines.aspx
National Sleep Foundation—http://www.sleepfoundation.org/
Sleep.com—http://www.sleep.com/
Willis-Ekbom Disease Foundation—http://www.rls.org/

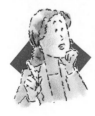

Quick quiz

1. REM sleep is characterized by:
   A. light sleep.
   B. paralysis of the muscles.
   C. restricted eye movements.
   D. nonvivid dreams.

Answer: B. During REM sleep, many muscles are effectively paralyzed so the sleeper won't act out dreams. Eye movements are rapid.

2. NREM sleep is regulated by the:
   A. pons.
   B. hypothalamus.
   C. basal forebrain.
   D. amygdala.

Answer: C. The basal forebrain controls NREM sleep. The pons and midbrain control REM sleep.

3. A classic feature of OSAHS is:
   A. snoring.
   B. sneezing.
   C. early morning awakening.
   D. bursts of energy.

Answer: A. Snoring is a hallmark of OSAHS. Sneezing, bursts of energy, and early morning awakening aren't common in this disorder.

4. Primary treatments for circadian rhythm sleep disorders include all of the following *except:*
   A. chronotherapy.
   B. short-acting sedative-hypnotics.
   C. relaxation techniques.
   D. luminotherapy.

Answer: C. Relaxation techniques aren't used as primary treatments for circadian rhythm sleep disorders.

5. Cataplexy is a symptom of:
    A.   REM sleep.
    B.   hypersomnia disorder.
    C.   OSAHS.
    D.   narcolepsy.

Answer: D. Cataplexy—a condition marked by sudden attacks of bilateral muscle tone loss—occurs in narcolepsy.

6. "Sleep drunkenness" is a common finding in patients with:
    A.   insomnia disorder.
    B.   hypersomnia disorder.
    C.   narcolepsy.
    D.   alcoholism.

Answer: B. "Sleep drunkenness" (difficulty awakening completely, confusion, disorientation, and poor motor coordination) on awakening occurs in hypersomnolence disorder.

7. Information typically gathered in a sleep diary includes:
    A.   usual bedtime.
    B.   foods consumed before bedtime.
    C.   daily weights.
    D.   fluid consumption.

Answer: A. In a sleep diary, the patient records sleep-related items, such as usual bedtime and awakening times, time elapsed before sleep onset, number of nightly awakenings, and total time spent in sleep. Food and fluid consumption and daily weights aren't relevant.

Scoring

☆☆☆ If you answered all seven items correctly, stupendous! Your study of snoozing and snoring has succeeded beyond our wildest dreams!

☆☆ If you answered five or six items correctly, remarkable. Your solid grasp of sleep disorders should make for a sweet slumber tonight.

☆ If you answered fewer than five items correctly, consider this your wake-up call. Read the chapter again—but try not to doze off this time.

13

Sexual disorders

Just the facts

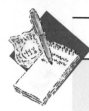

In this chapter, you'll learn about the following:

♦ stages of sexual development

♦ phases of the sexual response cycle

♦ categories and definitions of sexual disorders

♦ causes, diagnosis, and treatment of sexual disorders

♦ nursing interventions for patients with sexual disorders

A look at sex

Sex is something we all have in common, as none of us would be here without it. It is a universal experience and something which many believe motivates quite a bit of our human behavior. Sex is responsible for keeping us going as a species and it can bring much joy and pleasure to our lives. However, it is also true that sex can be problematic for some, creating a number of difficulties in their lives. In some cases, certain sexual behaviors or activities are against the law and as such are considered criminal offenses. And aside from legal sanctions, almost all societies and religions have sexual behaviors and activities which are considered at least immoral if not illegal as well. In many cultures, sex is something that is not often talked about, even in health care settings. It is important that anyone working in health care, especially in psychiatric and mental health nursing, realize that in addition to medical problems, a number of psychiatric disorders and medications can cause problems with an individual's sexual functioning and enjoyment. In 2011, a number of initiatives recognized sexual health as a key area for improving the lives of Americans so your understanding of some of the key areas related to sexual disorders will help you to better serve your patients (Ford, Barnes, Rompalo, & Hook, 2013; National Prevention Council, 2011).

A look at sexual disorders

Sexuality is expressed not just in a person's appearance but also in attitude, behaviors, and relationships. Influenced by ongoing biophysical and psychosocial factors, sexuality starts to take shape during early childhood and is reshaped throughout life.

A sexual disorder can cause distress and anxiety for the individual who has it and can create strife in intimate relationships. A global study early in the 2000 decade provided evidence of sexual dysfunction among 38% of the women and 29% of the men surveyed (Laumann et al., 2005). It is clear that sexual disorders are not uncommon problems among many populations (Cleveland Clinic, 2012).

We also know that sexual disorders can be caused by physical or psychological problems and in some cases even both. Physical causes can include various diseases and medical conditions such as heart problems, diabetes, or neurologic disorders; medications taken for whatever reason; endocrine disorders; or hormonal deficiencies. Psychological factors include, among others, depression, past sexual trauma, relationship problems, or sexual fears (Cleveland Clinic, 2012; Medline Plus, 2010).

> Dad's not gonna want to hear this, but my sexuality is already starting to take shape. Cowabunga!

Scrolling through sexual disorders

Sexual disorders described in the *Diagnostic and Statistical Manual of Mental Disorders*, 5th Edition (*DSM-5*) (American Psychiatric Association [APA], 2013), include the following:
- paraphilias (such as exhibitionism, fetishism, and voyeurism)
- sexual dysfunctions (which include sexual desire disorders, sexual arousal disorders, orgasmic disorders, and sexual pain disorders)
- gender identity disorders

Defining "abnormal" sexual behavior

The definition of "abnormal" sexual behavior depends largely on cultural and historical context. Accepted norms of sexual behavior and attitudes vary greatly within and among different cultures. In America, the work that defines what is abnormal or what can be considered a mental illness is the *Diagnostic and Statistical Manual of Mental Disorders*, also known as the *DSM*. Published by the American Psychiatric Association, the text is periodically revised.

In the past, many people believed that the only "normal" sexual behavior was intercourse between heterosexual partners for procreation. Even masturbation was widely seen as a perversion and a potential cause of mental disorders. Catholicism considered it a carnal sin, it was punishable by death in Orthodox Judaism, and some believed that it caused insanity (Townsend, 2012). Homosexuality was also previously viewed in an extremely negative light. In 1952, it was classified in the *DSM-I* as a mental disorder and it was not completely removed from the *DSM* until 1973 (Spitzer, 1981).

Today, a much broader range of attitudes toward sexuality exists. Homosexuality is now widely regarded as a normal variant of sexuality, and masturbation is accepted as a normal sexual activity.

Psychiatrists no longer consider homosexuality abnormal.

Other opinions on abnormality

Some authorities classify abnormal sexual behavior as any behavior that causes personal distress. Others view sexuality on a continuum from adaptive to maladaptive; in their view, normal sexuality is adaptive, whereas abnormal sexuality is maladaptive.

For example, sexual behavior is maladaptive for an individual if it prevents reaching goals and adapting to life's demands. It's maladaptive to society if it interferes with or disrupts social group functioning.

Stages of sexual development

Beginning in infancy, human beings progress through various phases of sexual and psychosexual development. Characteristic physical attributes and feelings related to sex develop during each phase.

Parents and puritans

Crucial factors affecting sexual development include early role models, religious and cultural teachings, early sexual experiences, and parental attitudes toward sex. A parent's puritanical rejection of sexuality, for example, can produce guilt and shame in a child, subsequently inhibiting the child's capacity to enjoy sex and develop healthy relationships as an adult. Similarly, a child who's treated with cruelty, hostility, or rejection may become sexually maladjusted.

Infancy to age 5

The combination of the mother's X chromosome and the father's X or Y chromosome creates either a male or a female child. Gender assignment of a healthy infant is reinforced by family members' interactions with the infant. These interactions may influence and reinforce either masculine or feminine behavior. For example, an infant girl may be rocked gently, whereas an infant boy may be played with more roughly. Young girls typically receive dolls as gifts, whereas boys may receive sports-related items and toy cars. By age 2, most children have a clear sense of their gender identity. (See *Components of sexual identity*.)

Age of discovery

Between ages 1 and 3, children start to observe body differences and show an interest in bathroom habits. Sexual discovery starts between ages 3 and 5. Curious and explorative, young children commonly ask where babies come from and what their sex organs

---

Components of sexual identity

Sexual identity encompasses four components: the biopsychosocial integration of biological sex gender role expression, gender identity, and sexual orientation or preference (Rainbow Access Initiative, n.d.).

Biological sex

Bisexual identity is the physical state of being either male or female. It results from genetic and hormonal influences.

Gender role expression

Gender role is the outward expression of one's gender—the behaviors, feelings, and attitudes appropriate for either a male or female. Labels attached to gender role include masculine or feminine, traditional or conforming, and gender-neutral. Learned by the individual, gender role is influenced by culture, religion, schools, peers, and social messages.

Gender identity

Gender identity is a person's private experience of gender—the sense of oneself as being male, female, or ambivalent. It's usually based on physical features, parental attitudes and expectations, and psychological and social pressures.

Various theories explain how gender identity develops.
• Biological theory proposes that gender identity develops in utero and contributes to the fetus's anatomic development.
• Psychodynamic theory sees gender identity as evolving from role modeling, during which the child learns to identify with the same-sex parent.
• Social learning theory holds that gender identity is learned and reinforced by environment and social expectations.
• Cognitive theory holds that a child can mentally construct male or female behavior and tell these behaviors apart.

Sexual orientation or preference

Sexual orientation or preference refers to a person's feelings about his or her sexual attraction and erotic potential.
• Heterosexuality is marked by sexual arousal from or sexual activity with people of the opposite gender.
• Homosexuality refers to sexual arousal from or sexual activity with people of the same gender.
• Bisexuality is characterized by sexual arousal from or sexual activity with both males and females.

are for. They're accepting and straightforward about sex and may comment on the differences between genders. At this age, they learn that touching feels good.

A topic apart

Toward the end of this stage, children pick up cues from others that sex is a "different" topic. They may become shy, ask fewer questions about sex, and show a desire for privacy about their bodies.

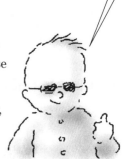

Mom and Dad better get their answers ready! When I turn 3, I'm gonna start asking where babies come from and what my sex organs are for.

Ages 5 to 10

Children ages 5 to 10 may think in terms of "good" and "bad" parts of their bodies. Aware of bodily functions and how these relate to sex, they're same-sex oriented.

Outwardly, they may seem unconcerned about sex or uncomfortable or apprehensive about discussing it. However, they're actually quite interested in it. Also, masturbation and sexual exploration are common at this stage.

Ages 10 to 14

Puberty begins at about age 11 for girls and age 12 for boys. Young adolescents may be confused, embarrassed, and self-conscious about their bodily changes and may be uncomfortable with, or unaware of, their social roles.

Sexual responsiveness develops during this stage, as does the ability to reproduce. In response to peer pressure and other influences, some young adolescents become sexually active.

Ages 14 and older

From age 14 on, children develop more adult characteristics. This may be apparent physically, emotionally, and socially. They are easily influenced by peer pressure and media messages. They want to be in control of themselves and are forming their identities and self-concepts.

Active but uncertain

According to a 2011 survey among U.S. high school students, 47.4% have had sexual intercourse, 33.7% had had sexual intercourse within 3 months of the survey, and 15.3% have had sex with four or more people by the time they were surveyed (Centers for Disease Control and Prevention, 2012). Broken down by grade, 32% of 9th graders and 62% of 12th graders reported to be sexually active, which included oral and anal sex in addition to intercourse (Chandra, Mosher, Copen, & Sionean, 2011; Centers for Disease Control and Prevention, 2010; Centers for Disease Control and Prevention, n.d.-a; U.S. Department of Health and Human Services, 2013). However, they're still uncertain about sex. They may feel that it's a part of the adult world.

Adults

By adulthood, sex and sexuality are a part of a person's life. An estimated 90% of adults are sexually active. Adults hold views on sexuality that have been influenced by society and its standards of normal behavior.

> By adulthood, sex and sexuality are a part of a person's life. An estimated 90% of adults are sexually active.

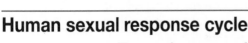

Human sexual response cycle

The sexual response cycle refers to the progressive mental, physical, and emotional changes that occur during sexual stimulation. Although the sexual response is highly individualized, nearly everyone experiences certain basic physiologic changes.

The sex scientists

Different researchers have proposed various models of the sexual response cycle, describing three, four, or five distinct phases. For example, Helen Singer Kaplan's model (1979) encompasses three stages—desire, excitement, and orgasm. William Masters and Virginia Johnson (1966) describe four phases—excitement (arousal), plateau, orgasm, and resolution. Using instruments that monitor changes in heart rate and muscle tension, Masters and Johnson 1996 identified the physiologic changes that take place during each phase.

Currently, many experts conceptualize a four-phase cycle that begins with desire.

Desire phase

The desire phase is marked by a strong urge for sexual stimulation and satisfaction, either by oneself or with another person. Cultural and societal values affect the range of stimulation that provokes sexual desire.

Potential sexual partners may communicate desire either verbally or through behavior and body language (e.g., flirting). Such communication may be subtle and easily misread. (See *Flirting across cultures.*)

Desire is mental, not physical. Without further mental or physical stimulation, the desire phase may not progress to sexual excitement.

Memory jogger

Think DEOR to remember the main phases of the sexual response cycle.

D Desire

E Excitement

O Orgasm

R Resolution

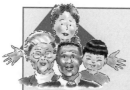

Bridging the gap

Flirting across cultures

In different cultures, behaviors meant to communicate sexual desire may vary greatly along gender lines. Some cultures disapprove of women expressing overt communication of their sexual desire—but expect such communication from men. In other cultures, women have more leeway to be flirtatious.

Culturally defined behaviors can also influence perceptions of what is—and what isn't—flirting. In some cultures, especially Latin American, Southern European, and Arabian cultures, people tend to stand relatively close to each other and make frequent physical contact. Americans might misinterpret this behavior as flirting.

In other cultures, such as the British, Australian, and East Asian cultures, people tend to stand farther away and make less physical contact. Someone who isn't aware of these social customs might misconstrue them as a lack of romantic interest—even when such interest is present.

Nice—but not always needed

Desire doesn't have to be present for sex to occur. For example, a couple trying to conceive a child may have intercourse even on days when they lack sexual desire. Also, a person can respond to a partner's sexual advances even if he or she doesn't feel desire to begin with.

Excitement or arousal phase

The excitement or arousal phase prepares both partners for intercourse. Muscle tension increases, the heart rate quickens, the skin becomes flushed or blotchy (called *sexual flush*), and the nipples grow hard or erect.

Congested, lubricated, and swollen

Vasocongestion begins during this phase, causing the female's clitoris, vagina, and labia minora to swell. The vaginal walls start to produce a lubricating fluid, the uterus and breasts enlarge, and the pubococcygeal muscle surrounding the vaginal opening tightens.

In the male, the penis becomes erect, the testes become elevated and swollen, the scrotal sac tightens, and the Cowper glands secrete a lubricating fluid.

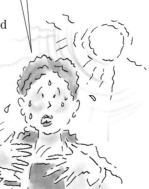

It's getting hot in here! I'm glad I'm wearing clothes so that no one can see my sexual flush.

Plateau

With continued stimulation (especially stroking and rubbing of the erogenous zones or sexual intercourse) during full arousal, the plateau stage may be reached. Actually, a person may achieve, lose, and regain a plateau several times without orgasm occurring.

During the plateau stage, the heart and respiratory rates and blood pressure rise further, sexual flush deepens, and muscle tension increases. A sense of impending orgasm occurs. In the female, the clitoris withdraws, vaginal lubrication increases, the labia continue to swell, and the areolae enlarge. The lower vagina narrows and tightens.

In the male, the ridge of the glans penis becomes more prominent, the Cowper glands secrete preejaculatory fluid, and the testes rise closer to the body.

If this were a movie, you'd see fireworks or a wave crashing on the beach right about now.

Orgasm phase

The orgasm phase is the peak of sexual excitement. Physiologic changes include involuntary muscle contractions; elevated heart rate and blood pressure; rapid oxygen intake; sphincter muscle contraction; and sudden, forceful release of sexual tension.

Describing the indescribable

Orgasm is the shortest phase of the sexual response cycle, typically lasting just a few seconds. (It may be slightly longer in women.) For men, orgasm usually climaxes with the ejaculation of semen. For women, orgasm involves rhythmic muscle contractions of the uterus, which put pressure on the penis and promote male orgasm. Unless a sexual dysfunction is present, orgasm is intensely pleasurable for both sexes.

Resolution phase

During the resolution phase, the body returns to its normal, unexcited state. The heart and respiratory rates slow, blood pressure decreases, and muscle tone slackens. Swollen and erect body parts return to normal, and skin flushing disappears. Some of these changes occur rapidly, whereas others take longer. This phase is marked by a general sense of well-being and enhanced intimacy.

Refractory period

For a male, the resolution phase includes a refractory period during which he can't reach orgasm—although he may be able to maintain a partial or full erection. This period lasts a few minutes to several days, depending on such factors as age and frequency of sexual activity. Many females, in contrast, can return rapidly to the orgasmic phase with minimal stimulation.

Paraphilias

Paraphilias are complex psychosexual disorders marked by repetitive sexual urges, fantasies, or behaviors that center on:
- inanimate and nonhuman objects (such as clothing)
- suffering or humiliation
- children or other nonconsenting persons.

Certain unusual psychosexual behaviors are similar to paraphilias but aren't officially designated as such.

Forbidden fruits

Paraphilias involve an attraction to a nonsanctioned source of sexual satisfaction. The source may be a behavior, as with exhibitionism or sadism, or a forbidden object of attraction, as with pedophilia or fetishism.

Paraphilias commonly involve sexual arousal and orgasm, usually achieved through masturbation and fantasy. (See *Puncturing some paraphilia myths,* page 492.) In most people with these disorders, the paraphiliac urge, fantasy, or behavior is always present, although its frequency and intensity may vary. Usually, a paraphilia is chronic and lifelong, although it may diminish with age.

> For some people, the paraphilia is destined to diminish as they get older.

Like other mental disorders, paraphilias may worsen during times of increased psychological stress, when other mental disorders are present, or when opportunities to engage in the paraphilia become more available.

Pinning down prevalence

Reliable statistics on the prevalence of paraphilias are hard to come by. These disorders are rarely diagnosed in clinical settings—most likely because people with paraphilias are secretive about them. Although some experts believe paraphilias are relatively rare, large commercial markets in paraphiliac pornography and paraphernalia suggest otherwise.

Myth busters

Puncturing some paraphilia myths

Like other sexual topics, paraphilias aren't well-understood by the public—and even by some health care professionals. Here are some examples.

Myth: Exhibitionism is the act of masturbating in front of peers or family members.

Reality: Exhibitionism is an intense sexual urge to expose one's genitals to an unsuspecting person. Masturbation may occur during an exhibitionist act.

Myth: Pedophilia is defined as exhibitionism in front of a prepubescent child.

Reality: Pedophilia is defined as having sexually arousing fantasies, sexual urges, or behaviors involving sexual activity with a prepubescent child.

In clinics specializing in paraphilia treatment, the most commonly seen disorders include pedophilia, voyeurism, and exhibitionism. Sexual masochism and sexual sadism are much less common.

The majority of paraphiliacs are males. Sexual masochists are the exception; female masochists outnumber male masochists by 20 to 1.

Criminal compulsions

Some paraphilias are crimes in many jurisdictions. Those that involve or harm another person—particularly pedophilia, exhibitionism, voyeurism, frotteurism, and sexual sadism—are commonly considered criminal acts, leading to arrest and possible incarceration.

Exhibitionists, pedophiles, and voyeurs make up the majority of apprehended sex offenders. Sex offenses against children, as in pedophilia, constitute a significant portion of reported criminal sex acts.

Specific paraphilias

The *DSM-5* recognizes eight paraphilias. This chapter discusses four of them in detail. For information on the other four, see *Learning about other paraphilias.*

Exhibitionism

One of the most common paraphilias, exhibitionism is marked by sexual fantasies, urges, or behaviors involving surprise exposure of the male genitals to strangers—primarily female passersby in public places. The behavior is usually limited to genital exposure, with

Learning about other paraphilias

In addition to the paraphilias described in the chapter, the *DSM-5* provides diagnostic criteria for four other paraphilias—frotteurism, sexual masochism, sexual sadism, and voyeurism. Rare paraphilias also exist.

Frotteurism

A person with frotteurism becomes sexually aroused from touching or rubbing against a nonconsenting person. For example, he may rub his genitals against a woman's thigh or fondle her breasts. The behavior frequently occurs in crowded places, where it's easier to avoid detection. Frotteurism is most common between ages 15 and 25.

Sexual masochism

With sexual masochism, a person gets sexual gratification from being physically or emotionally abused. The term masochism comes from Leopold von Sacher-Masoch, a 19th-century writer whose novels describe a man who becomes a slave to a woman and encourages her to treat him in progressively more degrading ways.

Infantilism, another form of sexual masochism, is a desire to be treated as a helpless infant, including wearing diapers.

One dangerous form of sexual masochism, called *sexual hypoxyphilia*, relies on oxygen deprivation to induce sexual arousal. The person uses a noose, mask, plastic bag, or chemical to temporarily decrease brain oxygenation. Equipment malfunction or other mistakes can cause accidental death.

Sexual sadism

With sexual sadism, a person achieves sexual gratification by inflicting pain, cruelty, or emotional abuse on others. The term dates back to 18th-century French writer and libertine, Donatien Alphonse François. Known as the Marquis de Sade, he engaged in violent and scandalous behavior and published erotic writings.

The sexual sadist may verbally humiliate his or her partner and abuse him or her physically through torture, whipping, cutting, binding, beating, burning, stabbing, or rape.

Both sadism and masochism may start in adolescence or early adulthood. The behaviors are chronic and usually grow more severe over time.

Voyeurism

The voyeur derives sexual pleasure from looking at sexual objects or sexually arousing situations, such as an unsuspecting couple engaged in sex. He or she may experience an orgasm during the voyeuristic activity or later, in response to the memory of what he or she witnessed.

The onset of voyeurism occurs before age 15. The disorder tends to be chronic.

Rare paraphilias

Rare paraphilias not included in the *DSM-5* include:
• coprophilia—sexual attraction to feces
• emetophilia—sexual attraction to vomit
• hybristophilia—sexual arousal by people who have committed crimes, particularly cruel or outrageous crimes
• klismaphilia—sexual pleasure from enemas
• necrophilia—sexual attraction to corpses
• plushophilia—sexual attraction to stuffed toys
• urolagnia—sexual attraction to urine
• zoophilia—sexual attraction to animals.

no harmful advances or assaults made toward the victim. The exhibitionist is considered more of a nuisance than an actual danger.

Exhibitionism has three characteristic features:
• It's typically performed by men for unknown women.
• It occurs in a place where sexual intercourse is impossible such as a crowded shopping mall.
• It's meant to be shocking; otherwise, it loses its power to produce sexual arousal in the paraphiliac.

Exhibitionism is the most prominent sexual offense leading to arrest, accounting for approximately one-third of sexual crimes.

Post-40 fadeout

Exhibitionism usually begins during adolescence and continues into adulthood. Although it may be a lifelong problem if untreated, it commonly becomes less severe by about age 40.

Fetishism

Fetishism is characterized by sexual fantasies, urges, or behaviors that involve the use of a fetish—a nonhuman object or a nonsexual part of the body—to produce or enhance sexual arousal.

Fetishism may involve a partner. Sometimes, focusing on certain parts of the body, such as the feet, hair, or ears, can become a fetish. In some cases, the person can achieve sexual gratification *only* when using the fetish. Usually, fetishes begin during adolescence and persist into adulthood.

Forms of fetishism

Fetishism typically has two forms. The first form involves a partner and associates sexual activity with some object such as an article clothing. In the extreme form of fetishism, a nonliving object completely replaces a human partner. The object may be underwear, boots, shoes, or fabric such as velvet or silk. The person achieves orgasm when alone and fondling the object.

Transvestic fetishism

In transvestic fetishism, a heterosexual male dresses in female clothes (called *cross-dressing*) to produce or enhance sexual arousal. He may only wear a single item of clothing, such as a garter or stockings, under masculine clothing. Alternatively, he may dress entirely as a woman, including full make-up and a feminine hairstyle to achieve a female appearance.

When not cross-dressing, they may behave in a stereotypical—or even exaggerated—masculine fashion. (See *The truth about transvestites*.)

Transvestic fetishism is commonly accompanied by masturbation and mental images of other men being attracted to the patient as a "woman."

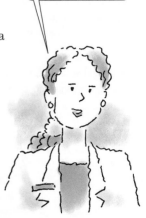

Cross-dressing allows a man to display the feminine side of his personality.

Pedophilia

Pedophilia is marked by sexual fantasies, urges, or activity involving a child, usually age 13 or younger. (In adolescent pedophilia, typically, the child is 5 years younger than the adolescent is.) The pedophile is erotically aroused by children and seeks sexual gratification with them. This urge is his preferred

Myth busters

The truth about transvestites

Let's lay to rest some common myths about transvestites—that is, people with transvestic fetishism.

Myth: Transvestites are homosexuals.

Reality: Most transvestites—by some estimates, 90%—are heterosexual. (In fact, *only* heterosexual males qualify for the official diagnosis established in the *DSM-5.*) Many are or have been married. Only a small minority are bisexual or exclusively homosexual.

Myth: Transvestites act like women even when wearing men's clothes.

Reality: Because many transvestites fear they'll be discovered, they consciously try to act as traditionally masculine as possible when not cross-dressing. For most, this isn't difficult because they're "masculine" men.

Myth: Transvestites are effeminate.

Reality: Transvestites are no more effeminate than any other males. While wearing men's clothes, most don't stand out from the crowd. In fact, out of fear that others will discover their secret, some transvestites adopt exaggerated masculine mannerisms and may appear extremely macho when not cross-dressing.

Myth: Transvestites want to be women.

Reality: Few transvestites wish to change sexes. Although both transvestites and transsexuals (people with gender dysphoria, who wish to live as or become the opposite gender) cross-dress, their motives differ. Transvestites gain sexual gratification from dressing as women but always revert back to and maintain their male gender identity. They identify primarily as males and usually feel and behave like normal males.

Myth: Transvestites cross-dress because they were dressed as girls when they were children.

Reality: Although many transvestites first experienced cross-dressing as young children, in many cases, they initiated these experiences themselves to play out fantasies involving their gender role. Typically, their parents strongly disapproved of cross-dressing.

or exclusive sexual activity, although some pedophiles are also attracted to adults. It should be noted that engaging in sex with a child or person younger than the age of 18 is considered a criminal offense and can result in prison time for convicted perpetrators.

Activity agenda

During sexual activity with a child, the pedophile may:
- undress the child
- encourage the child to watch him masturbate
- touch or fondle the child's genitals
- forcefully perform sexual acts on the child.

Types of victims

Prepubertal children are the most common targets of pedophiles. Attraction to girls is almost twice as common as attraction to boys. The pedophile may sexually abuse his own children or those of a friend or relative.

Behavior profile

Many pedophiles never come to the attention of authorities. Relatively few engage in violent behavior. Even more rarely, they kidnap or murder their victims. When this occurs, it is probably to prevent the victims from reporting their predatory behavior. It is also the case that most abusers offend against children they know and already have a relationship with (U.S. Department of Veterans Affairs, n.d.). In fact, it has been reported that 90% of child victims know the person violating them and that almost half of the offenders are family members (California Department of Justice, 2001).

More typically, the pedophile behaves seductively, showering the child with money, gifts, drugs, or alcohol. The pedophile may be quite attentive to the child's needs to gain loyalty and prevent the child from reporting the encounters. The pedophile will frequently tell the child to keep their activities a secret and will spend an inordinate amount of time doing things with the child. Nurses or health care providers who suspect that any child is being sexually abused are mandated reporters.

> Caution should be taken when an adult is giving a young person excessive gifts of money, other items of value, drugs and/or alcohol, and the like.

Causes

The specific cause of paraphilias is unknown, but experts have proposed behavioral, psychoanalytical, biological, and learning theories to explain these disorders. Behavioral models suggest that a child who was the victim or observer of inappropriate sexual behaviors learns to imitate such behavior and later gains reinforcement for it. Biological models, on the other hand, focus on the relationship among hormones, behavior, and the central nervous system (CNS)—especially the role of aggression and male sexual hormones.

Contributing factors

Based on common patient history findings, some experts have identified factors that may contribute to paraphilia. For example, many paraphiliacs come from dysfunctional families marked by isolation and sexual, emotional, or physical abuse. Some have concurrent mental disorders, such as psychoactive substance use or personality disorders.

Other factors that may contribute to paraphilias include:
- closed head injury
- CNS tumors
- history of emotional or sexual trauma
- lack of knowledge about sex
- neuroendocrine disorders
- psychosocial stressors.

Signs and symptoms

The patient's history reveals the particular pattern of abnormal sexual fantasies, urges, or behaviors associated with one of the eight recognized paraphilias.

General assessment findings may include:

• anxiety
• depression
• development of a hobby or an occupation change that makes the paraphilia more accessible
• disturbance in body image
• guilt or shame
• ineffective coping
• multiple paraphilias at the same time
• purchase of books, videos, or magazines related to the paraphilia or frequent visits to paraphilia-related Web sites
• recurrent fantasies involving a paraphilia
• sexual dysfunction
• social isolation
• troubled social or sexual relationships.

Diagnosis

Penile plethysmography may measure the patient's sexual arousal in response to visual imagery. However, the results of this procedure can be unreliable.

The diagnosis of paraphilia is confirmed if the patient meets the criteria established in the *DSM-5*. (See *Diagnostic criteria: Paraphilias*, page 498.)

Some paraphiliacs may enter the health care system only because they're forced to by legal authorities.

Treatment

Paraphiliacs seldom seek help because of their guilt, shame, fear of social ostracism, and/or legal problems. Those who encounter the health care system usually do so only at the behest of their family or when forced to by legal authorities. Treatment is mandatory if the patient's sexual behavior is deemed harmful to others or is of a criminal nature.

Depending on the specific paraphilia, treatment may involve a combination of psychotherapy, cognitive therapy, behavioral therapy, sex therapy, the use of antilibido medications, the use of psychopharmacologic medications such as selective serotonin reuptake inhibitors (SSRIs) and tricyclic antidepressants (TCAs), hormonal therapy, and rarely, surgery (Cleveland Clinic, 2012; "Sexual Dysfunction Disorder," 2012; Thibaut, De La Barra, Gordon, Cosyns, & Bradford, 2010).

Diagnostic criteria: Paraphilias

The diagnosis of a paraphilia is confirmed when the patient's symptoms meet the criteria established in the *DSM-5*. The criteria below apply to the specific paraphilias discussed in the chapter.

Exhibitionism
• Over a period of at least 6 months, the patient has experienced recurrent, intense, sexually arousing fantasies; urges; or behaviors involving the exposure of his genitals to an unsuspecting stranger.
• These fantasies, urges, or behaviors cause clinically significant distress or impairment in his social, occupational, or other areas of functioning.

Fetishism
• Over a period of at least 6 months, the patient has experienced intense, recurrent, sexually arousing fantasies; urges; or behaviors involving the use of nonliving objects (such as female undergarments).
• The fetish objects aren't limited to items of female clothing used in cross-dressing or devices used for tactile genital stimulation (for instance, a vibrator).
• The patient's fantasies, urges, or behaviors cause clinically significant distress or impairment in his social, occupational, or other important areas of functioning.

Transvestic fetishism
• Over a period of at least 6 months, a heterosexual male has experienced recurrent, intense, sexually arousing fantasies; urges; or behaviors involving cross-dressing (dressing in feminine clothing).

• These fantasies, urges, or behaviors cause clinically significant distress or impairment in his social, occupational, or other important areas of functioning.
    Transvestic fetishism occurs with gender dysphoria if the patient has persistent discomfort with his gender identity or role.

Pedophilia
• Over a period of at least 6 months, the patient has experienced recurrent, intense, sexually arousing fantasies; urges; or behaviors involving sexual activity with one or more prepubescent children (generally age 13 or younger).
• The patient has acted on these urges, or the urges or fantasies cause marked distress or interpersonal difficulty.
• The patient is at least age 16 and at least 5 years older than the child or children who are the object of his fantasies, urges, or behaviors. (*Note:* A person in his late teens who's involved in an ongoing sexual relationship with a 12- or 13-year-old *isn't* considered a pedophile.)

Subtypes
• A pedophile may be sexually attracted to males, females, or both.
• The pedophilia may be limited to incest.
• The pedophilia may be of the exclusive type, in which the patient is attracted only to children, or the nonexclusive type, in which he's also attracted to adults.

Shock treatment

In behavioral therapy, the patient may be subjected to aversive stimuli, such as bad odors or electric shocks, when he engages in the paraphiliac behavior.

To succeed, treatment should include teaching the patient alternatives to the forbidden behaviors. The effectiveness of treatment varies. In nearly all cases, treatment must be long-term to be effective.

Improving social skills

Some patients with paraphilias (especially pedophilia) have deficient social skills, which are required to obtain sexual satisfaction with consenting adults. Thus, social skills training is an essential part of treatment.

Treatment programs for sex offenders

Treatment for paraphiliacs who are sex offenders may include:
• a specialized sex offender program
• group therapy
• a 12-step sexual addiction or compulsion recovery program
• a rational thinking group
• a structured sexual disorder process group
• educational sessions focusing on the offender's psychological factors, victim impact, and human sexuality
• therapeutically structured recreational activities, adventure-based programming, arts and crafts, team sports, and experimental games
• resident and parent participation in treatment reviews
• alcohol and drug awareness programs
• values clarification
• independent living skills
• vocational exploration.

Pharmacologic therapy

Certain drugs may be used to reduce the compulsive thinking associated with paraphilias. Occasionally, hormones are prescribed if the patient experiences intrusive sexual thoughts or urges or demonstrates frequent abnormal sexual behaviors.

Nursing interventions

For nursing actions appropriate for patients with paraphilias, see *Nursing interventions for patients with sexual disorders*, pages 500 and 501. Most patients are not hospitalized primarily for sexual disorders so it is likely nurses will work with patients in settings that are not focused on treating these disorders.

Hormones may be used to treat paraphiliacs with intrusive sexual thoughts or urges or frequent abnormal sexual behavior. However, there is some question as to the effectiveness of treatment of sex offenders.

Advice from the experts

Nursing interventions for patients with sexual disorders

You can use the general interventions below when caring for a patient with any sexual disorder.

Ensure a therapeutic relationship
• Arrange to spend uninterrupted time with the patient. Encourage him to express his feelings, and accept what he says.
• Explain all treatments and procedures, and answer the patient's questions to allay his fear and help him regain a sense of control.
• Never say anything that would make the patient feel ashamed. It's his needs and feelings—not your opinions—that matter.
• Realize that treating the patient with empathy doesn't threaten your sexuality.

Promote self-knowledge
• Initiate a discussion about how the need for self-esteem, respect, love, and intimacy influence a person's sexual expression. This helps the patient understand his disorder.
• Encourage the patient to identify feelings—such as pleasure, reduced anxiety, increased control, or shame—associated with his sexual behavior and fantasies.
• Help the patient distinguish between practices that are distressing because they don't conform to social norms or personal values and those that may place him or others in emotional, medical, or legal jeopardy. Doing this reinforces the need for him to stop behaviors that could harm himself or others.
• Encourage him to express his sexual preferences as well as his feelings about them.

Increase the level of interaction
• Spend specific, non-care-related time with the patient during each shift to encourage social interaction. Start with one-on-one interaction and increase to group interaction when his social skills indicate he's ready. Increasing social interaction gradually eases his feeling of being overwhelmed and minimizes sensory input that may renew cognitive or perceptual disturbances.

• Give positive reinforcement for appropriate and effective interaction behaviors, both verbal and nonverbal.

Promote participation in care
• Encourage the patient to make decisions about his care, to enhance his self-esteem, and increase his sense of mastery over the current situation.
• Assist the patient and his family or close friends in progressive participation in care and therapies.
• Have the patient increase his self-care performance levels gradually so he can progress at his own pace.
• Initiate or participate in multidisciplinary patient-centered conferences to evaluate progress and plan discharge. These conferences should involve the patient and his family in a cooperative effort to individualize his care plan.

Improve coping skills
• Encourage the patient to use support systems to assist with coping, thereby helping to restore psychological equilibrium and prevent crises.
• Try to identify factors that cause or exacerbate poor coping ability, such as a fear of being fired.
• Help the patient look at his current situation and evaluate various coping behaviors to encourage a realistic view of the crisis.
• Urge the patient to try new coping behaviors. A patient in crisis tends to accept interventions and develop new coping behaviors more readily than at other times.
• Request feedback from the patient about behaviors that seem to work. This encourages him to evaluate the effect of these behaviors.
• Praise the patient for making decisions and performing activities to reinforce coping behaviors.

Provide referrals
• Refer the patient for professional psychological counseling. If his maladaptive behavior has high crisis potential, formal counseling can help ease your frustration, increase your objectivity, and foster a collaborative approach to patient care. As appropriate, refer the patient

Nursing interventions for patients with sexual disorders (continued)

to a physician, nurse, psychologist, social worker, or counselor trained in sex therapy.

Other actions

• Be aware that whenever possible, a primary nurse should be assigned to the patient to ensure continuity of care and promote a therapeutic relationship.

• Initially, allow the patient to depend partly on you for self-care because he may regress to a lower developmental level during the initial crisis phase.

• If the patient poses a threat to himself and others, institute safety precautions, according to facility protocol.

• Identify and reduce unnecessary environment stimuli.

Sexual dysfunctions

Sexual dysfunctions are characterized by pain during sex or by a disturbance in one of the phases of the sexual response cycle. (See *Sexual pain disorders*, page 502.) These dysfunctions may cause marked distress and interpersonal problems. They can impair intimate relationships by reducing the enjoyment of normal sex or preventing the normal physiologic changes of the sexual response cycle.

In some people, a sexual dysfunction is present at the onset of sexual functioning and activity. In others, it follows a period of normal sexual functioning.

Sexual dysfunctions have high rates of prevalence both here and in other countries. One study estimated a 24% rate of dysfunction for the U.S. population (Robins et al., 1984) and as previously mentioned, a global study found a 38% rate for women and 29% for men (Laumann et al., 2005). Sexual dysfunction can be classified as primary or secondary. If the condition is caused by a psychiatric disorder, physical conditions, or medications, then it is considered to be secondary (Bhugra & Colombini, 2013). Sexual dysfunctions are commonly linked to psychological factors, medical conditions, substance use, or a combination of these factors.

Categorizing sexual dysfunctions

Sexual dysfunctions fall into several categories:
• sexual arousal disorders
• sexual desire disorders
• orgasmic disorders
• sexual dysfunction caused by a medical condition
• sexual pain disorders. (See *Types of sexual dysfunctions*, page 503.)

Generalized versus situational dysfunction

A sexual dysfunction may be generalized or situational. In the generalized type, the dysfunction occurs with all types of stimulation,

Sexual pain disorders

The two main types of sexual pain disorders are dyspareunia and vaginismus.

Dyspareunia

With dyspareunia, which can occur in both males and females, unexplained genital pain occurs before, during, or after intercourse. The condition may be mild—or may be severe enough to restrict the enjoyment of sex.

Causes

Physical conditions that can cause dyspareunia include:
- acute or chronic infections of the genitourinary tract
- allergic reactions (as from diaphragms, condoms, or other contraceptives)
- benign or malignant reproductive system growths or tumors
- deformities or lesions of the vagina or its opening
- disorders of the surrounding viscera (including the residual effects of pelvic inflammatory disease and disease of the adnexal and broad ligaments)
- endometriosis
- genital, rectal, or pelvic scar tissue
- insufficient lubrication (as from medications, estrogen loss, or radiation to the genital area)
- intact hymen
- local trauma (such as hymenal tears or bruising of the urethral meatus)
- retroversion of the uterus.

Psychological causes of dyspareunia include a history of sexual abuse and problems in intimate relationships.

Treatment

When dyspareunia has a physical cause, treatment may include:
- creams and water-soluble jellies for inadequate lubrication
- medications for infections
- excision of hymenal scars
- gentle stretching of painful scars at the vaginal opening
- a change in coital position to reduce pain on deep penetration.

When the condition has a psychological cause, interventions may include psychotherapy or sensate focus exercises. With these exercises, each partner takes turns paying increased attention to his own physical sensations.

Vaginismus

With vaginismus, involuntary spasmodic muscle contractions occur at the entrance to the vagina when the male tries to insert his penis. Pain occurs if intercourse is attempted despite these contractions.

This condition makes intercourse extremely painful or impossible. However, women with vaginismus are capable of becoming sexually aroused and achieving lubrication and orgasm through clitoral or other alternative stimulation.

Vaginismus can be primary or secondary. With primary vaginismus, the patient has never been able to have intercourse with penetration (resulting, e.g., in an unconsummated relationship). In secondary vaginismus, the patient previously experienced normal intercourse before developing the condition.

Causes

Most authorities believe vaginismus is a learned response commonly stemming from dyspareunia. Women who have had frightening, unsatisfying, or painful sexual experiences may fear that penetration and intercourse will cause pain. A strict cultural or religious background can have the same effect. This fear and anticipation of pain may lead to a pattern of sexual anxiety, causing vaginal dryness and tightness before intercourse.

Other psychological factors that may cause or contribute to vaginismus include fears of pregnancy, of being controlled by a man, or of losing control.

Physical causes of vaginismus include vaginal infection, physical aftereffects of childbirth, and fatigue.

Treatment

Treatment for vaginismus stemming from psychological causes may include a combination of:
- couples therapy
- Kegel exercises to strengthen the pubococcygeal muscle
- sensate focus exercises for the couple
- progressive use of a plastic dilator or finger, which is inserted into the vaginal opening to progressively stretch the contracted muscles.

When treated by a professional using these or similar techniques, vaginismus has a cure rate of about 80% to 100% (Schuiling & Likis, 2013).

Types of sexual dysfunctions

The *DSM-5* classifies sexual dysfunctions (other than paraphilias and gender dysphoria) as described below.

Sexual desire disorders: Hypoactive sexual desire disorder, sexual aversion disorder
The key feature of hypoactive sexual desire disorder is a deficiency or absence of sexual fantasies or desire for sexual activity. The patient rarely initiates sexual activity but may engage in it reluctantly when the partner initiates it.

With sexual aversion disorder, the patient dislikes and avoids genital sexual contact with a sexual partner.

Sexual arousal disorders: Female sexual arousal disorder, male erectile disorder
With female sexual arousal disorder, the patient has a persistent or recurrent inability to attain or maintain (until the completion of sexual activity) an adequate lubrication–swelling response of sexual excitement.

With male erectile disorder, the patient has a persistent or recurrent inability to attain or maintain (until the completion of sexual activity) an adequate erection.

Orgasmic disorders: Female orgasmic disorder, male orgasmic disorder, premature ejaculation
With male and female orgasmic disorders, the patient experiences a persistent or recurrent delay in, or absence of, orgasm following a normal sexual excitement phase.

Premature ejaculation refers to a persistent and recurrent onset of orgasm and ejaculation with minimal sexual stimulation.

Sexual dysfunction due to a general medical condition
With sexual dysfunction due to a general medical condition, the patient's sexual dysfunction is fully explained by the direct physiologic effects of a general medical condition. This category includes sexual dysfunction caused by substance use, such as alcohol, prescription drugs, or street drugs.

Sexual pain disorders: Dyspareunia, vaginismus
The essential feature of dyspareunia is genital pain associated with sexual intercourse. Vaginismus refers to a recurrent or persistent involuntary contraction of the perineal muscles surrounding the outer third of the vagina when vaginal penetration is attempted. With some patients, even the anticipation of vaginal insertion may result in muscle spasm.

situation, and partners. In the situational type, the dysfunction is limited to certain types of stimulation, situations, or partners.

Prognosis

The prognosis is good for temporary or mild sexual dysfunctions stemming from misinformation or situational stress. It's guarded for dysfunctions that result from intense anxiety, chronically discordant relationships, psychological disturbances, or drug or alcohol abuse in either partner (Schuiling & Likis, 2013).

Female sexual arousal disorder and female orgasmic disorder

Defined as the inability to achieve or maintain an adequate lubrication–swelling response of sexual excitement, female sexual arousal disorder is one of the most severe sexual dysfunctions in women.

Female orgasmic disorder, the most common sexual dysfunction in women, is the inability to achieve orgasm (Schuiling & Likis, 2013). Unlike a woman with sexual arousal disorder, one with orgasmic disorder may desire sexual activity and become aroused but feels inhibited as she approaches orgasm.

Primary and secondary categories

These disorders can be primary or secondary. They're primary when they occur in someone who has never experienced sexual arousal or orgasm. They're secondary when a physical, mental, or environmental condition inhibits or prevents previously normal sexual functioning.

Causes

Factors that may cause or contribute to female sexual arousal or orgasmic disorder include:
• depression
• drug use (such as CNS depressants, antidepressants, hormonal contraceptives, alcohol, or street drugs)
• discordant relationships (poor communication, hostility or ambivalence toward the partner, or fear of abandonment or of asserting independence)
• diseases (general systemic illness, endocrine or nervous system disorders, or diseases that impair muscle tone or contractility)
• fatigue
• gynecologic factors (chronic vaginal or pelvic infection or pain; congenital anomalies; or genital cancer, trauma, or surgery)
• inadequate or ineffective sexual stimulation
• lifestyle disruptions
• psychological factors (such as stress, anxiety, anger, hostility, boredom with sex, guilt, depression, unconscious conflicts about sexuality, or fear of losing control of one's feelings or behavior)
• pregnancy
• religious or cultural taboos that reinforce guilt feelings about sex (Schuiling & Likis, 2013).

Signs and symptoms

Assessment findings in patients with sexual dysfunctions vary with the specific dysfunction.

Female sexual arousal disorder

A woman with sexual arousal disorder usually reports limited or absent sexual desire and little or no pleasure from sexual stimulation. Her history may include:
- decreased sexual desire
- individual or family stress or fatigue, as occurs in many working mothers with children younger than age 5 who are too exhausted to care about sex
- misinformation about sex and sexuality
- a pattern of dysfunctional sexual response
- conceptual problems during childhood and adolescence about sex in general and, specifically, about masturbation, incest, rape, sexual fantasies, and homosexual or heterosexual practices
- concerns about contraception and reproductive ability
- problems in the current sexual relationship
- poor self-esteem and body image.

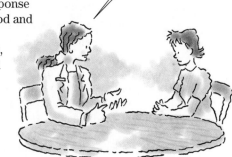

Sexual arousal disorder commonly occurs in working mothers with young children. Maybe you're just too exhausted to care about sex.

Physical indications of sexual arousal disorder include the lack of vaginal lubrication and the absence of signs of genital vasocongestion (Schuiling & Likis, 2013).

Female orgasmic disorder

A woman with orgasmic disorder may report an inability to achieve orgasm, either totally or under certain circumstances.

Diagnosis

A thorough physical examination, laboratory tests, and medical history can rule out physical causes of female sexual arousal or orgasmic disorder.

A sexual dysfunction is diagnosed if the patient fulfills the criteria in the *DSM-5*.

Treatment

Treatment varies with the specific dysfunction.

Treating sexual arousal disorder

Female sexual arousal disorder can be challenging to treat—especially if the patient has never experienced sexual pleasure. The goal of therapy is to help her relax, become aware of her feelings about sex, and eliminate guilt and fear of rejection. Some women and their partners need reassurance about their activities, whereas others need suggestions and more intensive therapy.

For some patients, psychotherapy or behavioral therapy is indicated. Psychotherapy may consist of free association, dream analysis, and discussion of life patterns to achieve greater sexual awareness. One behavioral approach attempts to correct maladaptive patterns through systematic desensitization to situations that provoke anxiety—for example, by encouraging the patient to fantasize about these situations. Hormonal treatment may also improve sexual desire in some women (Cleveland Clinic, 2012).

> To treat sexual arousal disorder, I recommend that you fantasize about the situations that cause you anxiety.

Sensate focus exercises

Many patients with sexual arousal disorder benefit from sensate focus exercises. These exercises minimize the importance of intercourse and orgasm while emphasizing touching and awareness of sensual feelings over the entire body (not just genital sensations).

Sensate focus exercises are done with a partner. Each partner takes turns giving and then receiving touch and massage. At first, they're instructed to give pleasure without touching the breasts or genitals. The person receiving the pleasure places his or her hand over the giver's to show where the touch should be and what it should feel like. This improves communication and teaches the couple what they *can* achieve rather than what they *can't*.

Later, the ban against genital touching and orgasm is reduced as the couple realizes that mutual pleasure can be derived from simple touching. A sensate focus program may also include masturbation, either alone or together.

> Focusing on breathing patterns or muscle contractions is therapeutic for some patients with primary orgasmic disorder.

Treating orgasmic disorder

In treating orgasmic disorder, the goal is to decrease or eliminate involuntary inhibition of the orgasmic reflex. Treatment may include experiential therapy, psychoanalysis, or behavior modification. Individual therapy, marital or couples therapy, or sex therapy may be indicated.

Medications may be prescribed to decrease symptoms, if appropriate. Any underlying physical disorder should be treated.

Managing primary orgasmic disorder

For primary orgasmic disorder, treatment may include teaching the patient self-stimulation and distraction techniques, such as focusing on fantasies, breathing patterns, and muscle contractions to relieve anxiety.

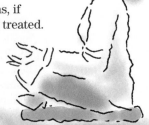

Thus, the patient learns new behavior through exercises she does at home between sessions. Eventually, the therapist involves the patient's sexual partner in treatment sessions (although some therapists treat the couple as a unit from the beginning).

Strategies for secondary orgasmic disorder

For secondary orgasmic disorder, the goal of treatment is to decrease anxiety and promote the factors necessary for the patient to experience orgasm. The therapist communicates an accepting and permissive attitude and helps the patient understand that satisfactory sexual experiences don't always require coital orgasm.

Nursing interventions

Nursing interventions for female sexual arousal or orgasmic disorder are the same for other sexual disorders. (See *Nursing interventions for patients with sexual disorders*, pages 500 and 501.)

Premature ejaculation

Premature ejaculation refers to a male's inability to control the ejaculatory reflex during sexual activity. The condition causes ejaculation to occur before or immediately after penetration or before the wishes of both partners.

This disorder affects men of all ages. Unlike male erectile disorder, premature ejaculation doesn't affect the ability to have or maintain an erection. (See *Understanding male erectile disorder*, page 508.) Premature ejaculation can seriously disrupt intimate relationships. It may lead to generalized anxiety disorder or pervasive feelings of inadequacy, guilt, and self-doubt.

Causes

Psychological factors, such as stress, performance anxiety, or limited sexual experiences, typically play a key role in premature ejaculation. Other psychological factors that may cause or contribute to this disorder include:
- ambivalence toward or unconscious hatred of women
- negative sexual relationships in which the patient unconsciously denies his partner sexual fulfillment
- guilt feelings about sex.

However, the disorder can occur in emotionally healthy men with stable, positive relationships.

In some men, premature ejaculation is linked to an underlying degenerative neurologic disorder such as multiple sclerosis or an inflammatory process, such as posterior urethritis or prostatitis. Other physical factors associated with premature ejaculation include drug or alcohol use and genital surgery or trauma.

Understanding male erectile disorder

Male erectile disorder (commonly called *impotence*) refers to the inability to attain or maintain penile erection long enough to complete sexual intercourse. The patient's history may reveal a long-standing inability to achieve erection, sudden loss of erectile function, or a gradual decline in function. It may also include a medical condition, drug therapy, or psychological trauma that could contribute to erectile disorder.

When the cause of the disorder is psychogenic rather than organic, the patient may report that he can achieve erection through masturbation but not with a partner. He may show signs of anxiety when discussing his condition, such as sweating and palpitations—or he may appear disinterested. Depression, another common complaint, may be either a cause or an effect of erectile disorder.

Treatment

Sex therapy designed to reduce performance anxiety may effectively cure psychogenic impotence.

Treatment for organic impotence focuses on eliminating the underlying cause. If this isn't possible, counseling may help the couple deal with their situation realistically and explore alternatives for sexual expression. Some patients may benefit from a surgically inserted inflatable or semirigid penile prosthesis. Others may benefit from such medications as sildenafil (Viagra), from the use of vacuum pumps or constriction rings, or from intracorporeal injections into the penis (Cleveland Clinic, 2012; Medline Plus, 2010; "Sexual Dysfunction Disorder," 2012).

Signs and symptoms

The patient's history may reveal that he can't prolong foreplay or that he ejaculates as soon as he inserts his penis into the vagina. In some cases, the partner seeks psychiatric treatment, complaining that the patient is indifferent to her sexual needs.

Other assessment findings may include:
- anxiety
- depression
- disturbance in body image
- frustration and feelings of being unattractive
- ineffective coping
- pain during sexual intercourse
- poor self-concept
- social isolation.

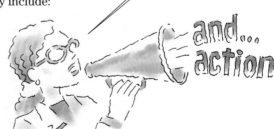

Next time, wait until I yell "Action!"

and... action

Diagnosis

Diagnostic tests can rule out medical causes of premature ejaculation. The disorder is diagnosed if the patient meets the criteria in the *DSM-5*. The patient with premature ejaculation can cause marked distress or interpersonal difficulty and may be lifelong, generalized, situational, or caused by psychological factors (APA, 2013).

Treatment

Although the SSRIs are known to cause problems with sexual functioning (Montgomery, 2008; Smith, 2007), they can be therapeutic in other areas and are often used to treat male premature ejaculation. Aside from medication, Masters and Johnson (1966) developed a highly successful intensive treatment program for premature ejaculation that helps the patient focus on sensations of impending orgasm. The program combines insight therapy, behavioral techniques, and experiential sessions involving both partners.

Therapy Types

Therapy sessions, which last 2 weeks or longer, typically include:
• mutual physical exploration to enhance the couple's awareness of anatomy and physiology while reducing shameful feelings about sexual body parts
• sensate focus exercises, which allow each partner to caress the other's body without intercourse and to focus on pleasurable touch sensations
• the squeeze technique, which helps the patient gain control of ejaculatory tension. (See *Squeeze play for premature ejaculation*, page 510.)

Start, stop, start, stop

The stop-and-start technique also helps to delay ejaculation. Performed with the woman in the superior position, this method involves pelvic thrusting until orgasmic sensations begin. Thrusting then stops and is restarted to promote control of ejaculation. Eventually, the couple is allowed to achieve orgasm.

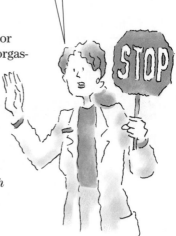

In the stop-and-start technique, the couple starts and stops pelvic thrusting repeatedly to help the man learn to control his ejaculation.

Nursing interventions

Nursing interventions for patients with premature ejaculation resemble those used for other sexual disorders. (See *Nursing interventions for patients with sexual disorders*, pages 500 and 501.)

Advice from the experts

Squeeze play for premature ejaculation

The squeeze technique, used to overcome premature ejaculation, may be practiced either with a partner or alone during masturbation. Advise the patient or his partner to position the fingers correctly around the penis and apply the right amount of pressure. When the patient feels the urge to ejaculate, he or his partner should place a thumb on the frenulum of the penis and place the index and middle fingers above and below the coronal ridge, as shown here.

Then the patient or partner should squeeze the penis from front to back—more firmly for an erect penis and less firmly for a partially flaccid one. They should apply and release pressure every few minutes during a touching exercise. The goal is to delay ejaculation by keeping the patient at an earlier phase of the sexual response cycle.

The patient should feel pressure but no pain. After several squeezes, he should have a more intense ejaculation than usual.

Anatomic structures

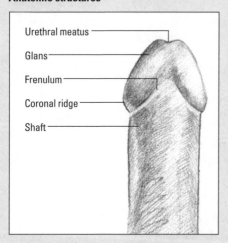

- Urethral meatus
- Glans
- Frenulum
- Coronal ridge
- Shaft

Hand position

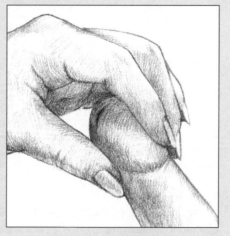

Gender dysphoria

Gender dysphoria is marked by discomfort with one's apparent or assigned gender and a strong, persistent identification with the opposite sex. Someone with this disorder (sometimes called a *transsexual*) wants to be like or wants to become the opposite sex and is extremely uncomfortable with his or her assigned gender role.

Gender identity—the intimate, personal feeling one has about being male or female—includes three components: self-concept, perception of an ideal partner, and external presentation of masculinity or femininity through behavior, dress, and mannerisms. Patients with gender dysphoria may have a problem with one or all of these components. Typically, they behave and present themselves as a person of the opposite sex.

Gender dysphoria shouldn't be confused with the far more common phenomenon of feeling inadequate in meeting the expectations normally associated with a particular sex.

Impaired and despairing

Gender dysphoria may seriously impair social and occupational functioning—not just because of the psychopathology but also because of the problems associated with trying to live as the opposite sex. Anxiety and depression are common among those with this disorder and may lead to suicide attempts.

Prevalence and onset

Gender dysphoria is known to appear beginning in infancy and the prevalence among children and adolescents is believed to be less than 1%. It is estimated at 1 in 30,000 in men and 1 in 100,000 in women (Black and Andreasen, 2011; Korte et al., 2008; Townsend, 2012).

Causes

Current theories about the cause of gender dysphoria suggest a combination of predisposing factors, including:
- chromosomal anomalies
- hormonal imbalances (particularly in utero during brain formation)
- pathologic defects in early parent–child bonding and child-rearing practices. For example, parents who treat their child as a member of the opposite sex may contribute to gender dysphoria.

Contributing factors may include:
- concurrent paraphilias, especially transvestic fetishism
- feelings of sexual inadequacy
- generalized anxiety disorder
- personality disorders.

> Parents who treat their child like a member of the opposite sex may contribute to gender dysphoria.

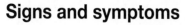

Signs and symptoms

Signs and symptoms of gender dysphoria differ among adults, adolescents, and children.

Assessment findings in adults and adolescents

Adults and adolescents with this disorder typically believe they were born the wrong sex. They're preoccupied with eliminating primary and secondary sex characteristics. Some people request hormones, surgery, or other procedures to physically alter their sexual characteristics.

Males may describe a lifelong history of feeling feminine and pursuing feminine activities. Females exhibit similar propensities for opposite-sex activities and discomfort with the female role.

Other assessment findings may include:
- anxiety
- attempts to mask or remove the sex organs
- cross-dressing
- depression
- disturbances in body image
- dreams of cross-gender identification
- fear of abandonment by family and friends
- finding one's genitals "disgusting"
- ineffective coping strategies
- peer ostracism
- preoccupation with appearance
- self-hatred
- self-medication such as with hormonal therapy
- strong attraction to stereotypical activities of the opposite sex
- suicide attempts or ideation.

In both sexes, the crisis seems especially acute during puberty. Development of secondary sex characteristics (breasts and pubic hair in the female, enlarged penis and testes in the male) may trigger intense distress or intensify the feeling that one is a misfit.

Assessment findings in children

Children with gender dysphoria may express the desire to be—or insist that they are—the opposite sex. They may express disgust with their genitalia, along with an ardent hope to become the opposite sex when they grow up.

> The criteria in the DSM-5 determine whether the patient qualifies for an official diagnosis of gender dysphoria.

Diagnosis

Diagnostic test results suggesting gender dysphoria include:
- karyotyping for sex chromosomes, which may show abnormalities
- psychological tests, which reveal cross-gender identification or behavior patterns
- sex hormone assay, which may reveal an abnormality.

The diagnosis of gender dysphoria is confirmed if the patient meets the criteria in the *DSM-5*.

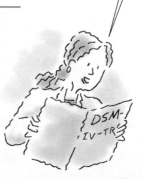

Treatment

Individual and couples therapy may help an adult patient cope with the decision to live as the opposite sex or, depending on the circumstances, to cope with the knowledge that he or she *won't* be able to live as the opposite sex.

Psychiatric management, including hospitalization, may be indicated if the patient has the potential for violence, such as suicidal ideation or self-mutilation fantasies. Group or individual psychotherapy may also be appropriate.

For a child, individual and family therapy are indicated. Having a therapist of the same sex may be useful for role-modeling purposes. The earlier the problem is diagnosed and treatment begins, the better the prognosis.

Sex reassignment surgery

For some patients, sex reassignment through hormonal therapy and sex change surgery may be an option. However, sex reassignment hasn't been as beneficial as first hoped. Severe psychological problems may persist afterward.

Nursing interventions

Nursing interventions for patients with gender dysphoria resemble those for other sexual disorders. (See *Nursing interventions for patients with sexual disorders*, pages 500 and 501.)

Mental health and medications

It is important to remember that sexual problems, including a lack of desire and interest in sex and intimacy and inability or difficulty with performance, can be directly related to the individual's mental health (Bhugra & Colombini, 2013). Any of the mental health disorders can adversely impact how a person feels about sex and their level of interest, particularly if someone is experiencing a mood or anxiety disorder. In addition, a number of illegal drugs as well as medications prescribed to treat behavioral disorders are known to cause problems related to sexual interest and performance. (See *Categories of psychotropics that can cause sexual dysfunction*, page 514.) Included among drugs that create problems with performance are alcohol and opioids. In terms of prescribed psychotropic medications, a number of antidepressants, antipsychotics, and anxiolytics can impair erection and ejaculation in males and inhibit or prevent orgasm in women (Crenshaw & Goldberg, 1996;Montgomery, 2008). A thorough assessment will ask about the patient's mental health and medications he or she is taking. Most importantly, among the first steps in managing sexual

Categories of psychotropics that can cause sexual dysfunction

Antidepressants

TCAs can cause erectile failure and ejaculation problems in men and anorgasmia and dyspareunia in women. Examples include imipramine (Tofranil), amitriptyline (Elavil), and clomipramine (Anafranil).

SSRIs are the class of antidepressants most commonly associated with sexual dysfunction. They can cause a lack of interest in sex, erectile dysfunction, ejaculatory delay or failure, and anorgasmia. They are also associated with dyspareunia and priapism. Examples include fluoxetine (Prozac), paroxetine (Paxil), and sertraline (Zoloft).

Monoamine oxidase inhibitors (MAOIs) can cause erection difficulties and can delay and inhibit ejaculation and female orgasm. Examples include phenelzine (Nardil), tranylcypromine (Parnate), and isocarboxazid (Marplan).

Antipsychotics

Antipsychotics, both first and second generation, are known to cause a number of problems with sexual functioning such as decreased sexual desire, diminished or lack of orgasm, a variety of ejaculation disorders, difficulty in achieving an erection, and priapism. Examples include haloperidol (Haldol), thioridazine (Mellaril), fluphenazine (Prolixin), and chlorpromazine (Thorazine).

Anxiolytics

Benzodiazepines can reduce desire because they can cause drowsiness, although in some cases, they can and do increase desire and libido. Examples include diazepam (Valium), chlordiazepoxide (Librium), lorazepam (Ativan), and oxazepam (Serax) (Sadock & Sadock, 2007; Smith, 2007; Stahl, 2009).

problems is to live as healthy a lifestyle as possible. Simple steps such as watching one's weight; exercising and eating right; and refraining from smoking, drinking to excess, and using drugs can help improve an individual's general health thus making the road to sexual health a smoother one to travel.

References

American Psychiatric Association. (2013). *Diagnostic and statistical manual of mental disorders* (5th ed.). Washington, DC: American Psychiatric Publishing.

Bhugra, D., & Colombini, G. (2013). Sexual dysfunction: Classification and assessment. *Advances in Psychiatric Treatment, 19*(1), 48–55.

Black, D. W., & Andreasen, N. C. (2011). *Introductory textbook of psychiatry* (5th ed.). Washington, DC: American Psychiatric Publishing.

California Department of Justice. (2001). *Megan's law—Facts about sex offenders*. Retrieved from http://www.meganslaw.ca.gov/facts.htm

Centers for Disease Control and Prevention. (2010). Youth risk behavior surveillance survey—United States, 2009. *MMWR Surveill Summ, 59*(5), 1–142. Retrieved from http://www.cdc.gov/mmwr/pdf/ss/ss5905.pdf

Centers for Disease Control and Prevention. (2012). Youth risk behavior surveillance—United States, 2011. *MMWR Surveill Summ, 61*(4), 1–162.

Centers for Disease Control and Prevention. (n.d.-a). *1991-2013 high school youth risk behavior survey data*. Retrieved from http://www.nccd.cdc.gov/YouthOnline/App/Default.aspx

Chandra, A., Mosher, W. D., Copen, C., & Sionean, C. (2011). *Sexual behavior, sexual attraction, and sexual identity in the United States: Data from the 2006-2008 National Survey of Family Growth*. Retrieved from http://www.cdc.gov/nchs/data/nhsr/nhsr036.pdf

Cleveland Clinic. (2012). *Diseases and conditions: An overview of sexual dysfunction*. Retrieved from http://www.my.clevelandclinic.org/health/diseases_conditions/hic_An_Overview_of_Sexual_Dysfunction

Crenshaw, T. L., & Goldberg, J. P. (1996). *Sexual pharmacology: Drugs that affect sexual functioning*. New York, NY: W.W. Norton and Company.

Ford, J. V., Barnes, R., Rompalo, A., & Hook, E. W., III. (2013). Sexual health training and education in the U.S. *Public Health Reports, 128*(Suppl. 1), 96–101.

Kaplan, H. S. (1979). *Disorders of sexual desire and other new concepts and techniques in sex therapy*. Delran, NJ: Simon and Schuster.

Korte, A., Lehmkuhl, U., Goecker, D., Beier, K. M., Krude, H., & Grüters-Kieslich, A. (2008). Gender identity disorders in childhood and adolescence. *Deutsched Arzteblatt International, 105*(48), 834–841.

Laumann, E. O., Nicolosi, A., Glasser, D. B., Paik, A., Gingell, C., Moreira, E., & Wang, T. (2005). Sexual problems among men and women aged 40–80 years. *International Journal of Impotence Research, 17*, 39–57.

Masters, W. H., & Johnson, V. E. (1966). *Human sexual response*. Boston, MA: Little Brown.

Medline Plus. (2010). *Sexual problems overview*. Retrieved from http://www.nlm.nih.gov/medlineplus/ency/article/001951.htm

Montgomery, K. A. (2008). Sexual desire disorders. *Psychiatry, 5*(6), 50–55.

National Prevention Council. (2011). *National prevention strategy: America's plan for better health and wellness*. Washington, DC: U.S. Department of Health and Human Services, Office of the Surgeon General. Retrieved from http://www.healthcare.gov/prevention/nphpphc/strategy/index.html

Rainbow Access Initiative. (n.d.). *Components of sexual identity*. Retrieved from http://www.rainbowaccess.org/FreeCourse/components.html

Robins, L. N., Helzer, J. E., Weissman, M. M., Orvaschel, H., Guenberg, E., Burke, J. D., Jr., & Regier, D. A. (1984). Lifetime prevalence of specific psychiatric disorders in three sites. *Archives of General Psychiatry, 41*, 949–958.

Sadock, B. J., & Sadock, V. A. (2007). *Kaplan and Sadock's synopsis of psychiatry* (10th ed.). Philadelphia, PA: Lippincott Williams and Wilkins.

Schuiling, K. D., & Likis, F. E. (2013). *Women's gynecologic health* (2nd ed.). Burlington, MA: Jones & Bartlett Learning.

Sexual dysfunction disorder and paraphilias 4. Treatment flashcards. (2012). Retrieved from http://quizlet.com/13941198/sexual-dysfunction-disorder-and-paraphilias-4-treatment-flash-cards/

Smith, S. (2007). Drugs that cause sexual dysfunction. *Psychiatry, 6*(3), 111–114.

Spitzer, R. (1981). The diagnostic status of homosexuality in DSM III: A reformation of the issues. *American Journal of Psychiatry, 138*(2), 210–215. Retrieved from http://ajp.psychiatryonline.org/article.aspx?Volume=138&page=210&journalID=13

Stahl, S. M. (2009). *The prescriber's guide: Stahl's essential psychopharmacology* (3rd ed.). New York, NY: Cambridge University Press.

Thibaut, F., De La Barra, F., Gordon, H., Cosyns, P., & Bradford, J. M. (2010) The World Federation of Societies of Biological Psychiatry (WFSBP) guidelines for the biological treatment of paraphilias. *The World Journal of Biological Psychiatry, 11*, 604–655.

Townsend, M. (2012). *Psychiatric mental health nursing: Concepts of care in evidence based practice.* Philadelphia, PA: F.A. Davis.

U.S. Department of Health and Human Services. (2013). *Adolescent sexual behaviors.* Retrieved from http://www.hhs.gov/ash/oah/resources-and-publications/info/parents/just-facts/adolescent-sex.html

U.S. Department of Veterans Affairs. (n.d.). *Child sexual abuse.* Retrieved from http://www.ptsd.va.gov/public/pages/child-sexual-abuse.asp

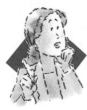

Quick quiz

1. The phase of the sexual response cycle involving fantasy and expectation is the:

    A.   desire phase.

    B.   excitement phase.

    C.   orgasm phase.

    D.   resolution phase.

Answer: A. The desire phase of the sexual response cycle involves fantasy and expectation.

2. The nurse understands that which of the following may cause or contribute to sexual dysfunction?

    A.   Drug use

    B.   Dissociative disorders

    C.   Supplemental vitamin use

    D.   Exercise

Answer: A. Sexual dysfunctions sometimes stem from transient conditions, such as drug or alcohol use.

3. A nurse is caring for a patient with a paraphilia diagnosis. The nurse understands that a persistent urge to show one's private parts to a stranger occurs in which of the following?
  A. Fetishism
  B. Pedophilia
  C. Exhibitionism
  D. Transsexualism

Answer: C. An exhibitionist has sexual fantasies, urges, or behaviors involving exposing the genitals to strangers.

4. Treatments the nurse could recommend when caring for female with orgasmic disorder include:
  A. taking soothing bubble baths.
  B. touching her partner.
  C. having sexual intercourse more often.
  D. increasing the degree of sexual arousal.

Answer: B. Sensate focus exercises are recommended for female orgasmic disorder. These exercises emphasize touching and awareness of sensual feelings throughout the entire body while minimizing the importance of intercourse and orgasm. The couple takes turns giving and receiving touch.

5. A nonliving object may replace a human partner in a patient with:
  A. fetishism.
  B. gender dysphoria.
  C. transsexualism.
  D. sexual desire disorder.

Answer: A. In one form of fetishism, a nonliving object completely replaces a human partner. The object may be undergarments, shoes, or a fabric, such as velvet or silk.

6. Gender dysphoria should be suspected if the patient:
  A. has a strong desire to be of the same sex.
  B. insists that he or she is of the opposite sex.
  C. prefers the opposite sex.
  D. engages in games with the same sex.

Answer: B. Gender dysphoria is marked by a repeatedly stated desire to be the opposite sex or an insistence that one is the opposite sex.

7. Sexual attraction to children is termed:
   A.   sadism.
   B.   necrophilia.
   C.   exhibitionism.
   D.   pedophilia.

Answer: D. In pedophilia, the patent has sexual fantasies, urges, or activity involving a child.

Scoring

☆☆☆   If you answered all seven items correctly, intense! Your dedication to understanding sexual disorders has climaxed in a perfect score!

☆☆   If you answered five or six items correctly, you deserve a pat on the back, if not a full-body massage! You've nearly mastered Masters' and Johnson's favorite topic.

☆   If you answered fewer than five items correctly, that's OK. We're sure you have the desire to understand sexual disorders and may even find the subject arousing. To reach peak comprehension, just read the chapter again.

Appendices and index

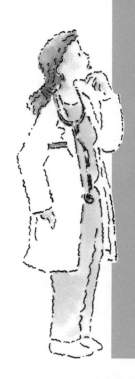

Glossary

abreaction
verbalization of a repressed memory, idea, or emotion

abuse
self-administration of any drug in a culturally disapproved manner that causes adverse consequences

acetylcholine
a neurotransmitter in the autonomic nervous system

acting out
repeatedly performing actions without weighing the possible results of those actions

addiction
a behavioral pattern of drug abuse characterized by overwhelming involvement with the use of a drug (compulsive use), the securing of its supply, and a strong tendency to relapse after discontinuation

age-related cognitive decline (ARCD)
deficits in memory that do not significantly impact daily function; also called *age-associated cognitive decline*

Alzheimer
a progressive, degenerative disorder that attacks the brain's nerve cells, or neurons, resulting in loss of memory, thinking and language skills, and behavioral changes

ambivalence
coexisting, strong positive and negative feelings, leading to emotional conflict

amphetamine
stimulant drugs used to increase alertness, relieve fatigue, and feel stronger and more decisive; used for euphoric effects or to counteract the "down" feeling of tranquilizers or alcohol

anhedonia
a diminished capacity to experience pleasure; may be reflected by a lack of interest in activities with substantial time spent in purposeless activity

antisocial personality disorder
a pervasive lack of remorse or lack of exhibiting feelings that leads to a total disregard for the rights of others

asociality
a lack of interest in relationships

attention level
ability to concentrate on a task for an appropriate length of time

aversion therapy
application of a painful stimulus that creates an aversion to the obsessed thought leading to the undesirable behavior

avoidant personality disorder
negativity, poor self-esteem, and issues surrounding social interaction; difficulty looking at situations and interactions in an objective manner

Beck Depression Inventory
a tool that helps diagnose depression and determine its severity

blunted affect
a flattening of emotions in which the person's face may appear immobile with poor eye contact and lack of expressiveness

body dysmorphic disorder
preoccupation with an imagined or an actual slight defect in physical appearance; perceived thoughts are often distorted, making the problem, or perceived problem, bigger than it actually is; in many cases, the flaw doesn't exist

borderline personality disorder
a pattern of instability or impulsiveness in a person's mood, interpersonal relationships, self-esteem, self-identity, behavior, and cognition; originates in early childhood

clang association
words that rhyme or sound alike used in an illogical, nonsensical manner—for example, "It's the rain, train, pain."

cocaine
a narcotic and stimulant which may be ingested, injected, sniffed, or smoked to obtain its effects; street names include *coke, dust, blow, white pony, line, flake, snow, nose candy, crack* (hardened form), and *hard rock*

cognition
conscious mental activities: the activities of thinking, understanding, learning, and remembering

cognitive assessment scale
measures orientation, general knowledge, mental ability, and psychomotor function

comorbidity
the coexistence of two disorders, such as mental and somatic disorders, occurring together in a person

compensation
hiding a weakness by stressing too strongly the desirable strength

comprehension
the ability to understand, retain, and repeat material

compulsion
a preoccupation that's acted out, such as constantly washing one's hands

concept formation
testing the patient's ability to think abstractly

concrete thinking
inability to form or understand abstract thoughts

confabulation
unconscious filling of gaps in memory with fabricated facts and experiences

conversion disorder
(previously called *hysterical neurosis*, *conversion type*) disorder in which patients resolve psychological conflicts through the loss of a specific physical function; examples include paralysis, blindness, or the inability to swallow; patients exhibit symptoms that suggest a physical disorder, but evaluation and observation can't determine a physiologic cause

delusions
false ideas or beliefs accepted as real by the patient; somatic illness, depersonalization, and delusions of grandeur, persecution, and reference are common in schizophrenia

dementia
description of a group of symptoms affecting memory, thinking, and social abilities severely enough to interfere with daily functioning

denial
protecting oneself from unpleasant aspects of life by refusing to perceive, acknowledge, or deal with them

dependence
the physiologic state of neuroadaptation produced by repeated administration of drug, necessitating continued administration to prevent the appearance of the withdrawal syndrome

dependent personality disorder
an extreme need to be taken care of that leads to submissive, clinging behavior and fear of separation; pattern begins by early adulthood, when behaviors designed to elicit caring from others become predominant

depersonalization
a persistent or recurrent feeling that one is detached from one's own mental processes or body

depression
a mood disorder that causes a persistent feeling of sadness and loss of interest

derailment
speech that vacillates from one subject to another; the subjects are unrelated; ideas slip off the track between clauses

derealization
the persistent or recurrent feeling of detachment from other persons, objects, or their surroundings

displacement
misdirecting pent-up feelings toward something or someone that's less threatening than that which triggered the response

dissociation
separating objects from their emotional significance

dyspareunia
painful sexual intercourse; although it occurs in both sexes, it is more common in women

echolalia
meaningless repetition of words or phrases

echopraxia
involuntary repetition of movements observed in others

exhibitionism
exposing one's sex organs and genitalia to strangers; classified as a form of paraphilia

fantasy
creation of unrealistic or improbable images to escape from daily pressures and responsibilities

fetishism
sexual attraction and arousal an individual feels in relation to a specific object, body part, context, or situation which is used to achieve sexual gratification; classified as a form of paraphilia

flat affect
unresponsive range of emotion, possibly an indication of schizophrenia or Parkinson disease

flight of ideas
rapid succession of incomplete and poorly connected ideas

flooding
a frequent full-intensity exposure, possibly through the use of imagination, to an object that triggers a symptom; produces extreme discomfort

fluid intelligence
a form of intelligence defined as the ability to solve novel problems

focusing
a technique in which the nurse assists the patient in redirecting attention toward something specific, especially if the patient is vague or rambling

frotteurism
touching or rubbing against a nonconsenting or unaware person to achieve sexual satisfaction

fugue
travel away from home with no memory of what happened on these trips

functional dementia scale
measures orientation, affect, and the ability to perform activities of daily living

gender
the behaviors, attitudes, and feelings that are culturally and socially compatible with a person's biological sex

gender identity
an individual's concept and experience of oneself as being male, female, or transgender

geropsychiatry
a discipline focused on the special needs of older adults with mental health concerns and psychiatric/substance misuse disorders

global deterioration scale
assesses and stages primary degenerative dementia based on orientation, memory, and neurologic function

grief
the normal process of reaction to a loss

hallucinations
false sensory perceptions with no basis in reality; usually visual or auditory, hallucinations also may be olfactory (smell), gustatory (taste), or tactile (touch)

hallucinogens
drugs that produce behavioral changes that are often multiple and dramatic; no known medical use; however, some block sensation to pain and use may result in self-inflicted injuries; an example is lysergic acid diethylamide that has street names such as *acid, green* or *red dragon, microdot, sugar,* and *big D*; mescaline, peyote, psilocybin, and phencyclidine; designer drugs (ecstasy-PCE) are made to imitate certain illegal drugs and are often many times stronger than the drugs they imitate

histrionic personality disorder
a pervasive pattern of excessive emotionality and attention-seeking; often begins in early adulthood and may be present in a variety of contexts

hypochondriasis
misinterpretation of the severity and significance of physical signs or sensations or the fear of contracting a disease; leads to the preoccupation with having a serious disease, which persists despite medical reassurance to the contrary; significant distress or impairment in functioning occurs

ideas of reference
misinterpreting acts of others in a highly personal way

identification
unconscious adoption of the personality, characteristics, attitudes, values, and behavior of another person

illusions
false sensory perceptions with some basis in reality; for example, a car backfiring mistaken for a gunshot

immature defense mechanisms
internal reactions to threats such as idealizing or devaluating others, projecting, and acting out

implicit memory
information that can't be brought to mind but can be seen to affect behavior

implosion therapy
a form of desensitization; requires repeated exposure (that increases in graduated levels) to a highly feared object, requires strong interpersonal support or anxiolytic medication

inappropriate affect
inconsistency between expression (affect) and mood (e.g., a patient who smiles when discussing an anger-provoking situation)

incoherence
incomprehensible speech

intellectualization
hiding feelings about something painful behind thoughts; keeping opposing attitudes apart by using logic-tight comparisons

introjection
adopting someone else's values and standards without exploring whether or not they actually fit; often responds to "should" or "ought to"

lability of affect
rapid, dramatic fluctuation in the range of emotion

loose associations
not connected or related by logic or rationality

magical thinking
belief that thoughts or wishes can control other people or events

magnetoencephalography
measures the brain's magnetic field

Minnesota Multiphasic Personality Inventory
helps assess personality traits and ego function in adolescents and adults

modeling
provides a reward when the patient imitates the desired behavior

narcissistic personality disorder
projecting an image of perfection and personal invincibility because of a fear of personal weakness and imperfection; often projecting an inflated sense of self to hide low self-esteem

negative reinforcement
involves the removal of a negative stimulus only after the patient provides a desirable response

neologisms
distorted or invented words that have meaning only for the patient

nonverbal communication
eye contact, posture, facial expression, gestures, clothing, affect, silence, and other body movements that can convey a powerful message

obsessions
intense preoccupations that interfere with daily living

obsessive-compulsive personality disorder
a lack of openness and flexibility in daily routines as well as in interpersonal relationships and expectations; a preoccupation with orderliness and perfectionism; treatment options that don't fit in with the patient's cognitive schema will be rejected quickly

opiates
narcotics and depressants used medicinally to relieve pain but have a high potential for abuse; cause relaxation with an immediate "rush" but also have initial unpleasant effects, such as restlessness and nausea; includes codeine, heroin, meperidine, and opium; street names include *junk*, *horse*, *H*, and *smack*

paranoid personality disorder
extreme distrust of others and an avoidance of relationships in which the person isn't in control or has the potential of losing control

paraphilia
objects or behaviors that sexually arouse and stimulate an individual—the person frequently becomes dependent on that object or behavior in order to achieve sexual gratification; more common in men than women; examples include pedophilia, exhibitionism, frotteurism, and voyeurism (observing private activities of unaware victims)

pedophilia
having sex or engaging in sexual activity with a minor

pharmacodynamics
the drug's effect on its target organ

phencyclidine or PCP
a hallucinogen that produces behavioral changes that are often multiple and dramatic; flashbacks may occur long after use; street names include *hog, angel dust, peace pill, crystal superjoint, elephant tranquilizer,* and *rocket fuel*

phobia
an irrational and disproportionate fear of objects or situations

positive reinforcement
increase of the likelihood of a desirable behavior being repeated by promptly praising or rewarding the patient when performing it

poverty of speech
diminution of thought reflected in decreased speech and terse replies to questions, creating the impression of inner emptiness

priapism
a painful and prolonged erection

processing capacity
understanding text, making inferences, and paying attention, which all depends on working memory capability

projection
displacement of negative feelings onto another person

prospective memory
remembering things that one needs

punishment
discouraging of problem behavior by inflicting a penalty, such as temporary removal of a privilege

rationalization
substitution of acceptable reasons for the real or actual reasons motivating behavior

reaction formation
conduct in a manner opposite from the way the person feels

recent memory
an event experienced in the past few hours or days

regression
return to an earlier developmental stage

remote memory
ability to remember events in the more distant past, such as birthplace or high school days

repression
unconsciously blocking out painful thoughts

response prevention
a form of behavior therapy that may require hospitalization as well as family involvement to be effective

schizoid personality
a pervasive pattern of detachment from social relationships and restricted range of expression of emotions in interpersonal settings

schizotypal personality disorder
a pervasive pattern of social and interpersonal deficits marked by acute discomfort with, and reduced capacity for, close relationships, as well as by cognitive or perceptual distortions and eccentricities of behavior; begins in early adulthood and is present in a variety of contexts

self-efficacy
a personality measure defined by the ability to organize and execute actions required to deal with situations likely to happen in the future

sex
a person's biological sex of being male, female, or intersex based on anatomy, chromosomes, and sex organs

sexual dysfunction
a broad term which includes disorders of sexual desire, sexual arousal, orgasmic disorders, and sexual pain disorders

sexual masochism
deriving sexual gratification through being physically and/or emotionally abused

sexual sadism
achieving sexual gratification by causing others pain through the use of cruelty and emotional and/or physical abuse

shaping
initially rewards any behavior that resembles the desirable one; then, step by step, the behavior required to gain a reward becomes progressively closer to the desired behavior

sharing impressions
a communication technique in which the nurse attempts to describe the patient's feelings and then seeks corrective feedback from the patient

somatization disorder
experiencing multiple signs and symptoms that suggest a physical disorder, but no verifiable disease or pathophysiologic condition exists to account for them; unexplained symptoms appear to represent an unconscious somatized plea for attention and care; often familial with unknown etiology

sublimation
transforming unacceptable needs into acceptable ambitions and actions; for instance, a person can funnel anger and resentment into an obsession to excel in a lucrative career

substance abuse
a maladaptive pattern of substance use coupled with recurrent and significant adverse consequences

substance dependence
physical, behavioral, and cognitive changes resulting from persistent substance use; persistent drug use results in tolerance and withdrawal

substance intoxication
the development of a reversible substance-specific syndrome due to the ingestion of or exposure to a substance; the clinically significant maladaptive behavior or psychological changes vary from substance to substance

tardive dyskenesia
a neurologic syndrome characterized by repetitive, involuntary, purposeless movements caused by the long-term use of certain drugs called *neuroleptics* used for psychiatric, gastrointestinal, and neurologic disorders

thematic apperception test
test in which, after seeing a series of pictures that depict ambiguous situations, the patient tells a story describing each picture

thought blocking
sudden interruption in the patient's train of thought

thought stopping
method that breaks the habit of fear-inducing anticipatory thoughts; to stop unwanted thoughts by saying the word *stop* and then focus attention on achieving calmness and muscle relaxation

tolerance
an increased need for a substance or need for an increased amount of the substance to achieve an effect

transgender
one whose sense of gender does not match the biological and anatomic sex; typically, the individual may have feelings of having been born into the wrong body

transvestite
an individual whose dress and behavior mirrors that traditionally associated with dress and behavior of the opposite sex

undoing
trying to superficially repair or make up for an action without dealing with the complex effects of that deed; also called *magical thinking*

voyeurism
the act of obtaining sexual gratification while secretly observing others engaged in such activities as sex, intimate acts, or undressing

withdrawal
becoming emotionally uninvolved by pulling back and being passive

word salad
illogical word groupings; the extreme form of loose associations; for example, "She had a star, barn, plant."

working memory
the part of the brain that enables not paying attention to irrelevancies

Index

Note: i refers to an illustration; t refers to a table.

Note: i refers to an illustration; t refers to a table.

Note: i refers to an illustration; t refers to a table.

Note: i refers to an illustration; t refers to a table.

Note: i refers to an illustration; t refers to a table.

Note: i refers to an illustration; t refers to a table.

Note: i refers to an illustration; t refers to a table.